MOLECULAR BIOLOGY AND PATHOGENESIS OF CORONAVIRUSES

ADVANCES IN EXPERIMENTAL MEDICINE AND BIOLOGY

MOLECULAR BIOLOGY AND PATHOGENESIS OF CORONAVIRUSES

Edited by

P. J. M. Rottier
B. A. M. van der Zeijst
W. J. M. Spaan
and
M. C. Horzinek
State University of Utrecht
Utrecht, The Netherlands

PLENUM PRESS • NEW YORK AND LONDON

Library of Congress Cataloging in Publication Data

EMBO Workshop on Molecular Biology and Pathogenesis of Coronaviruses (1983:
    State University of Utrecht)
    Molecular biology and pathogenesis of coronaviruses.

    (Advances in experimental medicine and biology; v. 173)
    "Proceedings of an EMBO Workshop on Molecular Biology and Pathogenesis of
Coronaviruses, held June 1983 at the State University of Utrecht, The
Netherlands." — T.p. verso.
    Includes bibliographical references and index.
    1. Coronaviruses — Congresses. 2. Virus disease — Congresses. 3. Molecular biology —
Congresses. I. Rottier, P. J. M. II. Title. III. Series. [DNLM: 1. Coronaviridae —
Congresses. 2. Coronavirus infections — Etiology — Congresses. W1 AD559 v.173/QW
168.5.C8 E53m 1983]
    QR399.E43   1983   636.089′60194   84-4710

Proceedings of an EMBO Workshop on Molecular Biology and Pathogenesis
of Coronaviruses, held June 1983 at the State University of Utrecht, The Netherlands

©1984 Plenum Press, New York
Softcover reprint of the hardcover 1st edition 1984

A Division of Plenum Publishing Corporation
233 Spring Street, New York, N.Y. 10013

ISBN 978-1-4615-9375-1   ISBN 978-1-4615-9373-7 (eBook)
DOI 10.1007/978-1-4615-9373-7

PREFACE

The present volume contains the Proceedings of an EMBO Workshop organized in June 1983 by the Institute of Virology, Veterinary Faculty, State University of Utrecht, The Netherlands. Some 70 scientists from 11 countries followed the invitation to present and discuss their recent data on the structure, replication, genetics and pathogenesis of coronaviruses. It was the second international meeting on these viruses; the Workshop, which was held in Zeist near Utrecht followed the example of the Wuerzburg symposium of October 1980.

At that time it became clear that coronaviruses are unique in many respects. Once a group of viruses that were defined merely on the basis of their characteristic peplomer morphology, Coronaviridae family members are known today

- to be constructed from essentially three polypeptides
- to use a "nested set" of 5-6 subgenomic mRNAs in the expression of their large, positive and single stranded RNA genome,
- to generate these subgenomic RNAs through specific fusion of non-contiguous sequences,
- to mature by budding from intracellular membranes,
- to cause persistent infection with neurological involvement and sometimes immunopathological conditons.

These and many other findings have been established only very recently. The articles collected in this book reveal and/or further detail these findings. Since these Proceedings contain the combined scientific presentations of representatives from virtually all laboratories engaged in the field, they provide a fairly comprehensive review of the state of the art in corona-virology.

The contents have been grouped into two main parts. The first part deals with the molecular biology of coronaviruses and contains contributions on viral proteins, virus maturation and on the structure and replication of viral RNAs. In the second part aspects of coronavirus pathogenesis are described including studies on genetic and immunological factors involved and on persistent infections in tissue culture. Both parts are preceded by synoptic papers compiled by B.W.J.Mahy and V. ter Meulen, respectively.

P.J.M.Rottier
B.A.M.van der Zeijst
W.J.M.Spaan
M.C.Horzinek

CONTENTS

MOLECULAR BIOLOGY OF CORONAVIRUSES

OVERVIEW

VIRAL PROTEINS AND MATURATION

PATHOGENESIS OF CORONAVIRUSES

OVERVIEW

BIOCHEMISTRY OF CORONAVIRUSES 1983

Brian W.J. Mahy

Division of Virology, Department of Pathology

University of Cambridge, England

INTRODUCTION

The first international symposium on coronaviruses was held in 1980. At that time the unique structural features of this virus family were recognised, and much of the discussion centred around evidence for an unusual replication strategy involving a 'nested set' of six subgenomic mRNA's (see Mahy, 1981). Most of the molecular biological studies then reported concerned avian or murine corona-viruses, and these still continue to dominate the field, with little new information available on the bovine, feline or porcine corona-viruses, for example. Major advances in 1983 have resulted from application of the new techniques of nucleic acid cloning and se-quencing to the avian and murine genomes, and although only two of the genes (N and E_1) have been analysed so far, the interpretation of experiments to study replication is already on a much firmer basis.

STRUCTURE AND SYNTHESIS OF VIRION PROTEINS

The major spike glycoprotein which forms the characteristic petal-like peplomers of the 'corona' is called the spike or S protein for avian infectious bronchitis virus (IBV) and the E_2 protein for mouse hepatitis viruses. D. Cavanagh (1983 and this volume) has clearly shown by gradient separation of the S protein in the absence of sodium dodecyl sulphate (SDS), that it consists of two polypep-tides, S_1 and S_2, of molecular weights 90K and 84K respectively. The molecular weight of the purified spike appears to be 354K ± 17K, and this is consistent with the spike being a tetramer of two S_1 and two S_2 polypeptides. These are apparently not dissociable by β-mercaptoethanol treatment, so are not held together by inter-peptide

1

disulphide bonds. Treatment of IBV particles with urea or low concentrations of SDS (0.01%) selectively removes the 90K S_1 polypeptide, leaving S_2 associated with the membrane of the virus.

Evidence that the spike protein of mouse hepatitis virus (strain
A59) also consists of two distinct polypeptides was reported by L.S.
Sturman (this volume), who terms the subunits, derived from E_2 by
trypsin cleavage, as 90A and 90B. He could detect differences in
amino-acid composition between the two polypeptides, and also found
that the 90A polypeptide contained covalently-bonded palmitic acid
in contrast to 90B which did not. Although this is a useful distin-
guishing marker, the significance of palmitic acid in association
with the spike glycoproteins is unclear; as pointed out by R.R.
Wagner, two related serotypes of vesicular stomatitis virus (VSV)
differ in that the Indiana strain has glycoprotein-associated palmitic acid whereas the New Jersey strain has none. It is tempting to
speculate, nevertheless, that the A59 and 90A polypeptide may be
membrane associated and so equivalent to the S_2 polypeptide of IBV.
Clearly there may also be analogies to the HA_2 portion of the influenza virus haemagglutinin spike, which is much more fully characteri-
sed (Wilson et al., 1981).

The preparation of monoclonal or polyclonal antibodies against
the murine hepatitis virus E_2 glycoprotein has facilitated further
studies of its function, and such antibodies block virus-mediated
cell fusion, in addition to neutralising virus infectivity (Collins
et al., 1982; Holmes et al., this volume). The application of monoclonal antibodies raised against the bovine enteric coronavirus
(Vautherot et al., this volume) has helped to distinguish the
105,000 dalton surface glycoprotein (gp 105) from the other surface
glycoprotein component (gp 125). It appears that gp 105 is involved
in infectivity and carries haemagglutinating activity in this virus;
it may therefore be functionally analogous to the IBV S_1 glycoprotein.

Sturman (this volume) presents evidence that trypsin treatment
of A59 virus, which cleaves the 180K E_2 to the 90A and 90B subunit
polypeptides, greatly increases the capacity of the virus to cause
cell fusion. Whether host cell-dependent protease activation is
essential for coronavirus infectivity is still not clear, although
there is good evidence in favour of this idea for the bovine enteric
coronavirus (Storz et al., 1981). It is possible that virus maturation may be defective in certain cell types which lack proteases of
the necessary specificity, and Garwes et al. (this volume) present
an interesting example of such a defect. Porcine transmissible
gastroenteritis virus grows well in secondary adult pig thyroid cell
cultures, but very low virus yields are produced from a pig kidney
cell line, LLC-PK1. No defects in virus-specific RNA synthesis were
apparent in the two culture systems, and a defect in viral glycoprotein processing seems the most likely explanation for the abort-
iveness in LLC-PK1 cells.

The second major envelope glycoprotein of coronavirus is known as the E_1 protein in murine viruses, and as the matrix or M protein in IBV. This protein provides the link between the nucleocapsid (N) protein and the envelope, and has been shown to interact directly with RNA of the A59 virus nucleocapsid in vitro (Sturman et al., 1980; Holmes et al., this volume). Use of the drug tunicamycin, which in murine virus-infected cells blocks formation of the E_2 but not the E_1 protein, shows that E_1 alone determines the formation of the virus envelope as well as the unusual site of virus budding from the endoplasmic reticulum. It is likely, though not formally proved, that in avian viruses the M protein serves the same function as E_1 in murine viruses. The original experiments with tunicamycin reported at the last meeting (see Mahy, 1981) as well as more formal analysis (Niemann and Klenk, 1981) showed that the carbohydrate moiety of E_1 in murine and in bovine coronaviruses is O-glycosydically linked. By contrast, it is now clear that the M protein of IBV is N-glycosidically linked (Cavanagh, 1983; Stern and Sefton, 1982b). Preliminary nucleotide sequence analysis of the IBV genome by M. Boursnell and T.D.K. Brown has confirmed that the predicted amino-acid sequence of the IBV M protein lacks potential O-glycosylation sites (serine and threonine residues) such as are found at the N-terminus of the murine virus E_1 protein (Armstrong, this volume, Niemann, this volume). Further comparative studies of other coronaviruses would be of interest in this respect, but clearly the existence of this unusual O-linked glycoprotein in the murine and bovine Coronaviridae cannot be used as a hallmark for all members of the family.

O-glycosylation of E_1 appears to be a late event, occurring in the Golgi apparatus, which is not essential for virus maturation. Addition of the glycoprotein transport inhibitor monensin to murine coronavirus-infected cells blocked the glycosylation of E_1 but allowed accumulation of enveloped virions in the endoplasmic reticulum (Niemann et al., 1982). Similar results were obtained in human embryo lung cells with the human coronavirus 229E (Kemp et al., this volume). It can be concluded from these in vivo experiments that glycosylation of E_1 is not co-translational, and further evidence for this has been obtained from the elegant in vitro study reported by Rottier et al. (this volume). Translation of A59 mRNA in a cell-free system containing dog pancreatic microsomes resulted in synthesis of E_1 protein, the bulk of which was buried in the membrane, only small portions from the N- and C-terminus being expressed in the lumenal and cytoplasmic domains respectively. No evidence for a cleavable N-terminal signal sequence for glycosylation was obtained. It is interesting that the microsomal preparation can be added at any stage during in vitro synthesis of the first 150 amino-acids, and the protein will still enter the membrane.

The complete amino-acid sequence of E_1 (predicted from the nucleotide sequence determined by Armstrong et al., this volume) con-

firms the strongly hydrophobic nature of this protein. The M protein of IBV has remarkably similar hydrophobic properties as judged
from the available nucleotide sequence data (Boursnell and Brown,
this volume). Presumably it is this hydrophobicity which restricts
the intracellular migration of E_1 and ultimately results in the occurrence of budding from the endoplasmic reticulum rather than the plasma membrane from where most other enveloped viruses are found to bud.

The third major virion protein of coronaviruses is the nucleoprotein (N) which has a molecular weight of 50-60,000. A nucleotide
sequence of the gene encoding this protein in murine A59 virus has
been published (Armstrong et al., 1983); two errors in this published
sequence were acknowledged and corrected at this meeting (Armstrong
et al., this volume). Since the NP gene is located at the extreme
3' end of virion RNA, proximal to the poly(A) tail, this is the eas-
iest gene to reverse transcribe, clone, and sequence, and an additional N gene sequence, that for the JHM strain of MHV, was reported at
this meeting (Skinner et al., this volume). The JHM sequence encodes
a basic protein of 455 amino-acids which is remarkably similar (94%
nucleotide homology in the coding region) to the corrected A59 virus
sequence (Armstrong et al., this volume) although two regions of lower homology occur at nucleotide positions 497-569 and 1271-1293
(Skinner et al., this volume). The first 83 nucleotides of the JHM
N gene sequence are non-coding, the same as the non-coding nucleotides in A59. As further sequence data become available, comparisons between the highly neurotropic JHM strain and less virulent MHV
strains such as A59 will be of considerable interest.

It has been reported that the JHM virion carries an associated
protein kinase activity (Siddell et al., 1981a) and this enzyme appears to phosphorylate mainly serine residues in the N protein of
murine coronaviruses (Stohlman and Lai, 1979; Siddell et al., 1981a).
The role of phosphorylation in the replication cycle is unknown, and
for the N protein at least it may be variable, leading to two forms
detectable by gel electrophoretic analysis in some systems (Garwes
et al., this volume). It has been suggested (Siddell et al., 1981a)
that phosphorylation may affect the interaction between N and E_1
protein which has been demonstrated in vitro (Sturman et al., 1980)
and this possibility would merit further study.

CORONAVIRUS-INDUCED NON-STRUCTURAL PROTEINS

Although a number of non-structural proteins have been detected
in murine coronavirus-infected cells, and were described at the last
meeting (Siddell et al., 1981b), progress in structural analysis or
in assigning functions to these intracellular polypeptides has been
disappointing, and they were hardly mentioned at this meeting. At
a minimum, the non-structural proteins comprise a 30K - 35K protein,
the product of murine coronavirus RNA 2, and a 14K - 17K protein

which has not been precisely mapped, but is encoded in either RNA
4 or RNA 5.   However the infectivity of coronavirion RNA means that
a further, presumed non-structural, polypeptide awaits identification as the product of RNA 1.   Mapping studies indicate that a protein of molecular weight greater than 200K, assumed to have RNA polymerase activity (reviewed by Siddell et al., 1983), is the likely
product of this mRNA.   Translation of genome RNA in an mRNA-dependent
rabbit reticulocyte cell-free system produces three structurally-
related proteins of the appropriate size to be the products of this
RNA (Leibowitz et al., 1982).

CORONAVIRUS RNA SYNTHESIS

     At the time of the last coronavirus meeting the following facts
emerged regarding coronavirus intracellular RNA synthesis:-

   (i)   Coronavirus virion RNA is infectious.

   (ii)   Up to seven intracellular virus-specific RNA species
           can be detected in infected cells, one of which is
           full-length genome-sized RNA, the others being smaller,
           subgenomic-sized RNAs.   All have the same positive
           polarity as genome RNA.

   (iii)   All the intracellular RNAs of both avian (Stern and
           Kennedy, 1980) and murine (Cheley et al., 1981; Lai
           et al., 1981; Leibowitz et al., 1981) coronaviruses
           are polyadenylated, have common sequences, and form a
           3'-coterminal nested sequence set.

   (iv)   Synthesis of each of the intracellular RNAs is initiated
           independently, and not by processing from a large pre-
           cursor molecule, as revealed by UV transcription map-
           ping experiments (Jacobs et al., 1981; Stern and Sefton,
           1982a).

   (v)   A major area of uncertainty concerned the role of the
           host cell nucleus in coronavirus RNA synthesis, since
           it has been suggested (Evans and Simpson, 1980) that
           IBV replication is α-amanitin- and actinomycin D-sensi-
           tive and requires host cell DNA-dependent RNA synthesis.

   (vi)   Apart from a report concerning porcine coronavirus
           (Dennis and Brian, 1981), no information on coronavirus-
           specified RNA polymerase activities was available.

     Since the 1980 meeting, the 'nested set' structure of the corona-
virus-induced intracellular RNAs has been confirmed (Spaan et al.,
1982; Weiss and Leibowitz, 1983) and it has been shown that the subgenomic RNAs, as well as genome RNA, contain 5'-cap structures (Lai

et al., 1982). These RNA molecules were also found to act as individual mRNAs, and to be translated into single proteins of a size
corresponding to the coding capacity of the unique 5'-terminal sequences not present in the next smallest RNA (Rottier et al., 1981;
Leibowitz et al., 1982; Siddell, 1983).

Summarising the last meeting, I suggested that although the
mRNAs appeared to be synthesised independently, the existence of a
short 5'-terminal sequence common to all the RNAs and derived by a
splicing or polymerase jumping mechanism could not be excluded (Mahy,
1981). Surprisingly, this has proved to be the case.

Lai et al. (1982a) first showed that the 5'-termini of most of
the MHV-A59 virus-specific RNAs induced in infected L2 cells contained a common tetranucleotide sequence, 5'-cap-N-UAAG, identical
to the 5'-terminal genome RNA sequence. In addition, T_1 oligonucleotide mapping of MHV-A59 mRNAs revealed one oligonucleotide, No.10,
which mapped at the 5' terminus of mRNAs 2, 3, 5, 6 and 7 but only
occurred once within the genome. This leads inescapably to the conclusion that a sequence containing oligonucleotide 10 is somehow
translocated from its position in genome RNA onto the 5' terminus
of each mRNA, and so must constitute a leader sequence. A consequence of such a translocation would be the formation of new T_1 oligonucleotides at the junction of the leader and the body sequence of
each mRNA, and such candidate oligonucleotides found in mRNA but not
in genome RNA, are oligonucleotides 19 and 19a (Lai et al., 1982a;
Lai et al., this volume). Similar results were reported by two other
groups (Leibowitz et al., 1981; Spaan et al., 1982).

The size of oligonucleotide 10 was determined to be 23 nucleotides (Lai et al., 1982a), and oligonucleotides 19 or 19a apparently
have 22 nucleotides (Lai et al., this volume). The total length of
the postulated leader sequence is not known, but can be estimated as
at least 40 nucleotides. These elegant and painstaking oligonucleotide mapping studies by Lai et al. (this volume) have been the stimu-
lus to two alternative approaches which have confirmed the existence
of leader RNAs on coronavirus mRNAs.

In the first of these approaches, single-stranded cDNA copied
from the smallest subgenomic mRNA (7), was hybridised with genome
RNA or subgenomic mRNAs then examined in the electron microscope after cytochrome spreading. The bulk of the cDNA (approximately 2000
nucleotides) hybridised to the 3' terminal region of genome RNA, but
large loops of RNA were also seen, consistent with a short region
(around 50 nucleotides) of homology between the cDNA and the 5' terminus of genome RNA (Spaan et al., this volume). Hybridisation of the
mRNA 7 cDNA to mRNA 6 also resulted in the formation of looped hybrid
structures.

The second approach has been direct sequence analysis of mRNA7 and the corresponding region of the genome. This confirmed the existence of a 'fusion-sequence' since the nucleotide sequence of the 5' region of mRNA 7 of A59 virus could be seen to diverge from the corresponding region of the genome upstream from the N gene iniatiation codon (Spaan et al., this volume). The 5'-terminus of mRNA 7, but not of the genome, contains sequences which correspond to oligonucleotides 10 and 19 as reported by Lai et al. (1982a). The fusion sequence of mRNA 7 was shown to be within oligonucleotide 19.

The RNA synthetic mechanism which generates these fused sequences is of considerable interest. Lai et al. (1982b) reported that the template for mRNA synthesis is a single, genome-length, negative-stranded RNA molecule, and no evidence for multiple negative-stranded RNAs has been obtained. Replication of murine coronaviruses, at least, seems to be confined to the cytoplasm since enucleated cells support A59 or JHM virus growth and inhibitors of cell DNA transcription such as α-amanitin or actinomycin D have no effect on virus yield (Brayton et al., 1981; Wilhelmsen et al., 1981; Mahy et al., 1983). (There remains some doubt concerning the role of the cell nucleus in avian coronavirus replication). From these data, the possibility that murine coronavirus mRNAs acquire leader sequences by splicing in the cell nucleus can be ruled out. Processing of a large precursor RNA in the cytoplasm is also excluded by the transcriptional mapping data which show that the UV target size of each mRNA corresponds to its physical size (Jacobs et al., 1981; Stern and Sefton 1982a). Thus each mRNA must be individually transcribed at its own initiation point on the negative strand template.

Two possible mechanisms by which the leader sequences could become fused to the mRNA body sequences during transcription were considered at the meeting. The first would involve the bringing together of non-contiguous sequences on the negative strand RNA template due to secondary structure alterations which lead to looping or folding of the molecule. The polymerase would then read the leader sequence and jump across a postulated gap in the template, joining the leader to mRNA body sequences in the process. Such a jumping mechanism, which involves the influence of ribonucleoprotein structure in bringing together non-contiguous sequences, is thought to be involved in the generation of defective interfering RNAs during influenza virus transcription (Fields and Winter, 1982; Jennings et al., 1983). The second mechanism involves reinitiation of the transcription process at a point near the start of each gene on the template; the leader RNA sequence would remain attached to the polymerase after its own synthesis, and serve to prime transcription at six different regions along the template. Although data is not yet available for murine coronavirus, it is interesting that Boursnell and Brown (this volume) have detected two regions of homology on the IBV genome which might be the primer attachment points.

Lai et al. (this volume) present further evidence in favour of the second mechanism. Only one size (full-length) of double-stranded replicative form (RF) molecule was found in infected cells after ribonuclease treatment. If the first mechanism were correct, multiple RF's would be expected to be generated by this procedure. Furthermore, they were able to isolate replicative intermediate (RI) structures containing single-stranded tails by precipitation with 2M lithium chloride. Only one species of RI, migrating faster than genome RNA, was found by gel electrophoresis. This species was 40-60% resistant to ribonuclease, and had a structure which suggested the existence of six single-stranded tails on each full-length template RNA. Evidence was also obtained that poly(A) is added to the mRNAs during synthesis and not post-transcriptionally.

The nature of the RNA-dependent RNA polymerase responsible for these events is still unclear. Since the report by Dennis and Brian (1981) on the induction of RNA polymerase activity by porcine corona-virus, two reports have appeared describing a similar enzyme activity in murine coronavirus-infected cells (Brayton et al., 1982; Mahy et al., 1983). No evidence for the existence of such an enzyme in cells infected with other coronaviruses, such as IBV, has been presented. Brayton et al. (1982) could distinguish two polymerase activities, one early (one hour post-infection) and the other late (six hours post-infection). The latter activity corresponds to the one detected by Mahy et al. (1983). The current hypothesis, presented by Lai et al. (this volume) would favour separate polymerase activities for the synthesis of negative and positive strands, and since the early polymerase activity declines rapidly, the negative-stranded RNA template would need to be rather stable. Considerable further work on the products of these enzymes is needed to establish the events involved in the unique RNA synthetic mechanism induced by coronavirus infection.

ACKNOWLEDGMENT

I wish to thank Mrs. Mary Wright for her excellent typing of the manuscript.

REFERENCES

Armstrong, J., Smeekens, S. and Rottier, P. (1983). Sequence of the nucleocapsid gene from murine coronavirus MHV-A59. Nucleic Acids Res. 11, 883-891.

Brayton, P.R., Ganges, R.G. and Stohlman, S.A. (1981). Host cell nuclear function and murine hepatitis virus replication. J. gen. Virol. 56, 457-460.

Brayton, P.R., Lai, M.M.C., Patton, C.D. and Stohlman, S. (1982). Characterization of two RNA polymerase activities induced by mouse heptatitis virus. J. Virol. 42, 847-853.

Cavanagh, D. (1983). Coronavirus IBV glycopolypeptides: size of
    their polypeptide moieties and nature of their oligosaccha-
    rides. J. gen. Virol. 64, 1187-1191.
Cheley, S., Anderson, R., Cupples, M.J., Lee Chan, E.C.M. and Morris,
    V.L. (1981). Intracellular murine hepatitis virus-specific RNAs
    contain common sequences. Virology 112, 596-604.
Collins, A.R., Knobler, R.L., Powell, H. and Buchmeier, M.J. (1982).
    Monoclonal antibodies to murine hepatitis virus 4 (strain JHM)
    define the viral glycoprotein responsible for attachment and
    cell fusion. Virology 119, 358-371.
Dennis, D.E. and Brian, D.A. (1981). Coronavirus cell-associated
    RNA-dependent RNA polymerase. Advances in Exp. Biol. Med. 142,
    155-170.
Evans, M.R. and Simpson, R.W. (1980). The coronavirus avian infec-
    tious bronchitis virus requires the cell nucleus and host trans-
    criptional factors. Virology 105, 582-591.
Fields, S. and Winter, G. (1982). Nucleotide sequences of influenza
    virus segments 1 and 3 reveal mosaic structure of a small viral
    RNA segment. Cell 28, 303-313.
Jacobs, L., Spaan, W.J.M., Horzinek, M.C. and van der Zeijst, B.A.M.
    (1981). The synthesis of the subgenomic mRNAs of mouse hepati-
    tis virus is initiated independently: evidence from UV transcrip-
    tion mapping. J. Virol. 39, 401-406.
Jennings, P.A., Finch, J.T., Winter, G. and Robertson, J.S. (1983).
    Does the higher order structure of the influenza virus ribo-
    nucleoprotein guide sequence rearrangements in influenza viral
    RNA? Cell. in press.
Lai, M.M.C., Brayton, P.R., Armen, R.C., Patton, C.D., Pugh, C. and
    Stohlman, S.A. (1981). Mouse hepatitis virus A59: mRNA struc-
    ture and genetic localization of the sequence divergence from
    hepatotropic strain MHV-3. J. Virol. 39, 823-834.
Lai, M.M.C., Patton, C.D. and Stohlman, S.A. (1982a). Further chara-
    cterization of mRNAs of mouse hepatitis virus: presence of
    common 5'-end nucleotides. J. Virol. 41, 557-565.
Lai, M.M.C., Patton, C.D. and Stohlman, S.A. (1982b). Replication of
    mouse hepatitis virus: negative-stranded RNA and replicative
    form RNA are of genome length. J. Virol. 44, 487-492.
Leibowitz, J.L., Weiss, S.R., Paavola, E. and Bond, C.W. (1982).
    Cell-free translation of murine coronavirus RNA. J. Virol.
    43, 905-913.
Leibowitz, J.L., Wilhelmsen, K.C. and Bond, C.W. (1981). The virus-
    specific intracellular RNA species of two murine coronaviruses:
    MHV-A59 and MHV-JHM. Virology 114, 39-51.
Mahy, B.W.J. (1981). Biochemistry of coronaviruses 1980. Advances
    in Experimental Medicine and Biology 142, 261-270.
Mahy, B.W.J., Siddell, S., Wege, H. and ter Meulen, V. (1983). RNA-
    dependent RNA polymerase activity in murine coronavirus-infec-
    ted cells. J. gen. Virol. 64, 103-111.
Niemann, H. and Klenk, H.D. (1981). Coronavirus glycoprotein E1, a
    new type of viral glycoprotein. J. Mol. Biol. 153, 993-1010.

Niemann, H., Boschek, B., Evans, D., Rosing, M., Tamura, T. and
    Klenk, H.-D. (1982). Posttranslational glycosylation of coro-
    navirus glycoprotein El: inhibition by monensin. EMBO J. 1,
    1499-1504.
Rottier, P.J.M., Spaan, W.J.M., Horzinek, M. and van der Zeijst,
    B.A.M. (1981). Translation of three mouse hepatitis virus
    (MHV-A59) subgenomic RNAs in Xenopus laevis oocytes. J. Virol.
    38, 20-26.
Siddell, S.G. (1983). Coronavirus JHM: coding assignments of sub-
    genomic mRNAs. J. gen. Virol. 64, 113-125.
Siddell, S.G., Barthel, A. and ter Meulen, V. (1981a). Coronavirus
    JHM: a virion associated protein kinase. J. gen. Virol. 52,
    235-243.
Siddell, S.G., Wege, H., Barthel, A. and ter Meulen, V. (1981b).
    Coronavirus JHM: intracellular protein synthesis. J. gen.
    Virol. 53, 145-155.
Siddell, S., Wege, H. and ter Meulen, V. (1983). The biology of
    coronaviruses. J. gen. Virol. 64, 761-776.
Spaan, W.J.M., Rottier, P.J.M., Horzinek, M.C. and van der Zeijst,
    B.A.M. (1982). Sequence relationships between the genome and
    the intracellular RNA species 1, 3, 6 and 7 of mouse hepatitis
    virus strain A59. J. Virol. 42, 432-439.
Stern, D.F. and Kennedy, S.I.T. (1980). Coronavirus multiplication
    strategy. II. Mapping the avian infectious bronchitis virus
    intracellular RNA species to the genome. J. Virol. 36, 440-449.
Stern, D.F. and Sefton, B.M. (1982a). Synthesis of coronavirus mRNAs:
    kinetics of inactivation of infectious bronchitis virus RNA
    synthesis by UV light. J. Virol. 42, 755-759.
Stern, D.F. and Sefton, B.M. (1982b). Coronavirus proteins: struc-
    ture and function of the oligosaccharides of the avian infec-
    tious bronchitis virus glycoproteins. J. Virol. 44, 804-812.
Stohlman, S.A. & Lai, M.M.C. (1979). Phosphoproteins of murine he-
    patitis viruses. J. Virol. 32, 672-675.
Storz, J., Rott, R. and Kaluza, G. (1981). Enhancement of plaque
    formation and cell fusion of an enteropathogenic coronavirus
    by trypsin treatment. Infect. Immun. 31, 1214-1222.
Sturman, L.S., Holmes, K.V. and Behnke, J. (1980). Isolation of
    coronavirus envelope glycoproteins and interaction with the
    viral nucleocapsid. J. Virol. 33, 449-462.
Weiss, S.R. and Leibowitz, J.L. (1983). Characterization of murine
    coronavirus RNA by hybridization with virus-specific cDNA probes.
    J. gen. Virol. 64, 127-133.
Wilhelmsen, K.C., Leibowitz, J.L., Bond, C.W. and Robb, J.A. (1981).
    The replication of murine coronaviruses in enucleated cells.
    Virology 110, 225-230.
Wilson, I.A., Skehel, J.J. and Wiley, D.C. (1981). Structure of the
    haemagglutinin membrane glycoprotein of influenza virus at 3Å
    resolution. Nature 289, 366-373.

ORGANIZATION OF THE IBV GENOME

David F. Stern* and Bartholomew Sefton

Molecular Biology and Virology Laboratory
The Salk Institute
P.O. Box 85800
San Diego, CA 92138
*Center for Cancer Research
Massachusetts Institute of Technology
Cambridge, MA 02139

We have investigated how the information contained within the large RNA genome of IBV is expressed. We began by examining the structure of IBV-specified RNAs. Infected chicken embryo kidney (CEK) cells contain at least 6 IBV RNA species. These consist of the viral genome, RNA F, with an estimated complexity of 23 kb[1], and subgenomic RNAs A, B, C, D, and E, which range in size from 2.4 kb to 7.9 kb[2]. We have recently identified an additional IBV-specified RNA species, RNA M, by Northern blot analysis using a hybridization probe containing cloned IBV cDNA sequences (see below). RNA M is intermediate in size between RNAs B and C (Table 1). Structural analysis of RNAs A, B, C, D, E, and F by ribonuclease T_1 fingerprinting revealed that they comprise a 3' coterminal nested set[3]. Synthesis of 3' coterminal RNAs is now known to be a characteristic feature of coronavirus multiplication[4,5].

Since the IBV intracellular RNAs were single-stranded, of positive sense, and polyadenylated, they were likely to function as viral mRNAs. This raised the question of the location of translationally active sequences within each mRNA. It was possible that each is translated over most of its length, yielding polypeptides proportional in size to the mRNAs. Another possibility, suggested by the activities of the overlapping alphavirus mRNAs, was that only the "unique" 5' domain of each mRNA not contained in smaller mRNAs would be translated. The size of the polypeptides produced would be proportional to the difference in size between each mRNA and the next smaller species, rather than to its

Table 1.   Coding Capacities of IBV mRNAs Predicted
from Two Different   Models

RNA	length (kb)	total coding capacity (kd)[a]	"non-overlapping" coding capacity (kd)[b]	size of translation product (kd)[c]
A	2.4	80	80	51
B	2.7	90	10	
M	3.2	110	20	
C	3.9	130	20	23
D	4.5	150	20	
E	7.9	260	110	110
F	23.	800	540	

[a]The molecular weight of each RNA was divided by 10 to estimate the size of a polypeptide encoded by the entire RNA.

[b]From the molecular weight of each RNA species the molecular weight of the next smaller species was subtracted, yielding the size of the unique 5' domain. This figure was divided by 10 to determine the coding capacity of that region.

[c]Determined by cell-free translation of fractionated mRNA as described in the text.

absolute size[3]. The sizes of polypeptides predicted according to this non-overlapping translational scheme are listed in Table 1. We describe here the use of cell-free translation to identify the mRNAs that encode the major viral structural proteins.

IBV virions prepared according to our procedures contain P14, which has not been localized within virions, P51, the nucleocapsid protein, and three distinct membrane proteins, GP90, GP84, and the P23 family proteins[8,9,10,11,12,13]. One or both of the large glyco-proteins, GP90 and GP84, comprise the large virion surface projec-tions. The P23 family of proteins consists of P23, which is not glycosylated, and glycoproteins GP28, GP31, and GP36. These proteins all contain the same 23 kd core polypeptide and differ in the number and type of N-linked oligosaccharides which they bear[7].

The P23 family of proteins and P51 are synthesized without obvious post-translational proteolytic modification. However, GP90 and GP84 are derived by post-translational cleavage of a cell-associated precursor, GP155[14]. The approximate size of the core polypeptide of GP155 was determined by removal of most of the carbo-hydrate with endoglycosidase H. This digestion product had an approximate molecular weight of 115 kd[7]. P14 was not reliably de-tected in infected cells, so we were unable to determine the manner of its synthesis [14]. We were able to conclude that 7 virion proteins are derived by maturation of only three polypeptides, which have molecular weights of 23 kd, 51 kd, and approximately 115 kd.

To determine which mRNAs specify these polypeptides, polyadeny-lated RNA from infected cells was translated in a messenger-dependent rabbit reticulocyte lysate[15]. Fractionation of the RNA prior to translation permitted the correlation of messenger activity with the presence of particular mRNAs.

Cell-free translation of total polyadenylated RNA from IBV-infected cells yielded products which comigrated with virion pro-teins P23 and P51 (Fig. 1, lanes I and V). These proteins were not produced by translation of RNA from uninfected cells (Fig. 1, lane M). Maps of methionine-labelled tryptic peptides demonstrated the identity of the 23 kd and 51 kd translation products (Fig. 2, panels E and A, respectively) with their counterparts purified from infected cells (Fig. 2, panels F and C). A series of proteins just larger than P51 was also produced by translation of RNA from infected cells (Fig. 1, lane I). Two-dimensional tryptic peptide mapping (Fig. 2, panel B) and one-dimensional partial proteolytic mapping (data not shown) of these proteins showed that they are closely related to P51. The reason for the polymorphism of P51 synthesized in vitro is not clear. It could, in principle, result from the use of multiple sites for initiation or termination of translation.

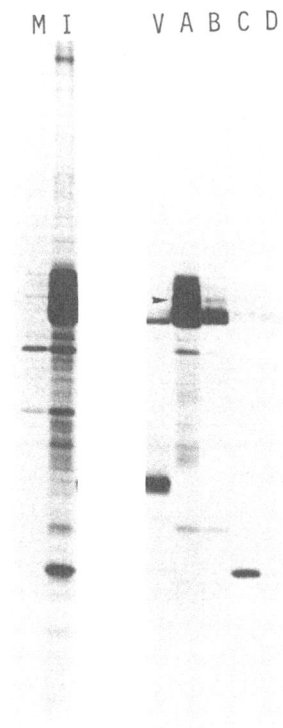

Fig. 1. In vitro translation of gel-purified IBV RNAs. Polyadenyl-
         ated RNA labeled biosynthetically with $^{32}P_i$ was purified
         from cells. The RNA was fractionated on a preparative 2%
         acrylamide-0.1% bisacrylamide gel. IBV intracellular RNAs
         were eluted and translated in a messenger-dependent rabbit
         reticulocyte lysate in the presence of ^{35}S-methionine. The
         products were analyzed by SDS-polyacrylamide gel electro-
         phoresis. Lane M, translation products of RNA from unin-
         fected cells; lane I, translation products of nonfraction-
         ated RNA from infected cells. Lane V, virion proteins;
         lanes A, B, C, and D, translation products of gel-purified
         IBV RNAs A, B, C, and D, respectively.

RNAs A, B, C, and D were purified by preparative acrylamide gel electrophoresis and translated in the reticulocyte lysate. P51 and P23 were produced by translation of RNAs A and C, respectively (Fig. 1, lanes A and C). There were no obvious virus-specific translation products associated with RNAs B and D. Because we were concerned about possible degradation of the mRNA during elution from the preparative gel, we also purified viral mRNA by a gentler technique. Infected cell RNA was labelled biosynthetically with ^{3}H-uridine in the presence of actinomycin D and fractionated by velocity sedimentation. The RNA in each fraction was analyzed by agarose gel electrophoresis (Fig. 3, upper panel) and compared with the corresponding cell-free translation products (Fig. 3, lower panel). Production of P51 and P23 again correlated with the presence of RNAs A and C. However, the resolution of this experiment was not sufficient to distinguish RNAs A and B.

The mRNA encoding GP155 remained to be identified. RNA E was an obvious candidate. RNA E, labelled biosynthetically with ^{3}H-uridine was purified by velocity sedimentation (Fig. 4, lane a). Translation of this RNA preparation yielded a 110 kd polypeptide designated P110 (Fig. 4, lane b). Comparison of maps of methionine-labelled tryptic peptides of P110 (Fig. 5, panel A) and GP155 (Fig. 5, panel B) demonstrated that they are closely related. Production of P51 by translation of this RNA preparation can perhaps be attributed to activation of the internal gene for P51 by degradation of the RNA during translation.

We concluded from these experiments that RNAs A, C, and E encode 51 kd, 23 kd, and 110 kd polypeptides, respectively, which are processed to produce P51, the P23 family proteins, and GP155. The sizes of proteins specified by RNAs C and E do not support a model in which each RNA is translated over its entire length, but are compatible with the non-overlapping translational model (Table 1). A map of the IBV genome based upon the non-overlapping scheme is depicted in the upper panel of Fig. 6. Viral genes are demarcated by loci corresponding to the 5' ends of the intracellular RNAs. The predicted sizes of unidentified products encoded by RNAs B, M, D, and F are listed in Table 1. A map of the mouse hepatitis virus (MHV) genome, determined by others[16,17,18,19] is shown in the lower panel of Fig. 6 for comparison.

There is a major difference between the transcription of MHV and IBV. IBV mRNA E and MHV RNA 3 encode the large virion glycoproteins of the two viruses. However, MHV produces an additional larger sub-genomic RNA which has no homologue in IBV. IBV and MHV thus differ in the means by which the gene upstream from that which encodes the large glycoprotein is expressed.

An additional potential difference between IBV and MHV is the location of genes which encode the small membrane protein. In MHV,

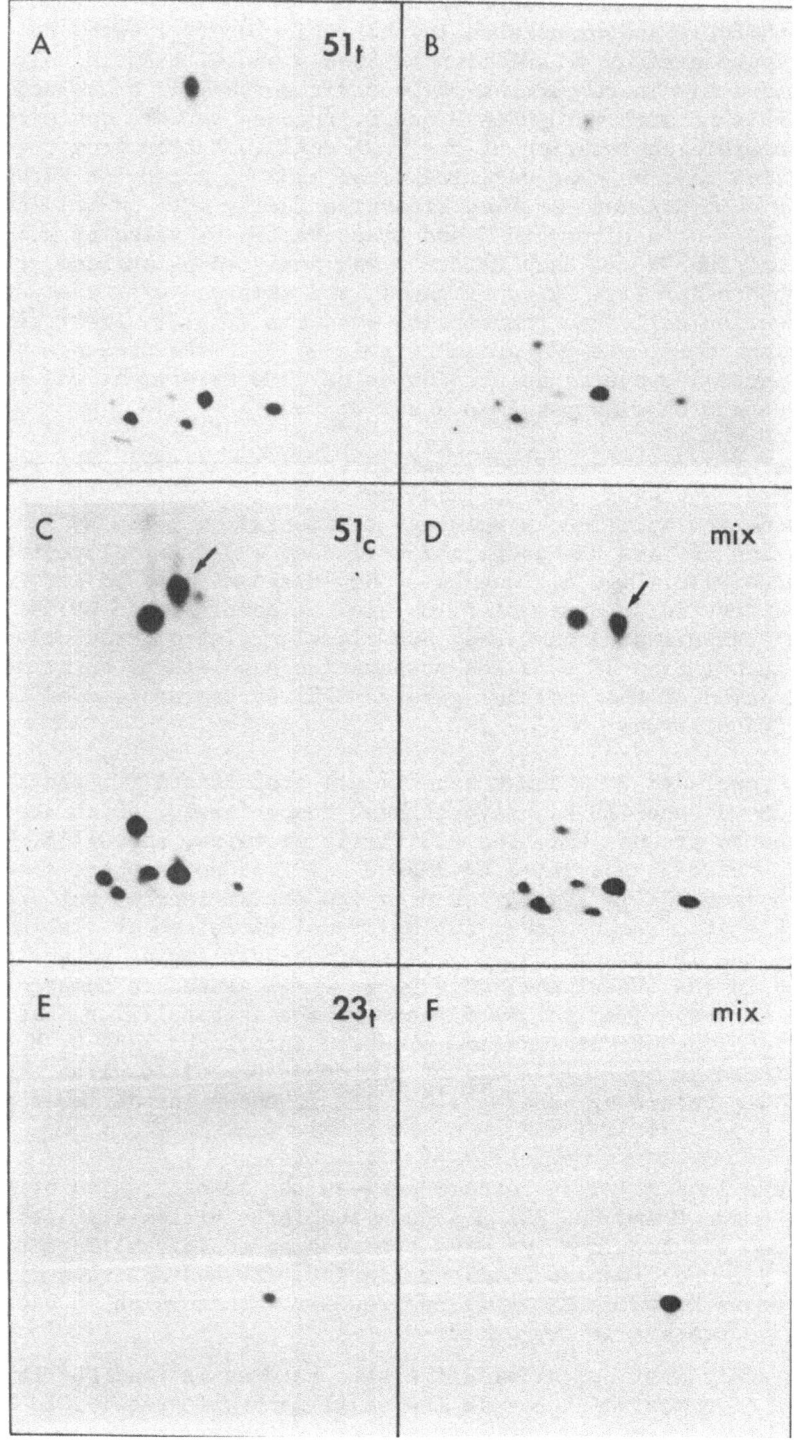

Fig. 2.   Tryptic peptide maps of P51 and P23 synthesized in vitro.
←——————   P23, P51, and a larger member of the P51 series, produced
           by cell-free translation of RNA from IBV-infected cells in
           the presence of ^{35}S-methionine, were purified in a prepar-
           ative gel. The proteins were eluted, digested with trypsin,
           and peptides were resolved in two dimensions on thin-layer
           cellulose plates^{6}. Electrophoresis in the first dimension
           was from left to right. Ascending chromatography in the
           second dimension was from bottom to top. The large member
           of the P51 series is marked in Fig. 1, lane A, with an
           arrow. Cell-associated forms of P51 and GP31 labeled with
           ^{35}S-methionine were mapped for comparison. A map of the
           preparation of GP31 used in the mixture in panel F has been
           published^{14}. Panel A, P51 synthesized in vitro; panel B,
           larger member of the P51 series, synthesized in vitro; panel
           C, P51 synthesized in vivo; panel D, mixture of peptides
           from P51 synthesized in vitro and in vivo; panel E, P23 syn-
           thesized in vitro; panel F, mixture of peptides from P23
           synthesized in vitro and GP31 synthesized in vivo.

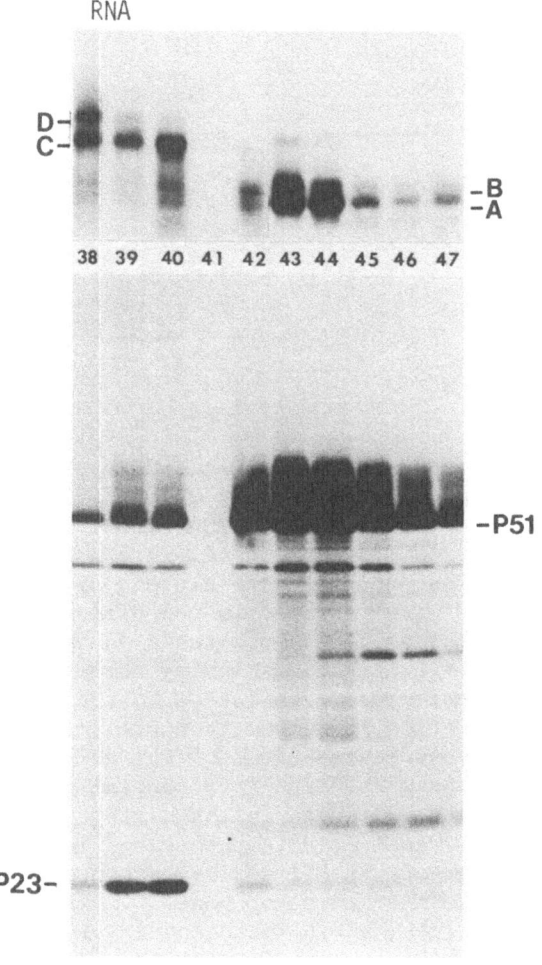

TRANSLATES

Fig. 3.   Translation in vitro of gradient-fractionated RNA. Polyadeny-
          lated RNA was purified from IBV-infected cells which had
          been labeled with ^{3}H-uridine in the presence of actinomycin
          D from 1 to 8 h post-infection. The RNA was fractionated by
          sedimentation in an 11.6 ml 15-30% sucrose-TLES gradient^3 at
          150,000 x g for 4.5 h at 10°C in a SW41 rotor. 56 fractions,
          numbered consecutively from bottom to top, were collected. A
          portion of the RNA from each fraction was analyzed by agarose
          gel electrophoresis (upper panel). Another portion was trans-
          lated in vitro and the products analyzed by SDS-polyacryl-
          amide gel electrophoresis (lower panel). RNAs and correspond-
          ing translation products from gradient fractions 38 to 47
          are shown. RNA in fraction 41 was evidently lost during
          handling.

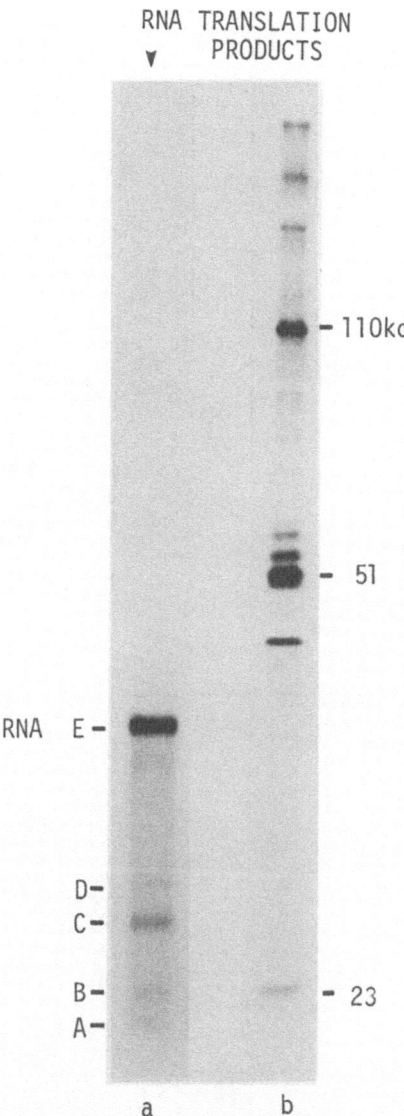

Fig. 4. In vitro translation of gradient-purified RNA E. Polyadenyl-
        ated RNA,   labeled with ^{3}H-uridine, was isolated from
        infected cells. The RNA was fractionated under the conditions
        described in the legend to Fig. 3. A portion of the RNA was
        analyzed by agarose gel electrophoresis and fractions con-
        taining RNA E were pooled. RNA in this pool was analyzed by
        agarose gel electrophoresis (lane a) and the in vitro
        translation products were analyzed by SDS-polyacrylamide
        gel electrophoresis (lane b).

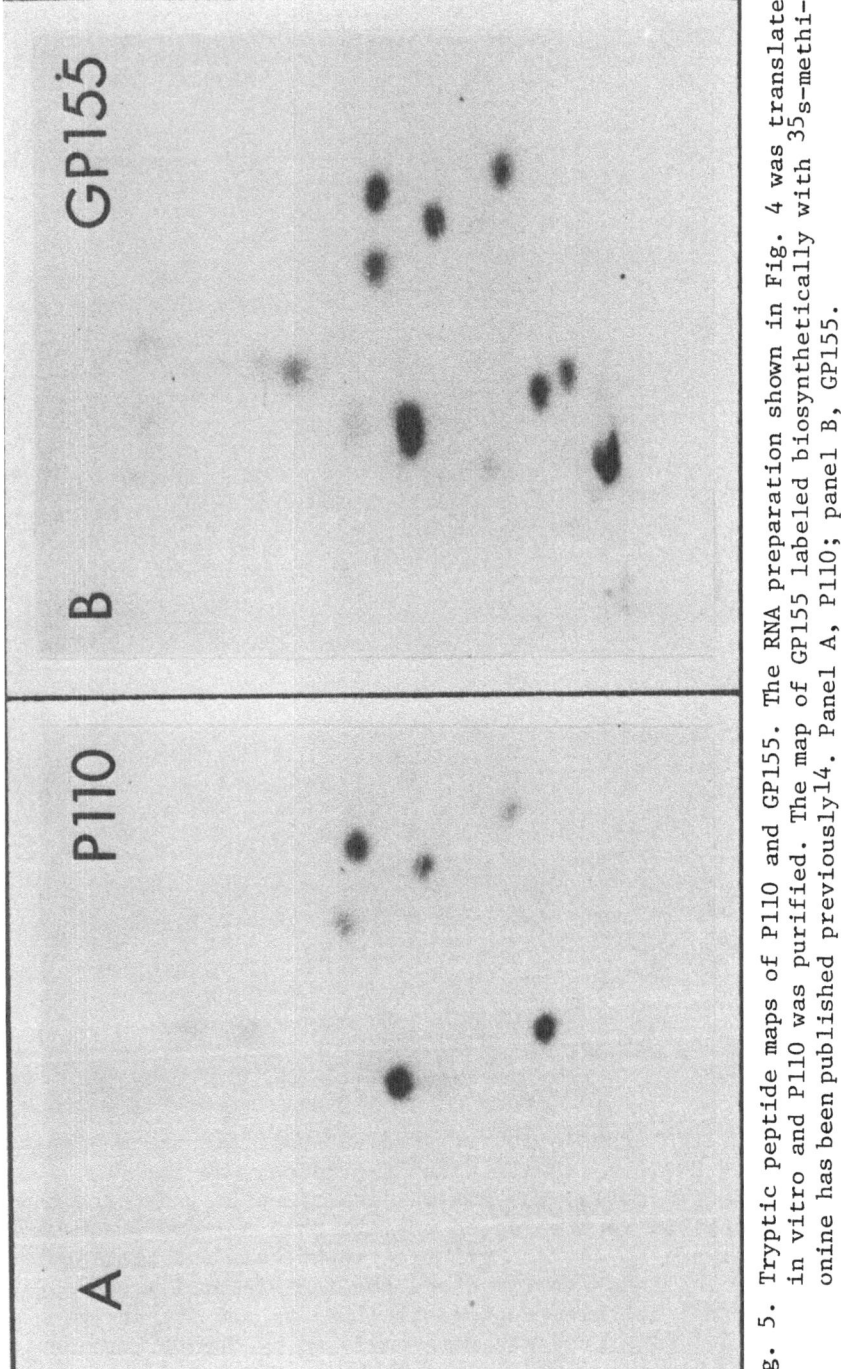

Fig. 5. Tryptic peptide maps of P110 and GP155. The RNA preparation shown in Fig. 4 was translated in vitro and P110 was purified. The map of GP155 labeled biosynthetically with 35-s-methionine has been published previously[14]. Panel A, P110; panel B, GP155.

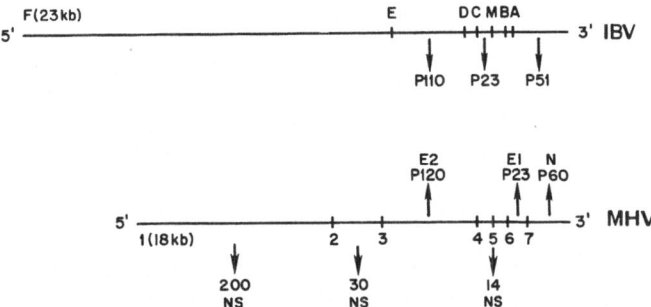

Fig. 6.   Genetic maps of IBV and MHV. The genomes of IBV and MHV are
depicted with the points corresponding to the 5' ends of
the intracellular RNAs marked. It was assumed that the
5' boundary of each viral gene is near a point corresponding
to the 5' terminus of a mRNA. The polypeptide encoded by
each gene is designated by its molecular weight in kd. The
map of MHV is based upon the work of others[16,17,18,19]

genes encoding E1 and the nucleocapsid protein are contiguous and expressed by translation of the two smallest mRNAs. In IBV, however, the locations of promoters for RNA B and RNA M suggest that two genes of unknown function separate the genes encoding P23 and the nucleocapsid protein.

Of the IBV virion proteins that are known to be structurally unique, only P14 remains unassigned to a mRNA. Completion of the genetic map of IBV will therefore depend upon identification of IBV nonstructural proteins.

We have obtained molecular clones of IBV sequences. These will greatly facilitate the detailed study of IBV multiplication. cDNA copies of the IBV genome were synthesized with virion RNA as a template and an oligo(dT) primer. Synthesis of the second strand, primed by spontaneous formation of hairpin loops, was catalyzed by the Klenow fragment of DNA polymerase I. The hairpin loop was opened with nuclease S_1 and deoxycytidylate tails were added with terminal transferase. The DNA was annealed to pBR322 that had been linearized by cleavage with Pst I (interrupting the ampicillin-resistance gene) and tailed with deoxyguanidylate. The recombinant plasmids were introduced into E. coli strain C600 by transformation. Plasmids were purified from 144 tetracycline-resistant, ampicillin-sensitive colonies and compared according to size. The largest, pIBV5, contained 3.3 kb of inserted sequences. In Northern blotting experiments, the insert hybridized to IBV mRNAs but not to RNA from uninfected cells. This confirms the viral origin of the inserted sequences. The presence of a deoxyadenylate tract at one end of the insert suggests that this terminus corresponds to the exact 3' end of the IBV genome. Preliminary data indicate that the 5'-most sequences contained in pIBV5 consist of an open reading frame which extends beyond the 5' end of the clone. This reading frame encodes an extremely hydrophobic protein which is almost certainly P23.

pIBV5 should prove useful in investigation of many problems pertaining to coronavirus multiplication. The nucleotide sequence of the plasmid may reveal open reading frames which indicate the structure of proteins encoded by RNAs B and M. These proteins could then be isolated with antisera directed against synthetic peptides homologous with the predicted sequence. Purification of viral RNA by hybrid selection and mapping cell-free translation products to the genome by hybrid arrest translation will also aid identification of additional viral gene products.

Recent reports indicate that the mechanism of coronavirus RNA synthesis differs from that of other RNA viruses. MHV RNAs contain identical 5' terminal leader sequences which are evidently joined to the bodies of mRNAs by transcription of non-adjacent sequences[20,21]. The use of primers derived from pIBV5 for determining the 5' terminal sequences of RNAs A, B, and M will permit their direct comparison to genomic sequences and reveal the structure of the leader-body junction. Further insight into IBV RNA synthesis may be gained by comparison of the promoters for synthesis of mRNAs A, B, and M, and of the negative-stranded template for mRNA synthesis, all of which should be contained in pIBV5.

REFERENCES

1. B. Lomniczi and I. Kennedy, J. Virol. 24:99-107 (1977).
2. D.F. Stern and S.I.T. Kennedy, J. Virol. 34:665-674 (1980).
3. D.F. Stern and S.I.T. Kennedy, J. Virol. 36:440-449 (1980).
4. S. Siddell, H. Wege, and V. ter Meulen, Curr. Topics in Microbiol. and Immunol. 99:131-163 (1982).
5. L.S. Sturman and K.V. Holmes, Adv. Virus Res. 28, in press (1983).
6. D.F. Stern, L. Burgess, and B.M. Sefton, J. Virol. 42:208-219 (1982).
7. D.F. Stern and B.M. Sefton, J. Virol. 44:804-812 (1982).
8. D. Cavanagh, J. Gen. Virol. 53:93-103, (1981).
9. J.A. Lanser and C.R. Howard, J. Gen. Virol. 46:349-361 (1980).
10. M.R. MacNaughton, M.H. Madge, H.A. Davies, and R.R. Dourmashkin, J. Virol. 24:821-825 (1977).
11. J.A. Lanser and C.R. Howard, J. Gen. Virol. 46:349-361 (1980).
12. H.A. Davies, R.R. Dourmashkin, and M.R. MacNaughton, J. Gen. Virol. 53:67-74 (1981).
13. C.N. Wadey and E.G. Westaway, Intervirology 15:19-27 (1981).
14. D.F. Stern and B.M. Sefton, J. Virol. 44:794-803 (1982).
15. H.R.B. Pelham and R.J. Jackson, Eur. J. Biochem. 67:247-256 (1976).
16. S. Siddell, H. Wege, A. Barthel, and V. ter Meulen, J. Virol. 33:10-17 (1980).
17. P.J.M. Rottier, W.J.M.Spaan, M.C. Horzinek, and B.A.M. Van der Zeijst, J. Virol. 38:20-26 (1981).
18. J.L. Leibowitz, S.R. Weiss, E. Paavola, and C.W. Bond, J. Virol. 43:905-913, (1982).
19. S. Siddell, J. Gen. Virol. 64:113-125 (1983).
20. M.C. Lai, C.D. Patton, R.S. Baric, and S.A. Stohlman, J. Virol. 46:1027-1033 (1983).
21. W. Spaan, P. Rottier, S. Smeekens, B.A.M. Van der Zeijst, H. Delius, J. Armstrong, M. Skinner, and S.G. Siddell, submitted for publication.

PROTEOLYTIC CLEAVAGE OF PEPLOMERIC GLYCOPROTEIN E2 OF MHV YIELDS TWO 90K SUBUNITS AND ACTIVATES CELL FUSION

Lawrence S. Sturman[1] and Kathryn V. Holmes[2]

[1]Center for Laboratories and Research
New York State Department of Health
Albany, New York 12201

[2]Department of Pathology, The Uniformed Services
University of the Health Sciences
Bethesda, Maryland 20814

INTRODUCTION

During the past decade our laboratories have been studying the structure and functions of coronavirus glycoproteins. Several years ago, based on our studies with mouse hepatitis virus (MHV)-A59, we proposed a schematic model of the molecular organization of the coronavirus particle (Sturman et al., 1980). This model appears to be valid for most other coronaviruses as well (Garwes, 1980; Siddell et al., 1982). Our current representation of the structure of MHV-A59 is shown in Fig. 1 (Sturman and Holmes, 1983).

The virion contains three structural proteins: N, E1, and E2. N is a phosphorylated nucleocapsid protein which forms the helical nucleocapsid in association with the RNA genome. E1 is a small, matrix-like, trans-membrane glycoprotein which is O-glycosylated in MHV and deeply embedded in the lipid bilayer. The viral peplomers, which are responsible for attaching the virus to cell-surface receptors, are composed of a large glycoprotein E2. It is not known how many oligomers of this N-linked glycoprotein made up each peplomer.

In this report we shall discuss the structure of E2 and its relation to an important biologic function, cell fusion. Fusion of cells by MHV-A59 will be correlated with trypsin-induced cleavage of the 180K form of E2 to two different 90K products.

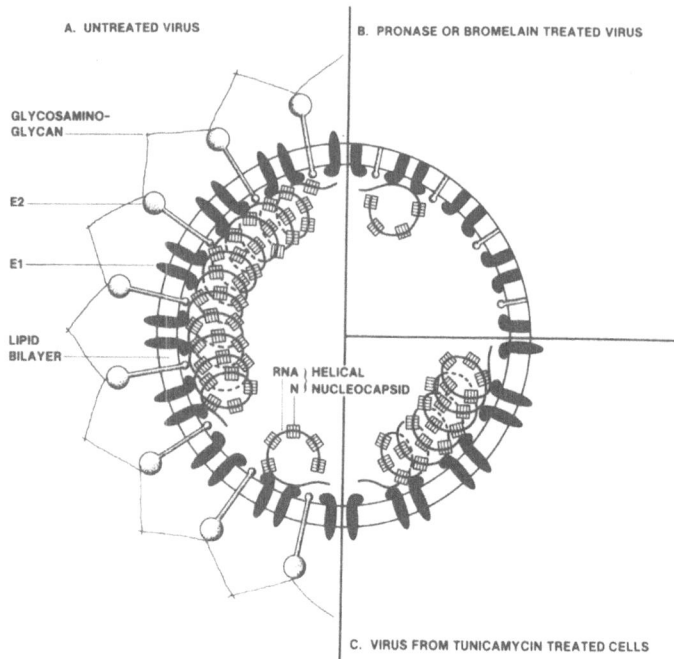

Fig. 1. Model for structure of MHV. (Copyright Academic Press; reprinted with permission from Sturman and Holmes, 1983)

EFFECTS OF TRYPSIN ON CORONAVIRUSES

The E2 peplomeric glycoprotein occurs in the virion in two forms with apparent molecular weights of 180,000 and 90,000 (Sturman and Holmes, 1977). We have shown previously that trypsin treatment of MHV quantitatively converts the 180K form of E2 to 90K forms and that the 180- and 90K components have identical tryptic peptide maps (Sturman and Holmes, 1977). At the time these observations were made, no functional role for proteolytic cleavage of E2 was known, and separation of the two 90K products was not achieved.

Trypsin influences in several ways the infection of cells by corona-viruses. Plaque formation of an enteropathogenic bovine coronavirus and several strains of infectious bronchitis virus (IBV) were enhanced by adding trypsin to the overlay (Storz et al., 1981; Otsuki and Tsubokura, 1981). In the presence of trypsin, infection with a bovine coronavirus was associated with cell fusion (Storz et al., 1981; Toth, 1982). Similar findings were obtained with some strains of MHV. Trypsin treatment of infected cells enable MHV-S to form fusion plaques on otherwise resistant cells and enabled MHV-2 to form fusion-type plaques (Yoshikura and Tejima, 1981).

The effects of trypsin on specific functions of coronavirus structural proteins have been more difficult to demonstrate. Initially trypsin treatment of virions appeared to be necessary for activation of IBV hemagglutinin (Corbo and Cunningham, 1959). Subsequently, however, the IBV hemagglutinin and the hemagglutinating activity of human coronavirus OC38/43 were shown to be inactivated by trypsin (Bingham et al., 1975; Kaye and Dowdle, 1969). Significant strain differences in IBV hemagglutination were noted, and the response of IBV to trypsin also differed according to the strain. Efforts to demonstrate an effect of trypsin on MHV infectivity gave equivocal results. Treatment of virions with low concentrations of trypsin enhanced infectivity two- to three-fold; treatment with high concentrations of trypsin reduced infectivity by a like amount (Sturman and Holmes, 1977).

ROLE OF E2 IN CELL FUSION

The role of E2 in induction of cell fusion was first indicated by the observations that (i) coronavirus-induced fusion was inhibited by mono-specific anti-E2 antibody and (ii) treatment of infected cells with tunicamycin simultaneously inhibited the synthesis of E2 and cell fusion (Holmes et al., 1981). Monoclonal antibodies to E2 also inhibit cell fusion (Collins et al., 1982).

Direct evidence for the role of proteolytic cleavage of E2 in cell fusion has recently been obtained. Although other viruses, such as paramyxoviruses, can cause fusion after adsorption of concentrated virus but in the absence of virus replication, efforts to demonstrate rapid fusion by concentrated coronavirus were unsuccessful until we employed virus which had been pretreated with trypsin. No rapid fusion of L2 cells was produced by direct action of concentrated MHV-A59 (500 pfu/cell) on the plasma membrane (Fig. 2a). In this experiment no fusion was demonstrated until the end of the virus latent period (6 h). However, if the virions were pretreated with trypsin, which cleaved the 180K E2 to 90K forms, extensive cell fusion was observed by 75 min (Fig. 2b). This response was not affected by inhibition of protein synthesis with cyclohexamide. The pH optimum for cell fusion by concentrated virus was pH 7.2 to 7.8.

PURIFICATION OF 90A AND 90B CLEAVAGE PRODUCTS OF 180K E2

To clarify the relationship between the 180- and 90K forms of E2, we made use of the fact that the E2 glycoprotein is acylated (Niemann and Klenk, 1981). Purified virions labeled with [^{3}H] palmitic acid and ^{14}C-labeled amino acids were treated with trypsin, repurified by ultracentrifugation, and applied to hydroxyapatite columns in sodium dodecyl sulfate (SDS) after the method of Moss and Rosenblum (1972). Three major peaks of MHV-A59 proteins were eluted by a gradient of phosphate buffer at pH 6.4 (Fig. 3) and were analyzed by SDS-polyacrylamide gel electrophoresis (PAGE; Fig. 4).

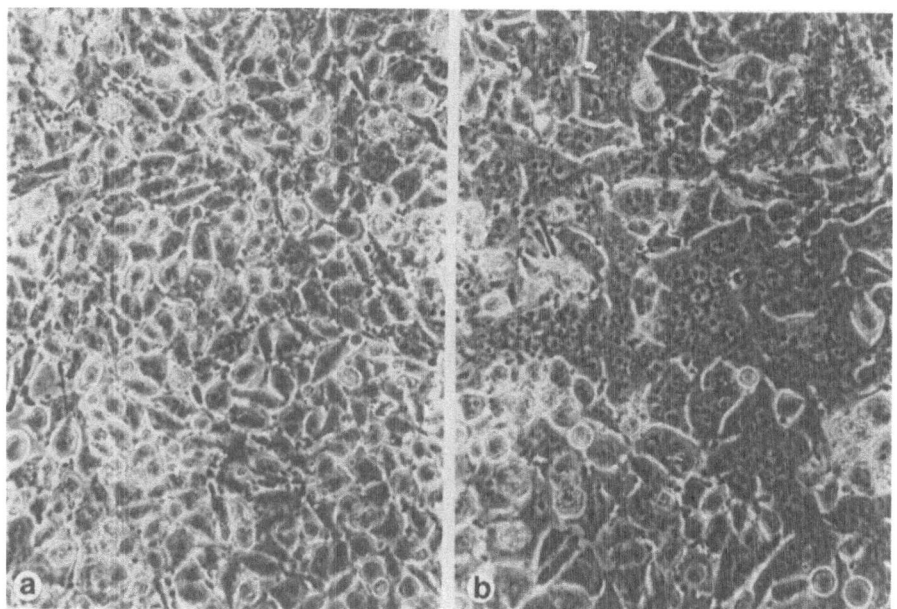

Fig. 2. Proteolytic activation of cell fusion by concentrated virus. (a)
No fusion of L2 cells by direct action of concentrated MHV-A59 (500 pfu/
cell) on the plasma membrane occurs within 2 h. (b) If the virions are pretreated with trypsin to cleave the 180K E2 to 90K forms, extensive fusion
of cells is observed in 75 min.

The first peak contained almost all of the palmitic acid label and a
90K protein (Fig. 4A). However, this fatty acid was not covalently bound
to the protein. The palmitic acid label from this peak migrated with the
dye front in the gel and was probably associated with lipids in the viral
envelope. The second peak contained the nucleocapsid protein N (Fig. 4B).
The third peak consisted of two glycoproteins: the 23K matrix glycoprotein
E1 and a 90K species which contained covalently bonded palmitic acid (Fig.
4C). Later fractions contained monomeric and aggregated forms of E1
(data not shown).

By analogy with other acylated viral glycoproteins, the fatty acid in
E2 is probably located in the region at which the protein is anchored to the
viral envelope. We have termed the 90K species which contained covalently bonded palmitic acid and which coeluted with E1, 90A. The other
90K species, which eluted first and did not contain palmitic acid label, we
have termed 90B.

To demonstrate that the separation of 90A from 90B does not depend
upon the interaction of 90A with E1 or the association of 90B with non-
covalently bonded lipid, the two subunits of E2 were purified on hydroxyapatite following removal of the nucleocapsid, E1, and lipid. Trypsin-
treated, purified virions were solubilized by NP40, the nucleocapsids were

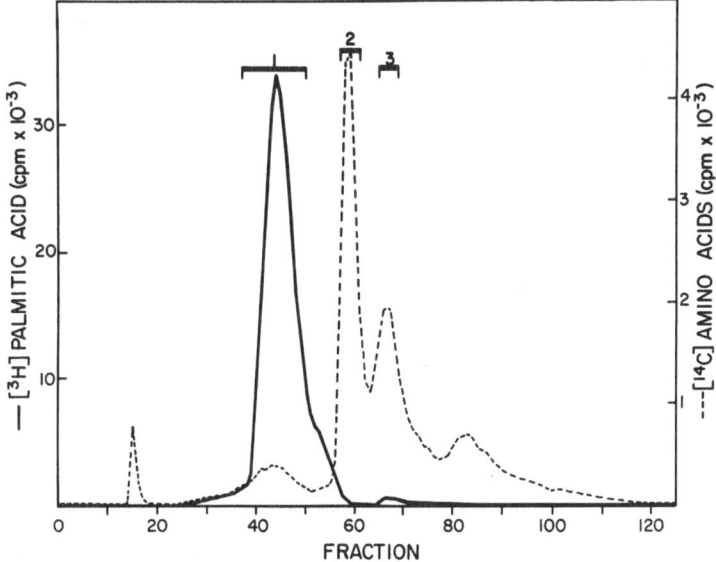

Fig. 3. Separation of structural proteins of MHV-A59 by chromatography on hydroxyapatite in SDS. Trypsin-treated MHV, labeled with ^{14}C-labeled amino acids and with [3H] palmitic acid, was eluted in a gradient containing 0.2 to 0.5 M sodium phosphate, pH 6.4, with 0.2% SDS, 1 mM dithiothreitol.

removed by sucrose density gradient centrifugation (Sturman et al., 1980), and E2 was separated from E1 and lipid by Fractogel chromatography. The separation of NP40-solubilized E2 from E1 on Fractogel TSK (HW-55S) in 1% SDS is shown in Fig. 5. The first peak contained all of the fucose label but only a small fraction of the methionine. SDS-PAGE analysis revealed that this peak consisted of 90K E2, while the second peak contained E1. E2 was then separated into its 90A and 90B components by chromatography on hydroxyapatite or Ultrogel HA, a form of hydroxyapatite bound to agarose. The flow rates with Ultrogel were 5-10 times faster than with hydroxyapatite. Elution of [3H] glucosamine and [35S] methionine-labeled 90A and 90B from Ultrogel HA in 1% SDS with a gradient of phosphate buffer at pH 6.4 is shown in Fig. 6. Part of the 90B form eluted in the void volume.

AMINO ACID COMPOSITIONS OF 90A and 90B

Separation of 90A from 90B permitted comparison of their amino acid compositions (Table 1). The peak fractions containing 90A and 90B were concentrated by ultrafiltration with Millipore CX-30 filter units, and the residual SDS was removed by ion-pair extraction according to the method of Henderson et al. (1979). The amino acid compositions of 90A and 90B were determined, in collaboration with Dr. Thomas Plummer of

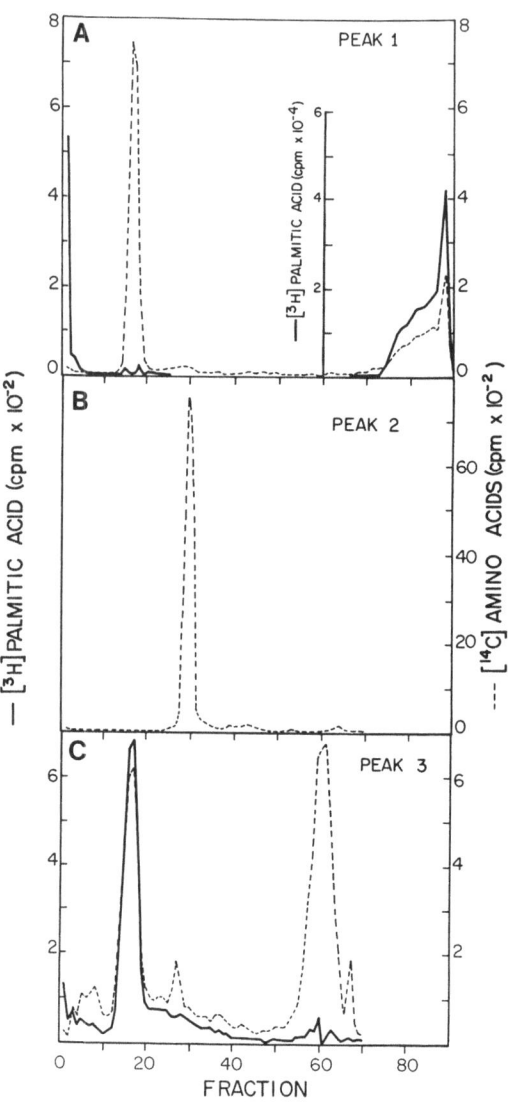

Fig. 4. SDS–PAGE profiles of peaks 1–3 from the hydroxyapatite column shown in Fig. 3.

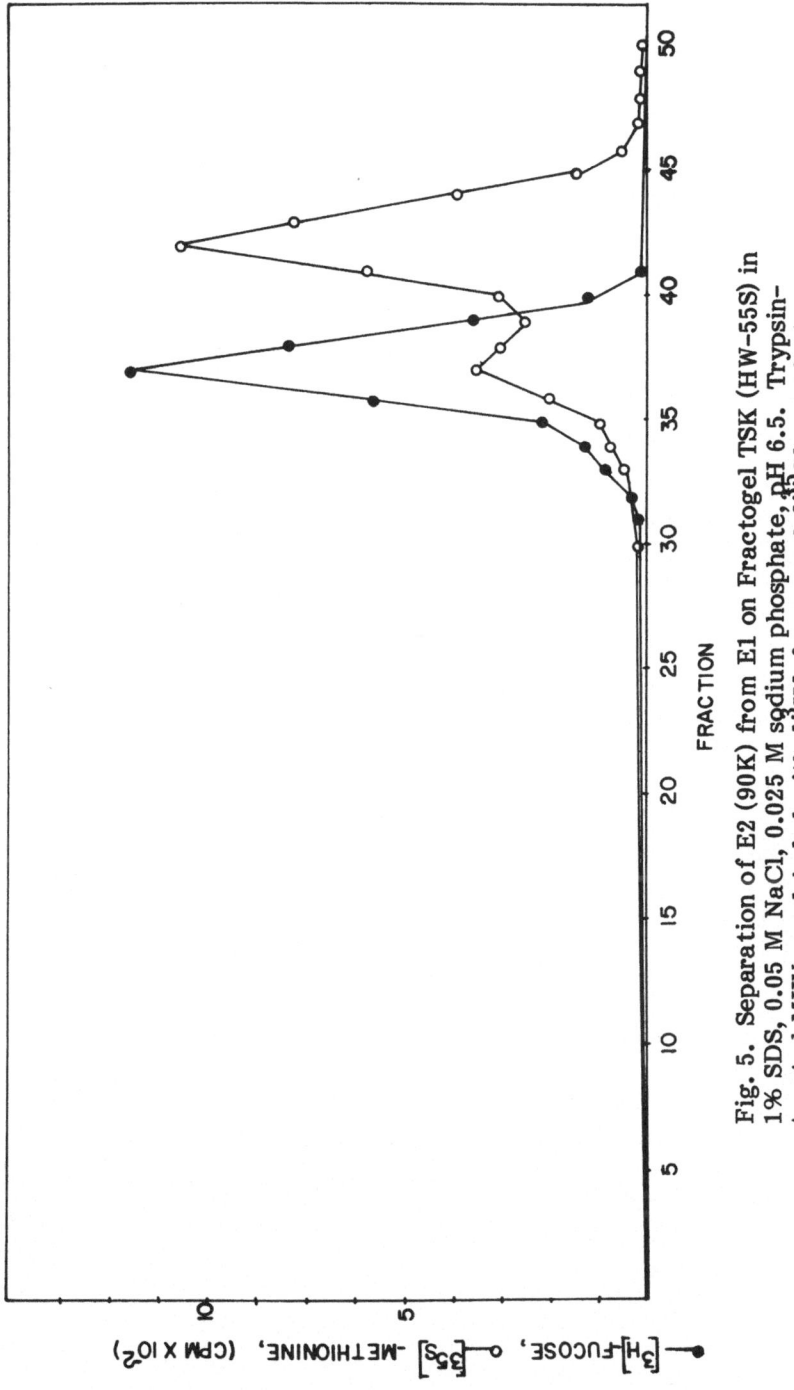

Fig. 5. Separation of E2 (90K) from E1 on Fractogel TSK (HW–55S) in 1% SDS, 0.05 M NaCl, 0.025 M sodium phosphate, pH 6.5. Trypsin-treated MHV was labeled with [^{3}H] fucose and [^{35}S] methionine.

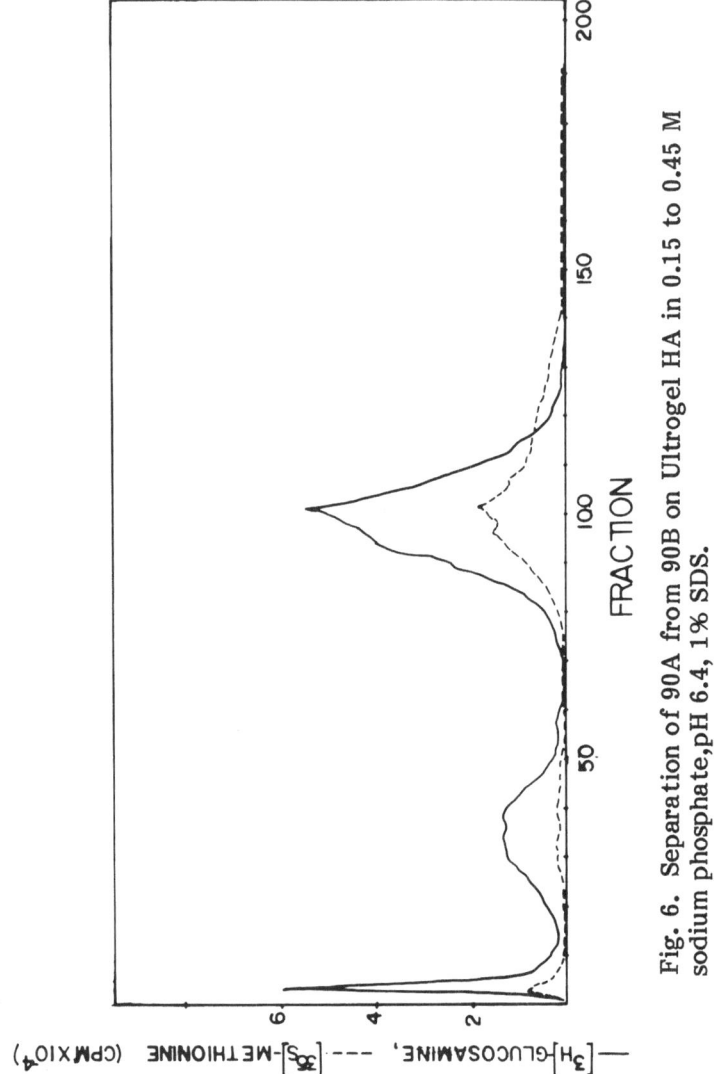

Fig. 6. Separation of 90A from 90B on Ultrogel HA in 0.15 to 0.45 M sodium phosphate, pH 6.4, 1% SDS.

this Center, on an amino acid analyzer after acid hydrolysis for 24 h.

As shown by the ratios of molar percentages (Table 1), threonine, serine, and glycine occurred in greater amounts in 90B, whereas the hydrophobic amino acids, valine, methionine, isoleucine, and leucine, were more abundant in 90A. These data support the conclusion that proteolytic cleavage of a large 180K form of E2 produces two different 90K products.

Table 1. Amino Acid Compositions of 90A and 90B Subunits of E2

Amino Acid[a]	Mole Percent[b]		90B/90A
	90A	90B	
Asx	11.06	11.51	1.04
Thr	6.63	7.97	1.20
Ser	6.67	8.40	1.26
Glx	11.30	11.25	1.00
Pro	4.29	4.06	0.95
Gly	8.96	11.46	1.28
Ala	7.81	6.78	0.87
Val	9.93	7.93	0.80
Met	1.33	0.87	0.65
Ile	4.64	3.78	0.81
Leu	9.31	7.63	0.82
Tyr	2.99	3.27	1.09
Phe	4.67	4.68	1.00
Lys	4.43	4.06	0.92
His	1.92	1.69	0.88
Arg	4.18	4.55	1.09

[a] Half-cysteine and tryptophan were not determined.
[b] Mean of three determinations.

CONCLUSIONS

The isolation of two different 90K cleavage products from the 180K E2 of MHV-A59 resolves the long-standing question of the relationship between the 90K and 180K forms of E2. Direct evidence for the role of proteolytic cleavage of E2 in activation of cell fusion suggests that cleavage of this large glycoprotein reveals a new active site, which has biologic functions in coronavirus infection and pathogenesis.

ACKNOWLEDGEMENTS

The authors thank C. Ricard, F. Baker, T. Plummer, C. Eastwood and M. Liebach, who participated in these studies. This work was supported by grants AI 18997 and GM 31698 from the National Institutes of Health and grant RO 7043 from the Uniformed`Services University of the Health Sciences. The opinions expressed are the private views of the authors and should not be construed as official or necessarily reflecting the views of the Uniformed Services University School of Medicine of the Department of Defense.

REFERENCES

Bingham, R.W., Madge, M.H., and Tyrrell, D.A., 1975, Hemagglutination by avian infectious bronchitis — a coronavirus, J. Gen. Virol., 28:381.

Collins, A.R., Knobler, R.L., Powell, H., and Buchmeier, M.J., 1982, Monoclonal antibodies to murine hepatitis virus-4 (strain JHM) define the viral glycoprotein responsible for attachment and cell-cell fusion, Virology, 119:358.

Corbo, L.J. and Cunningham, C.H., 1959, Hemagglutination by trypsin-modified infectious bronchitis virus, Am. J. Vet. Res., 20:876.

Garwes, D.J., 1980, Structure and physiochemical properties of corona-viruses, Colloq. Inst. Nat. Sante. Rech. Med., 90:141.

Henderson, L.E., Oroszlan, S., and Konigsberg, W., 1979, A micro-method for complete removal of dodecyl sulfate from proteins by ion-pair extraction, Anal. Biochem., 93:153.

Holmes, K.V., Doller, E.W., and Behnke, J.N., 1981, Analysis of the functions of coronavirus glycoproteins by differential inhibition of synthesis with tunicamycin, Adv. Exp. Med. Biol., 142:133.

Kaye, H.S. and Dowdle, W.R., 1969, Some characteristics of hemaggluti-nation of certain strains of "IBV-like" virus, J. Infect. Dis., 119:576.

Moss, B. and Rosenblum, E.N., 1972, Hydroxylapatite chromatography of protein-sodium dodecyl sulfate complexes, J. Biol. Chem., 247:5194.

Niemann, H. and Klenk, H.D., 1981, Coronavirus glycoprotein E1, a new type of viral glycoprotein, J. Mol. Biol., 153:993.

Otsuki, K. and Tsubokura, M., 1981, Plaque formation by avian infectious bronchitis virus in primary chick embryo fibroblast cells in the presence of trypsin, Arch. Virol., 70:315.

Siddell, S., Wege, H., and ter Meulen, V., 1982, The structure and replication of coronaviruses, Curr. Top. Microbiol. Immunol., 99:131.

Storz, J., Rott, R., and Kaluza, G., 1981, Enhancement of plaque formation and cell fusion of an enteropathogenic coronavirus by trypsin treatment, Infect. Immun., 31:1214.

Sturman, L.S., and Holmes, K.V., 1977, Characterization of a coronavirus. II. Glycoproteins of the viral envelope: Tryptic peptide analysis, Virology, 77:650.

Sturman, L.S., Holmes, K.V., and Behnke, J., 1980, Isolation of coronavirus envelope glycoproteins and interaction with the viral nucleocapsid, J. Virol., 33:449.

Sturman, L.S., and Holmes, K.V., 1983, The molecular biology of coronaviruses, Adv. Virus Res., 28:35.

Toth, T.E., 1982, Trypsin-enhanced replication of neonatal calf diarrhea coronavirus in bovine embryonic lung cells, Am. J. Vet. Res., 43:967.

Yoshikura, H., and Tejima, S., 1981, Role of protease in mouse hepatitis virus-induced cell fusion, Virology, 113:503.

CORONAVIRUS MATURATION

Kathryn V. Holmes, Mark F. Frana, Susan G. Robbins,
and Lawrence S. Sturman

Department of Pathology and Microbiology
Uniformed Services University of the Health Sciences
Bethesda, Md. 20814
          and
Center for Laboratories and Research
New York State Department of Health
Albany, N.Y. 12201

INTRODUCTION

Coronaviruses cause a wide variety of diseases which
includes both acute infections like infectious bronchitis of
chickens and persistent infections like infectious peritonitis of
cats. Current studies on the molecular biology of coronaviruses
will provide essential information on the nature of the
virus-cell interactions which can lead to such different outcomes
of viral infection. This article will analyze the interactions
of coronaviruses with host cells in order to identify host cell
dependent processes which are essential for coronavirus growth.
Coronavirus infection of a cell can have different results as
shown in Table 1.

Since coronaviruses usually exhibit very limited cell and
species tropisms, it is apparent that interactions of many cell
types with coronaviruses do not result in infection. The
molecular basis for this resistance to infection has not been
determined. One plausible explanation would be that
coronaviruses may require very specific receptors which are only
found on the plasma membranes of susceptible cells.

Several types of abortive infections with coronaviruses have
been identified. Abortive infection with mouse hepatitis virus
(MHV) occurs in macrophages or hepatocytes of mice from strains

37

Table 1. Possible Results of Coronavirus Infection

No infection
Abortive infection
Productive infection
    a. Leading to cell death
        1. By cell fusion
        2. By cell lysis
    b. Leading to persistent infection
        1. With continued viral replication
        2. Without continued viral replication

genetically resistant to MHV.[2,3] Little viral protein or RNA
synthesis can be detected in these cells, but the mechanism of
host cell restriction of viral replication has not yet been
identified. Abortive infections may also result from MHV
infection of a variety of differentiated host cell types in
genetically susceptible animals. For example, in primary
differentiated cultures of mouse spinal cord, virus production in
glial cells was abundant whereas only limited virus replication
could be detected in neurons.[4] The strain of virus is also
important in determining whether a given cell type will undergo
abortive infection with a coronavirus. The neurotropic JHM
strain of MHV can infect neurons _in vitro_ much more readily than
can the A59 strain of MHV.[4] Some types of abortive infection may
result in the accumulation of viral structural components within
the cytoplasm. A variety of coronavirus inclusions have been
described.[5]

Productive infection of a susceptible cell by a coronavirus
frequently results in cell death. Unlike many other types of
viruses, coronaviruses do not appear to induce rapid inhibition
of host cell macromolecular synthesis. Indeed, coronavirus
maturation appears to require continuation of many normal functions of the host cell. Death of infected cells is due to cell
fusion or cell lysis. It is not clear what viral factor leads to
cell lysis. Some coronaviruses such as bovine coronavirus (BCV)[6]
may induce lytic plaques without cell fusion in some cell types.
Coronavirus induced fusion occurs _in vitro_ and _in vivo_.[7] We have
recently shown that fusion of L2 cells by MHV-A59 depends on
proteolytic cleavage of the E2 peplomeric glycoprotein.[8]

Because of the lack of virus-induced inhibition of cellular
macromolecular synthesis and the non-lytic release of virions
from infected cells, persistent coronavirus infections can be
readily established _in vitro_ and _in vivo_. The virus-cell
interactions in persistent coronavirus infections vary
considerably. Some persistently infected cultures show active
virus production from all cells,[9] while in others such as our

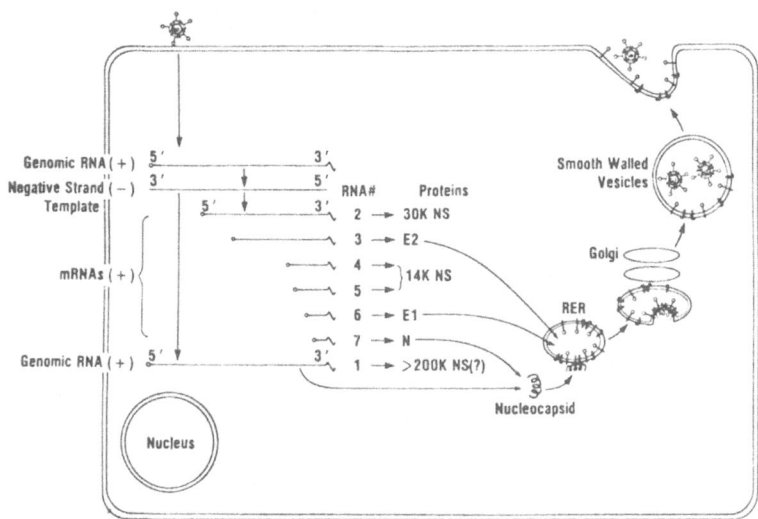

Figure 1.   Coronavirus Replication
(Reproduced from 5 with permission)

persistent infection of 17 Cl 1 cells by MHV-A59 only 10 to 20%
of the cells produce viral antigens and virions.[10]   In the
remaining cells some viral nucleic acid must be present since
infectious virus can be recovered after cloning and cocultivation
with susceptible cells. MHV can also induce a persistent
infection in which viral antigens are not detectable in any
cells, although virus can be rescued by cocultivation.[11]   During
persistent infection, virus mutants may be selected which are
less virulent (small plaque, temperature sensitive, and/or fusion
defective) and cells may be selected which are resistant to the
cytopathic effects of coronaviruses.[10,11]   The specific changes
in the viruses and cells during persistent infection have not yet
been characterized, but may elucidate important virus-host
control mechanisms.

HOST CELL PROCESSES REQUIRED FOR CORONAVIRUS MATURATION

The events that occur in a cell infected with a coronavirus
will be summarized in order to identify cellular processes that
are used for virus replication. These are illustrated in Figure 1.

Binding of coronaviruses to cells takes place by means of
the peplomeric glycoprotein E2 which binds to specific receptors
on the plasma membrane. Some cells such as spleen cells have
large numbers of receptors, whereas others have few or no
receptors. It is not yet clear whether coronaviruses enter cells

by fusion of the viral envelope with the plasma membrane or by an
endocytic pathway.

Virion RNA can apparently act as mRNA to direct the
synthesis of a viral specific RNA dependent RNA polymerase. This[12]
enzyme has been identified as early as 1 hour after infection.
The enzyme directs the synthesis of a full length negative strand
of RNA and then synthesis of genomic RNA and a nested set of 6
subgenomic mRNAs.[13]   No host dependent factors have yet been
identified in this aspect of coronavirus replication.

The synthesis of viral polypeptides does depend on many
cellular mechanisms. These include synthesis on free ribosomes
of the nucleocapsid protein, N, and synthesis on membrane bound
ribosomes of E1 and E2[14] and possibly some N.

Phosphorylation of the nucleocapsid protein, N,[15] may use a
cellular protein kinase. Acylation of the E2 glycoprotein but
not the E1 glycoprotein has been demonstrated.[16] This is
probably also a cell dependent modification.[17]

Glycosylation of the two viral glycoproteins of MHV-A59
appears to depend upon two different host cell pathways. Oligosaccharides of the E2 glycoprotein are attached to asparagine
residues by N-glycosidic bonds. The oligosaccharides of the E1
glycoprotein are markedly different, and are attached post-
translationally by a tunicamycin resistant mechanism to serine
and threonine residues via O-glycosidic bonds.[16,18,19] Thus
MHV-A59 may be a useful model system for study of the formation
of O-glycosidic bonds.

Proteolytic cleavage of viral proteins may depend either on
host cell or virus specific proteases. For coronaviruses, there
is no evidence to suggest viral specific protease activity. As
recently demonstrated in our laboratories,[8] the E2 glycoprotein
of the peplomers of MHV undergoes a proteolytic cleavage to yield
two cleavage products of identical molecular weight which we have
called 90A and 90B. This cleavage is critical for the activation
of MHV induced cell fusion.

Coronaviruses also make use of two different pathways for
the intracellular transport of glycoproteins. We have used[20]
monospecific antisera to the E1 and E2 glycoproteins[21] to study
the intracellular transport of these glycoproteins. We found
that E2 is rapidly dispersed throughout the cytoplasmic membrane
system and appears on the plasma membrane much like N-linked
glycoproteins of other enveloped viruses. In contrast, the E1[21]
glycoprotein did not migrate past the Golgi apparatus. These
two different patterns of intracellular transport are also
observed with monoclonal antibodies to E1 and E2 as shown in

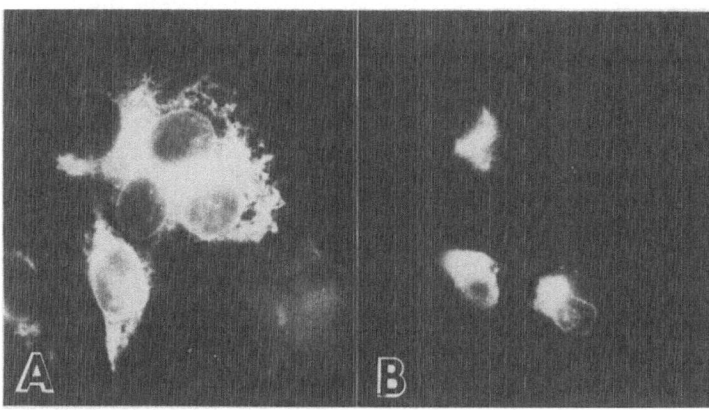

Figure 2.   Different patterns of intracellular transport of the
            two glycoproteins of MHV-A59. Fluorescent antibody
            labeling with monoclonal antisera to the peplomeric
            glycoprotein E2 (A) and to the membrane glycoprotein
            E1 (B) shows that E1 is limited to the Golgi apparatus
            while E2 migrates throughout the cytoplasmic
            membranes.

Figure 2. We have suggested that the localization of E1 to the
rough endoplasmic reticulum (RER) and Golgi apparatus determines
the intracellular location of virus budding.[21]

    A variety of experiments has suggested the functions of the
E1 and E2 glycoproteins that are listed in Table 2.

    To determine the order in which MHV-A59 glycoproteins are
synthesized, processed and incorporated into virions, cell
fractionation and pulse labeling studies have been
performed.[16,21] On the RER, E1 is not glycosylated and sugars
are added post-translationally in the Golgi apparatus.[16]
Although core sugars of E2 are apparently added to the 120K
apoprotein during translation on the RER, the trimming and
elaboration of the oligosaccharides probably occurs in the Golgi
apparatus. The proteolytic cleavage of E2 appears to be a host
dependent process which occurs at or near the plasma membrane.[21]
These processes are illustrated in Figure 3.

    We have observed that the proteolytic cleavage of the E2
glycoprotein is cell dependent. There is considerable variation
in the ratio of the 180K to the 90K forms of E2 in virions
released from different cell types as shown in Figure 4. Virions
released from 17 Cl 1 cells contain approximately equal amounts
of 180 and 90K E2. In contrast, virions released from Sac- cells
contain E2 almost totally in the 90K forms. This host cell

Table 2. Functions of Coronavirus Glycoproteins

E2, the Peplomeric Glycoprotein

1. Binding to receptors on the cell membrane
       (adsorption and/or hemagglutination)
2. Inducing neutralizing antibody
3. Eliciting cell-mediated cytotoxicity
4. Causing pH-dependent thermolability of
       coronaviruses
5. Inducing cell fusion;
       Activated by proteolytic cleavage
6. Fusing viral envelope with cell membrane;
       May be activated by proteolytic cleavage

E1, the Membrane Glycoprotein

1. Determining location of viral budding
2. Forming viral envelope
3. Interacting with viral nucleocapsid

dependent cleavage of E2 correlates with the different extent of
cell fusion induced in these cell types by infection with MHV-A59
as shown in Figure 5. In 17Cl 1 cells, MHV-A59 establishes a
moderate infection in which there is little fusion for 20 hours.
The same virus in Sac- cells produces rapid cell fusion and death
within 10 hours. We suggest that differences in the ability of
different cell types to incorporate viral glycoproteins
efficiently into virions or to transport them to the plasma
membrane as well as differences in the rate of cleavage of the E2
glycoprotein may determine whether the outcome of coronavirus
infection is moderate or cytocidal.

ASSEMBLY AND RELEASE OF VIRIONS

Budding of coronaviruses occurs in the RER and Golgi
apparatus but not at the plasma membrane. It appears likely that
this intracellular budding site for coronaviruses is determined
by the restricted intracellular transport of the E1 glycoprotein
which forms the viral membrane. In the budding virions, the
helical nucleocapsids appear as tubular structures in a regular
array under the viral envelope[4,10,21,23] and the virion has an
electron-lucent center. Virions isolated from within the cell
appear to have a normal complement of peplomers, suggesting that
the virus may be fully formed in the RER and Golgi and that the
glycoproteins may be processed on the virion as they migrate
through these cellular compartments. In 17 Cl 1 cells, the
virions change markedly in shape during this migration as shown

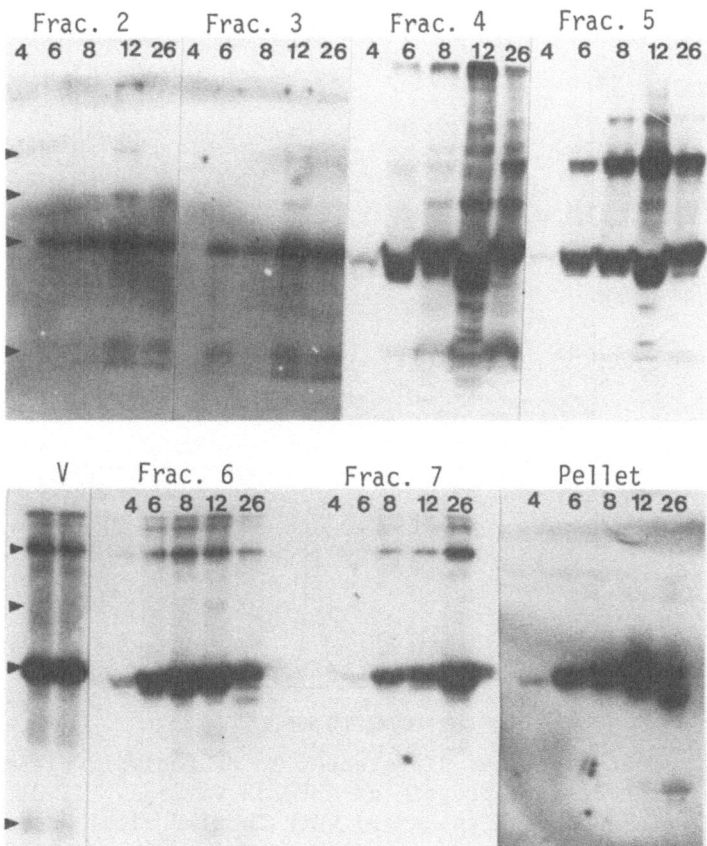

Figure 3.   Processing of MHV-A59 proteins in different cell
            membrane fractions. MHV infected cells were
            fractionated on sucrose density gradients[23] at 4, 6,
            8, 12 and 26 hours after inoculation. Proteins were
            analyzed by PAGE and Western blotting using
            anti-virion antibody and ^{125}I labeled protein A. In
            the pellet N accumulates and is processed into a
            faster migrating species. The glycoproteins El and E2
            are synthesized in the RER fractions 6 and 7. El
            appears to be glycosylated as it migrates into smooth
            membrane fractions 3, 4 and 5. Proteolytic cleavage
            of E2 from 180K to 90K appears to be a late step, as
            the 90K is most apparent in fraction 4 which contains
            mature virions as well as plasma membrane and Golgi
            membranes. Markers on virion proteins indicate E2
            (180 and 90K), N (50K), and El (23K).

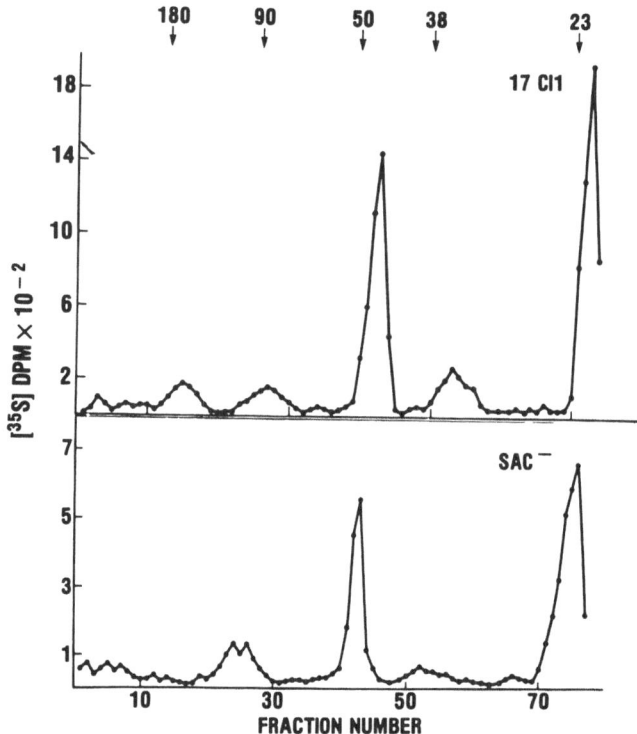

Figure 4.   Host dependent differences in proteolytic cleavage of
             the E2 glycoprotein of MHV-A59 virions.   17 Cl 1 cells
             (A) and Sac- cells (B) were labeled with ^{35}S-methionine
             for 15 min. and virus released from the cells 3 hr.
             later was pelleted and analyzed by PAGE.

in Figure 6.   In the smooth walled, post-Golgi vesicles, the
virions become flattened and disk shaped, and the nucleocapsid
appears as a rather homogeneous electron-dense mass within the
virion. This morphological change may be due to different ionic
conditions within the cellular compartments or to processing of
viral components in these compartments. These changes may be
similar to those seen in aggregates of cellular secretory
proteins which are condensed and concentrated in post-Golgi
vesicles of secretory cells. Thus, coronaviruses may make use of
the cellular secretory process for release from infected cells.[10]
Virions from 17 Cl 1 cells are also in the flattened mature shape
when they are released or readsorbed onto the plasma membrane as
shown in Figure 7.

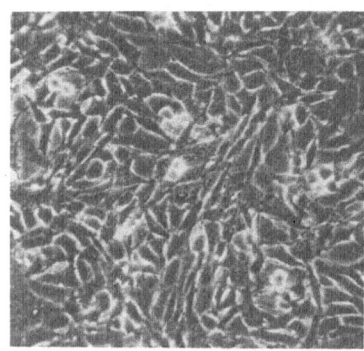 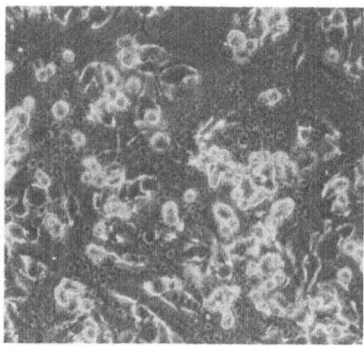

17 CL 1   SAC⁻

Figure 5.   Coronavirus induced fusion of different cell types.
            Infection with MHV-A59 causes much less fusion in 17
            Cl 1 cells than in Sac- cells.   Cell fusion correlates
            with the extent of cleavage of the cell dependent E2
            glycoprotein.

        Recently we have observed flattened disk-shaped virions on
the surface of 17 Cl 1 cells infected with MHV-A59 and prepared
for high voltage electron microscopy by the critical point drying
technique.   Late in the infectious cycle, many of the cells had
become detached from the substrate.   Adhering to the tiny bits of
cytoplasm remaining on the substrate were large numbers of disk
shaped virions as shown in Figure 8.   These probably represented
virions which had been released from the under surface of the 17
Cl 1 fibroblasts and remained adsorbed to the remnants of the
membrane left behind when the cells rounded up and peeled off.

        Late in the infectious cycle of coronaviruses, abnormal
formation of virions and acccumulations of structural elements of
virions may be observed in infected cells.   Inclusions consisting
of viral nucleocapsids have been observed in MHV infected
cultures of mouse spinal cord.[4]   Reticular inclusions formed of
highly convoluted membranes of the ER have been observed in
several cell types.[5]   A final type of intracellular structure
associated with coronavirus infection is the formation of long
tubules within the lumen of the RER as shown in Figure 9.[4,5]
These tubules have also been observed in infected cells treated
with tunicamycin.[18]   We believe that these may represent
accumulations of the matrix glycoprotein, E1.   Tubules somewhat
similar to these have been formed in vitro from the M protein of
parainfluenza virus which performs a similar function in the
formation of the viral membrane.[24]   We have recently found that

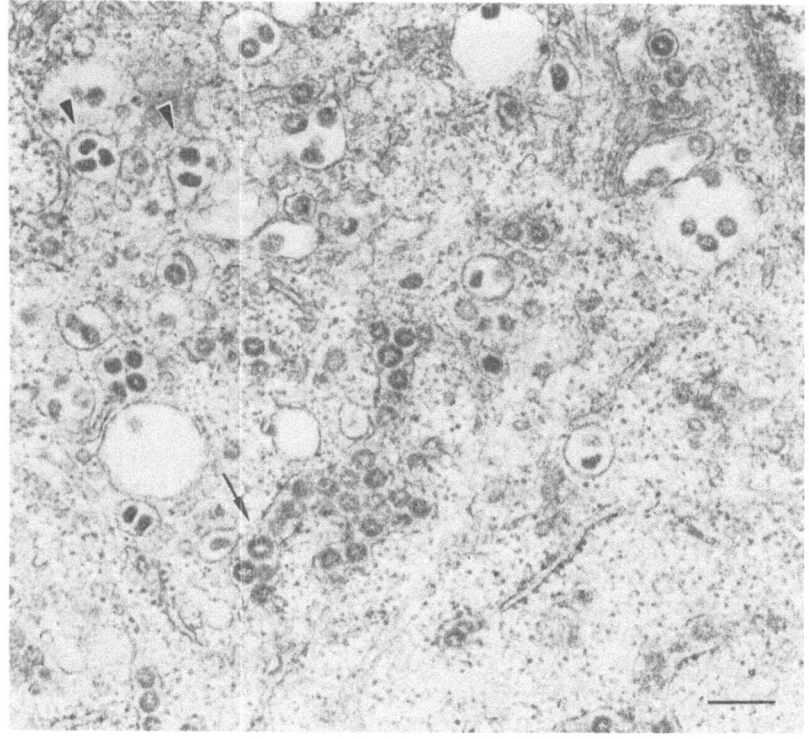

Figure 6.   Structure of mature and immature coronaviruses. In 17
            Cl 1 cells infected with MHV-A59 the virions in the
            RER are spherical with electron-lucent centers
            (arrow). Virions in smooth walled vesicles
            (arrowheads) or adsorbed to the plasma membrane are
            flattened and disk shaped with electron-dense
            nucleocapsids. Bar=200nm.

these tubular forms can be isolated from fractionated cells by
sucrose density gradient ultracentrifugation as shown in Figure
10. Experiments are now in progress to identify the components
of these tubular inclusions.

     In this manuscript, we have reviewed the many processes of
host cells which are required for the elaboration and release of
coronaviruses. These processes are summarized in Table 3. It is
apparent that the rate and extent of each of these processes may
vary from one cell to another. This may affect the outcome of
coronavirus infection. Thus 17 Cl 1 cells represent a cell type
which shows a good balance of synthesis and transport of viral
structural components, together with limited ability to cleave
the E2 glycoprotein which is required for cell fusion. Thus

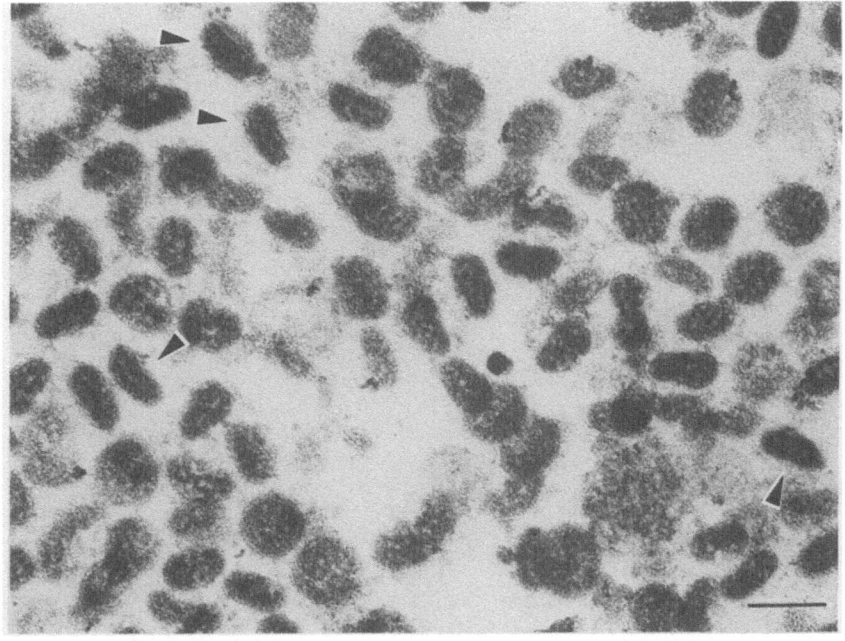

Figure 7.   Gradient purified MHV-A59 virions. Gradient purified
            virions released from 17 Cl 1 cells were pelleted and
            examined in thin sections. Many virions were
            flattened and disk-shaped (arrowheads). Bar=100nm.

MHV-A59 may cause moderate infection in these cells. Cells such
as Sac- or L2 cell lines, which cause rapid and extensive
cleavage of the E2 glycoprotein, undergo rapid cell fusion and
cell death. Because of the extensive dependence of coronavirus
maturation on the host cell processes, it appears likely that
host controlled modification of virus replication may determine
the outcome of coronavirus infection.

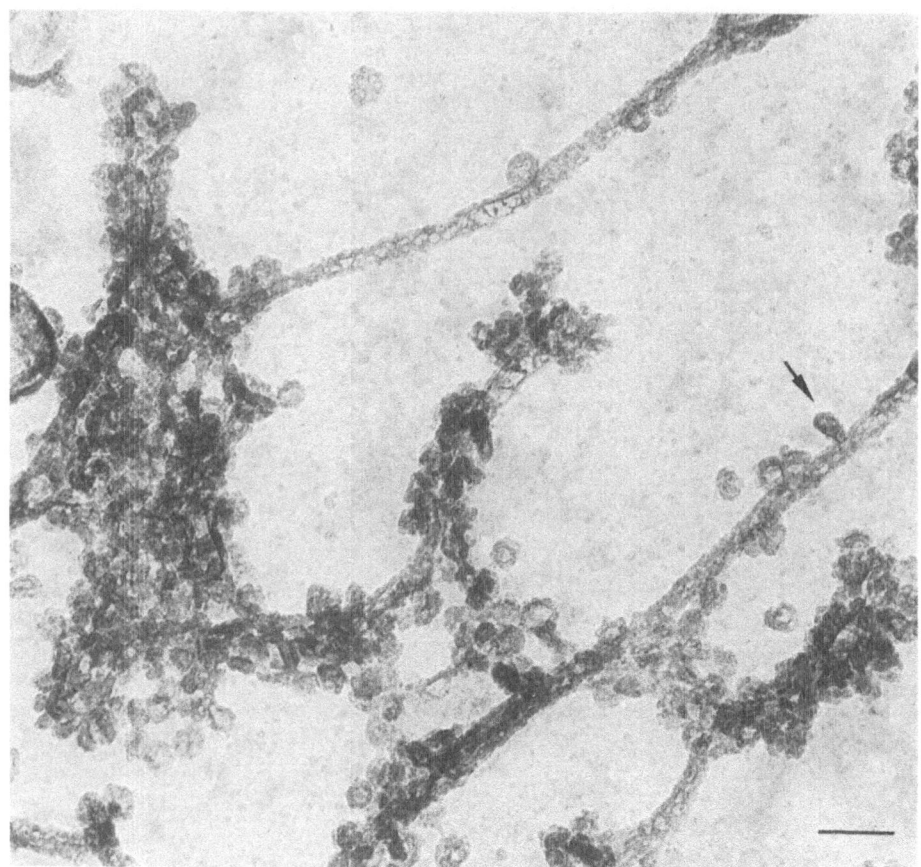

Figure 8. High voltage microscopy of mature virions. Cells
           grown on carbon films on grids were fixed, dehydrated
           by the critical point technique and examined with 1M
           KV. The virions released from the under side of the
           cells were flattened, disk shaped mature particles
           (arrow). Bar=200nm.

Table 3.   Cellular Functions Required for Coronavirus
           Replication

Uptake of virions (?)
Synthesis of proteins
Processing of proteins:
    N = phosphorylation (?)
    E1 = glycosylation with O-linked sugars
    E2 = glycosylation with N-linked sugars
        acylation
        proteolytic cleavage
Intracellular transport of proteins
    E1 = to Golgi
    E2 = through Golgi to plasma membrane

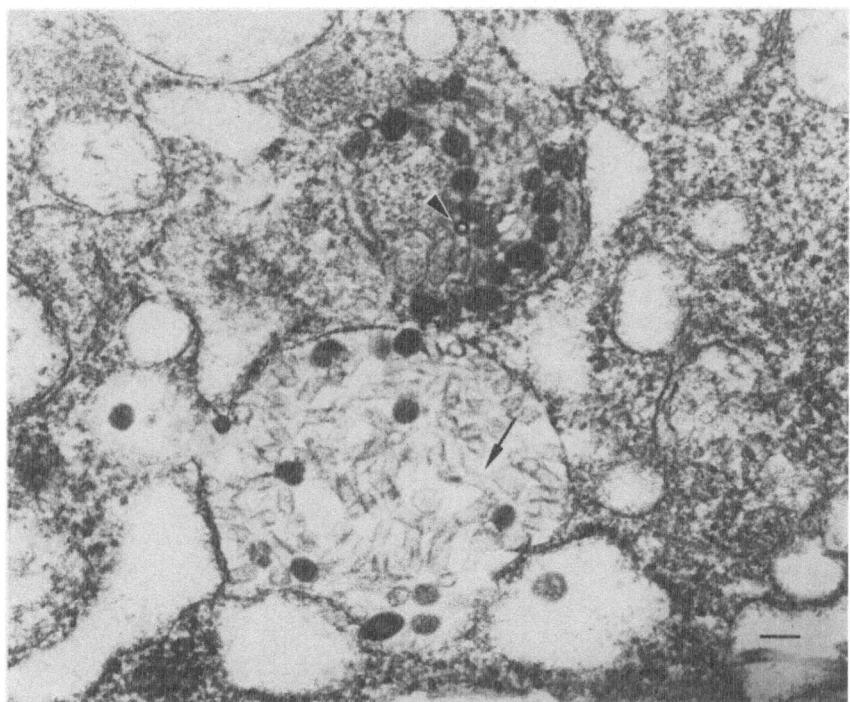

Figure 9.   Tubular inclusions in a coronavirus infected cell.   In
            a 17 Cl 1 cell infected with MHV-A59, long, rigid
            tubular inclusions are found in the lumen of the RER.
            Arrow shows tubule in longitudinal section; arrowhead,
            tubule in cross section.   Bar=100nm.

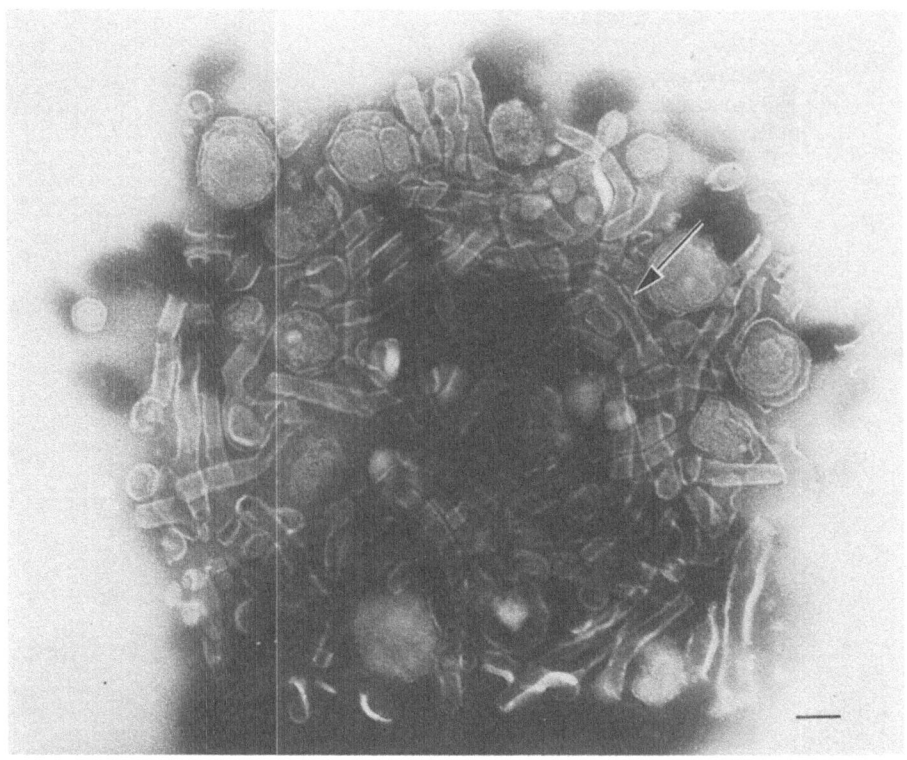

Figure 10.   Tubular inclusion isolated from coronavirus infected
             cells. The inclusion was released from cells by
             homogenization, isolated by sucrose gradient
             ultracentrifugation and examined in a negatively
             stained preparation. Arrow indicates tubule.
             Bar=100nm.

ACKNOWLEDGMENTS

    We are grateful for the excellent technical assistance of
Barbara O'Neill, Eileen Bauer, Cynthia Duchala, and Gus Boesch.
This work was supported by research grant GM 31698 from the
National Institutes of Health and #936-5592 from the U.S. Agency
for International Development. The opinions expressed are the
private views of the authors and should not be construed as
official or necessarily reflecting the views of the Uniformed
Services University of the Health Sciences or the Department of
Defense.

REFERENCES

1. Wege, H., Siddell, S., and ter Meulen, V. (1982). The
       biology and pathogenesis of coronaviruses. Curr. Top.
       Microbiol. Immunol. 99, 165-200.
2. Bang, F.B. (1981). Adv. Exptl. Med. Biol. 142, 359-373.
3. Arnheiter, H., Baechi, T., and Haller, O. (1982). Adult
       mouse hepatocytes in primary monolayer culture express
       genetic resistance to mouse hepatitis virus type 3. J.
       Immunol. 129, 1275-1281.
4. Dubois-Dalcq, M.E., Doller, E.W., Haspel, M.V., and Holmes,
       K.V. (1982). Cell tropism and expression of mouse
       hepatitis viruses (MHV) in mouse spinal cord cultures.
       Virology 119, 317-331.
5. Sturman, L.S., and Holmes, K.V. Adv. Virus Res. 28 (in
       press).
6. Brian, D.A. Personal communication.
7. Barthold, S.W., Smith, A.L., Lord, P.F.S., Bhatt, P.N.,
       Jacoby, R.O., and Main, A.J. (1982). In Epizootic
       Coronaviral Typhlocolitis in Suckling Mice. Lab. Animal
       Science, pp. 376-383.
8. Sturman, L.S., and Holmes, K.V. In "Coronaviruses:
       Molecular Biology and Pathogenesis," Plenum Publishing
       Company, London (in press).
9. Chaloner-Larsson, G., and Johnson-Lussenburg, C.M.
       Characteristics of a Long Term In Vitro Persistent
       Infection with human coronavirus 229E. Adv. Exp. Med.
       Biol. 146, 309-322.
10. Holmes, K.V., and Behnke, J.N. (1981). Evolution of a
       coronavirus during persistent infection in vitro. In
       "Biochemistry and Biology of Coronaviruses" (ter Meulen,
       V., Siddell, S., and Wege, H., eds.) Adv. Exp. Med. Biol.
       142, 287-299. Plenum Press, New York.
11. Stohlman, S.A., Sakaguchi, A.Y., and Weiner, L.P. (1979).
       Characterization of the cold sensitive murine hepatitis
       virus mutants rescued from latently-infected cells by
       cell fusion. Virology 98, 448-455.
12. Brayton, P.R., Lai, M.M.C., Patton, C.D., and Stohlman, S.A.
       (1982). Characterization of two RNA polymerase
       activities induced by mouse hepatitis virus. J. Virol.
       42, 847-853.
13. Lai, M.M.C., Patton, C.D., and Stohlman, S.A. (1982).
       Replication of mouse hepatitis virus: negative-stranded
       RNA and replicative form RNA are of genome length. J.
       Virol. 44, 487-492.
14. Niemann, H., Boschek, B., Evans, D., Rosing, M., Tamura, T.,
       and Klenk, H.-D. (1982). Posttranslational glycosylation
       of coronavirus glycoprotein E1: Inhibition by monensin.
       EMBO Journal 1, 1499-1504.

15. Stohlman, S.A., and Lai, M.M.C. (1979). Phosphoproteins of
    murine hepatitis viruses. J. Virol. 32, 672-675.
16. Niemann, H., and Klenk, H.-D. (1981). Coronavirus
    glycoprotein E1, a new type of viral glycoprotein. J.
    Mol. Biol. 153, 993-1010.
17. Schmidt, M.F.G., and Schlesinger, M.J. (1980). Relation of
    fatty acid attachment to the translation and maturation
    of vesicular stomatitis and Sindbis virus membrane
    glycoproteins. J. Biol. Chem. 255, 3334-3339.
18. Holmes, K.V., Doller, E.W., and Sturman, L.S. (1981).
    Tunicamycin resistant glycosylation of a coronavirus
    glycoprotein: Demonstration of a novel type of viral
    glycoprotein. Virology 115, 334-344.
19. Sturman, L.S. (1981). The structure and behaviour of
    coronavirus A59 glycoproteins. Adv. Exp. Med. Biol. 142,
    1-18.
20. Sturman, L.S., Holmes, and Behnke, J. (1980). Isolation of
    coronavirus envelope glycoproteins and interaction with
    the viral nucleocapsid. J. Virol. 33, 449-462.
21. Holmes, K.V., Doller, E.W., and Behnke, J.N. (1981).
    Analysis of the functions of coronavirus glycoproteins by
    differential inhibition with tunicamycin. Adv. Exp. Med.
    Biol. 142, 133-139.
22. Caliguiri, L.A., Tamm, I. (1972). The role of cytoplasmic
    membranes in poliovirus biosynthesis. Virology 42,
    110-111.
23. Massalski, A., Coulter-Mackie, M. Knobler, R.L., Buchmeier,
    M.J., and Dales, S. (1982). In vivo and in vitro models
    of demyelinating diseases. V. Comparison of the
    assembly of mouse hepatitis virus, strain JHM, in two
    murine cell lines. Intervirology 18, 135-146.
24. Heggeness, M.H., Smith, P.R., and Choppin, P.W. (1982). In
    vitro assembly of the nonglycosylated membrane protein
    (M) of Sendai virus. Proc. Natl. Acad. Sci (USA) 79,
    6232-6236.

IN VITRO ASSEMBLY OF THE MURINE CORONAVIRUS MEMBRANE PROTEIN E1

Peter Rottier, Dorothée Brandenburg, John Armstrong*, Ben van der Zeijst, and Graham Warren*
Institute of Virology, Veterinary Faculty, State University, Yalelaan 1, 3508 TD Utrecht, The Netherlands
*European Molecular Biology Laboratory, Postfach 10.2209, 69 Heidelberg, FRG

INTRODUCTION

One of the most striking differences between coronaviruses and other enveloped RNA viruses is that they bud into intracellular membranes. Only bunyaviruses behave similarly (1).

Coronavirions have been observed in the lumens of endoplasmic reticulum (ER) and Golgi apparatus from cells infected with various coronaviruses such as mouse hepatitis virus (MHV) (2-5), avian infectious bronchitis virus (IBV) (6) and porcine enteric coronavirus (7) The assembled virions then appear in smooth-walled vesicles en route to the plasma membrane (PM) where they are probably released from the cell by exocytosis (4,8).

The intracellular budding site of coronaviruses seems to be determined by one of its two envelope glycoproteins, E1, which stays in internal membranes after its synthesis on membrane-bound ribosomes (4,5). The other glycoprotein, E2, is also assembled in the rough ER, but is not needed for virus maturation and release. Incorporation of E2 into virions is, however, essential for virus infectivity (3,9). Some E2 passes to the cell surface where it fuses adjacent cells together thereby spreading the infection. E2 is similar to the spike glycoproteins of those viruses that bud at the PM in taking the same route through the cell, passing through the Golgi complex, being fatty acylated and having normal N-linked oligosaccharides (10). In contrast, the E1 protein has neither fatty acid groups nor N-linked oligosaccharides, instead it has O-linked oligosaccharides

(3,9,10) which are probably acquired in the Golgi complex (5,11) as the virions pass through the stacks of Golgi cisternae.

Viral glycoproteins have widely been used as models to study the biosynthesis and fate of those cellular membrane glycoproteins that are normally transported to the PM. The unusual behaviour of the coronavirus El glycoprotein implicates it as an intracellular transmembrane protein which can be used as a model to study the biogenesis of (proteins of) intracellular membranes. As a first step in characterization we report the assembly of this protein in microsomal membranes in cell-free extracts. The results show several striking differences between this glycoprotein and those that are normally transported to the cell surface.

MATERIALS AND METHODS

MHV strain A59 was grown in Sac(-) cells, labelled with ^{35}S-methionine, and purified as described previously (12,13). Iodination of the virus was carried out using Iodogen (14) and the final specific activity was 1.9 uCI/ug. Poly(A)$^+$-RNA from infected cells was prepared as described previously (13) except that poly(U)-Sepharose (15) was used to select the RNA. The RNA was translated in nuclease-treated rabbit reticulocyte lysates essentially as described by Pelham and Jackson (16). Incubations were for 1 h at 30°C. Where specified, dog pancreatic microsomes, prepared according to Blobel and Dobberstein (17) and treated with EDTA (18), were added. They were kindly provided by David Meyer (EMBL). N-formyl-^{35}S-methionyl-tRNA$_f$met was prepared essentially as described by Stanley (19). For immunoprecipitation, translation products were incubated overnight at 4°C with mouse anti-MHV-A59 serum (12), pre-immune mouse serum, or monoclonal anti-El (a kind gift from Marck Koolen, Institute of Virology, State University, Utrecht) and then treated for 5 h at 4°C with affinity-purified rabbit anti-mouse IgG, kindly provided by Brian Burke (EMBL). Immune-complexes were isolated essentially as described by Green et al. (20). Protease digestions were carried out by diluting the translation mixtures five-fold using 1.25 mg/ml proteinase K (Serva) in 50 mM Tris-HCl buffer pH 7.4, 100 mM NaCl and incubating at 37°C for 15 min in the presence or absence of 0.05% saponin (Sigma). After cooling on ice they were treated for 10 min with excess phenylmethylsulfonylfluoride (PMSF) to inhibit proteinase K activity. The samples were then precipitated with TCA or extracted with Triton X-114 (21). Proteins were analyzed by fractionation on 15% SDS-polyacrylamide gels with 4 or 5% stacking gel essentially as described previously (13, 20). Further details on the procedures used will be published elsewhere.

RESULTS

El assembled in microsomal membranes is neither cleaved nor lycosylated

Sac(-) cells were infected with coronavirus A59 and, 8-9 h later, poly(A)$^+$-RNA was extracted. When translated in a reticulocyte lysate many proteins were synthesized (cf lanes 1,2 and 3,4, Fig.1) and two (nucleocapsid (N) and El) were tentatively identified as viral proteins, the rest presumably being derived from host cellular mRNAs. The identity of the El protein was

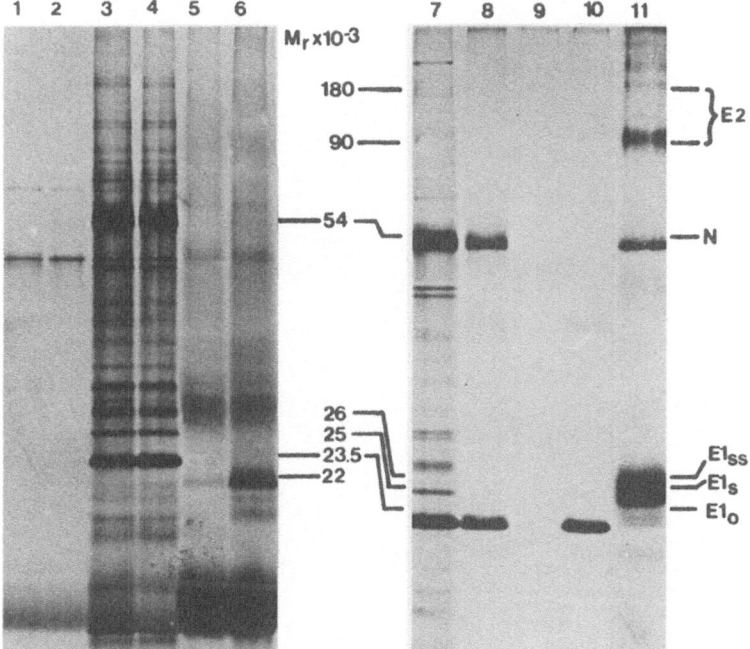

Fig.1. Synthesis of the El protein in the presence and absence of microsomal membranes. Samples of incubations in the absence (lanes 1,2) or presence (lanes 3,4) of poly(A)$^+$-RNA and in the absence (lanes 1,3) or presence (lanes 2,4) of microsomes were taken for direct analysis by SDS-PAGE. Samples of proteins synthesized in the absence (lane 3) or presence (lane 4) of microsomes were treated with proteinase K and applied to lanes 5 and 6, respectively. The identity of the capsid (N) and El protein was confirmed by immune precipitation from proteins synthesized in the presence of microsomes (lanes 4,7) using polyclonal anti-MHV-A59 antibodies (lane 8), pre-immune serum (lane 9) and monoclonal anti-El (lane 10). Lane 11 is iodinated virus. El$_o$ is unglycosylated El, whereas El$_S$ and El$_{SS}$ have sugars.

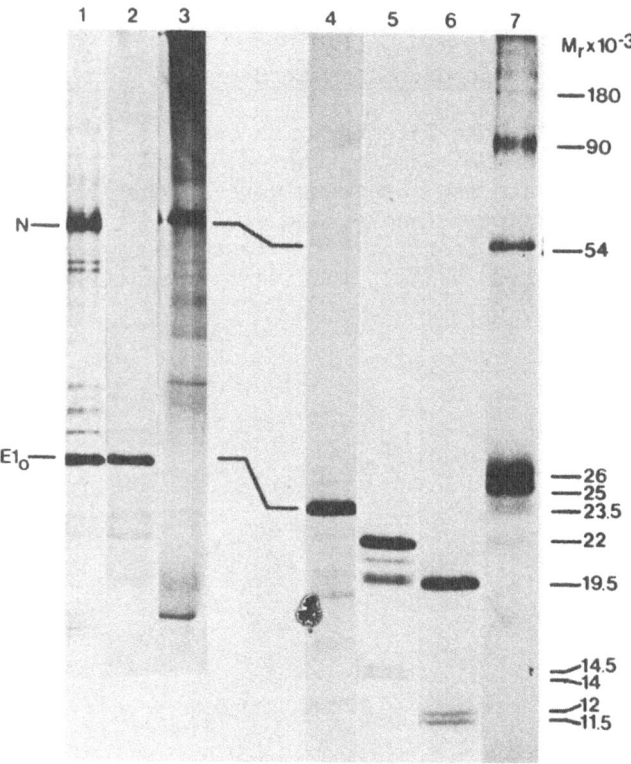

Fig.2. Protease digestion of the E1 protein synthesized in the presence of microsomes. Lanes 1-3, the E1 protein is purified by Triton X-114 extraction. After translation of poly(A)$^+$-RNA in the presence of microsomes (lane 1) a sample was extracted with Triton X-114 at 30°C and the detergent phase containing E1 (lane 2) was separated by centrifugation from the aqueous phase (lane 3). Lanes 4-6, protease digestion of E1 synthesized in the presence of microsomes and purified by Triton X-114 extraction. Lane 4, original incubation. Lanes 5 and 6, samples treated with proteinase K alone or in the presence of 0.05% saponin, respectively. Lane 7 is iodinated virus.

confirmed using specific antibodies. A 23.5 kD polypeptide was specifically precipitated from the total translation mixture by antiserum to the whole virus (Fig.1, lane 8) and a monoclonal anti-E1 (Fig.1, lane 10) but not by pre-immune serum (Fig.1, lane 9).

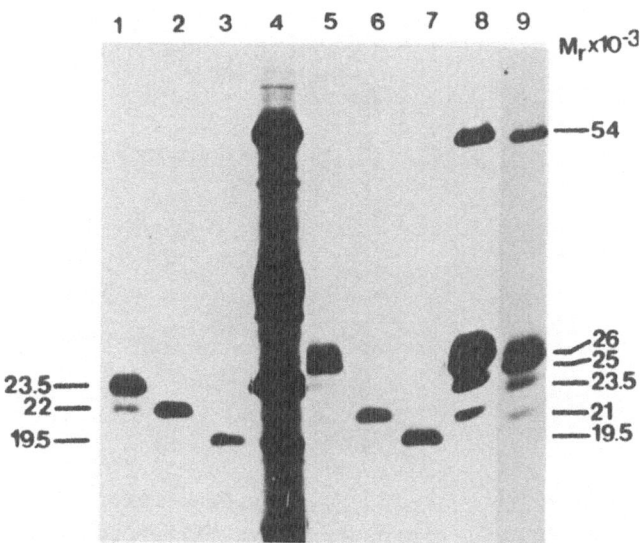

Fig 3. Protease digestion of labelled virions and of El
synthesized in the presence of microsomes. Lanes 1–4 are
directly comparable to lanes 4–6 and 1, respectively, of
Fig.2. Lanes 5–8, protease digestion of ^{35}S-methionine-
labelled virus. The virus (lane 8) was treated with
proteinase K in the presence (lane 5) or absence (lane 6)
of PMSF, or in the presence of 0.05% saponin (lane 7). Lane
9 is a shorter exposure of lane 8.

        El synthesized in the absence of dog pancreatic microsomes
(Fig.1, lane 3) could be digested completely by protease (Fig.1,
lane 5). Synthesis in the presence of microsomes (Fig.1, lane 4)
yielded an El protein of the same molecular weight but most of
this was resistant to protease digestion (Fig.1, lane 6)
indicating that assembly into the membrane had occurred. The
absence of any change in molecular weight after assembly into
microsomes strongly suggests that the signal sequence is
uncleaved, a suggestion strongly confirmed by N-terminal
labelling of the protein (see below). The assembled El protein
also co-migrated with unglycosylated El in virions (Fig.1, cf.
lanes 10 and 11) suggesting that addition of O-linked
oligosaccharides occurs after the completed protein has been
transported from the rough ER.

El spans the lipid bilayer
        El was separated from the background of non-viral proteins
by exploiting the phase separation properties of Triton X-114
(21). Since El behaves as an integral membrane protein (22) it was
selectively extracted into the detergent phase of a Triton X-114

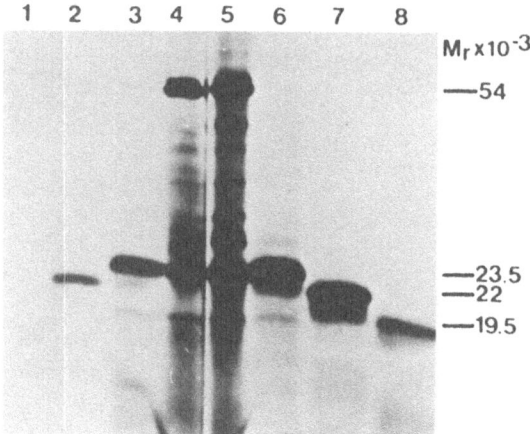

Fig.4. N-terminal labelling of E1. Poly(A) -RNA was translated in
the presence of microsomes in a mixture containing 0.1 mM
methionine and N-formyl- ^{35}S-methionyl-tRNA$_f$^{met}. A sample of
the original incubation (lane 4) was extracted with Triton
X-114 to purify E1 (lane 3). Two samples were treated with
proteinase K either in the absence (lane 2) or in the
presence (lane 1) of 0.05% saponin. For comparison a normal
translation using ^{35}S-methionine was performed and analyzed
in parallel. Lane 5, direct analysis; lanes 6-8, Triton X-
114 extracts before (lane 6) or after treatment with
proteinase K in the absence (lane 7) or presence of 0.05%
saponin (lane 8).

suspension at 30°C (Fig.2, lane 2) leaving soluble proteins such
as the nucleocapsid (N) and host cell proteins in the aqueous
phase (Fig.2, lane 3).

        After protease treatment of translation mixtures containing
microsomal membranes the 23.5 kD form of E1 was no longer visible
and the major product had a Mr of 22 kD (Fig.2, cf. lanes 4 and 5,
Fig.3, cf. lanes 1 and 2). A 1.5 kD fragment had thus been removed
from the equivalent of the cytoplasmic side of the ER membrane in
vivo. Previous studies have shown that E1 is accessible to
protease in intact virions (22). The different forms of E1, which
are presumably O-glycosylated to different extents (9) on that
part of the protein exposed on the virion surface, are all
digested to a common fragment of 21 kD (Fig.3, cf. lanes 5 and 6).
Since the virus buds into the ER lumen, the virion outer surface
is topologically equivalent to the lumenal side of the ER. E1 is
thus accessible to protease from the cytoplasmic and lumenal sides
of the ER membrane and must therefore span the bilayer.

This was demonstrated directly by permeabilizing the microsomal vesicles with the detergent saponin. When microsomal vesicles were treated with protease in the presence of 0.05% saponin the El protein was quantitatively converted into a fragment with a Mr of 19.5 kD (Fig.2, cf. lanes 4 and 6, Fig.3, cf. lanes 1 and 3). Treatment of intact virions under the same conditions gave a fragment of exactly the same size (Fig.3, cf., lanes 5 and 7), the size of which was that expected if El had been digested from both sides of the membrane. It would thus seem that saponin makes the membrane permeable to added protease but does not otherwise affect the protein. Complete disruption of the bilayer using Triton X-100 made the El protein completely sensitive to protease digestion (data not shown). An El fragment of the same mobility (Mr. 19.5 kD) was observed in some experiments in the absence of saponin (Fig.2, lane 5, Fig.4, lane 7). Since microsomal vesicles are known to be leaky to proteases to some extent (23) the fragment is probably derived by digestion of El from both sides of the bilayer. For analytical purposes, saponin treatment is advantageous in ensuring that all the microsomal vesicles are permeable to the protease.

The El fragment that is resistant to protease digestion from both sides of the membrane is large enough to contain up to seven polypeptide segments spanning the bilayer, although its precise topology in the membrane remains to be elucidated. The presence of minor proteolytic fragments of El does, however, suggest that one loop of this fragment is accessible to protease to a limited extent on the outside of microsomal vesicles. Depending on which part of the loop is cleaved the minor fragment has a Mr of 14 kD or 14.5 kD (Fig.2, lane 5). In the presence of saponin this drops to 11.5 and 12 kD (Fig.2, lane 6). The proposed topology that would result in these fragments is presented in Fig.6 and will be discussed below.

The N-terminus of El is on the lumenal side of the ER membrane
Since El is not proteolytically cleaved during assembly in microsomal vesicles it proved possible to label the N-terminus selectively using N-formyl-^{35}S -methionyl-tRNA$_f$met. This label was present on the assembled El protein (Fig.4, lane 3) and on the 22 kD fragment generated by protease digestion (Fig.4, lane 2) showing that the N-terminus was not on the cytoplasmic side of the membrane. Digestion in the presence of saponin resulted in complete loss of the label (Fig.4, lane 1), indicating that the N-terminus is on the lumenal side of the ER membrane. The presence of each of the proteolytically-derived forms of El was confirmed in parallel experiments using ^{35}S-methionine as the radiolabel (Fig.4, lanes 5-8).

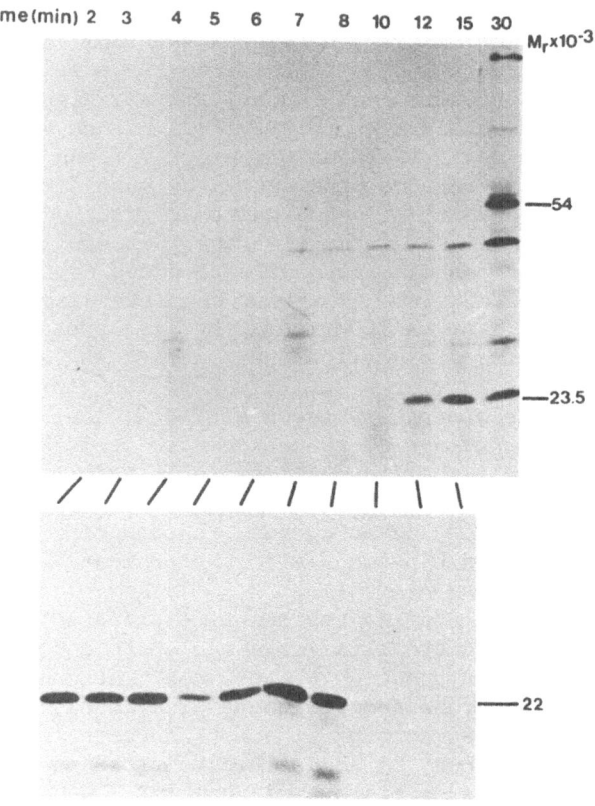

Fig.5. Addition of microsomes at different times after initiation
of protein synthesis. Poly(A)+-RNA was added at zero time
to initiate synthesis at 25oC. Two minutes later edeine
(final concentration 1.2 uM) was added and incubation
continued at 30 °C. At the times shown above the lanes
samples were removed either for direct analysis (top panel)
or for further incubation in the presence of microsomes
until t=30 min. These samples were then treated with
proteinase K, extracted with Triton X-114 and fractionated
by SDS-PAGE (bottom panel).

El can enter the membrane at late stages of synthesis
        Protein synthesis was started in the cell-free system by the
addition of poly(A)+-RNA. After two minutes, edeine was added to
prevent further initiation (24). At different times samples were
taken for direct analysis by SDS-PAGE or added to microsomal
membranes and incubated at 30°C until 30 min after the additon of
poly(A) + -RNA to allow assembly to occur. These samples were then
first protease-treated, to distinguish between soluble El and that
assembled in microsomal membranes, and then extracted with Triton

X-114 and fractionated by SDS-PAGE. As shown in Fig.5 (top), full-length E1 appeared after about 12 min synthesis at 30 °C corresponding to a synthetic rate of about 8 amino acids polymerized/min, a rate that was not affected when synthesis was carried out in the presence of microsomal membranes (data not shown). It proved possible to add microsomal membranes as late as 8 min after the start of synthesis and assembly would still occur (Fig.5, bottom). This corresponds to the synthesis of 65–70% of the E1 protein, or 140–150 amino acids.

DISCUSSION

Our study of the in vitro assembly of MHV-A59 envelope protein E1 into membranes reveals new and unusual features of this protein in addition to those previously known. One striking observation was that this protein, once assembled into microsomal membranes, appears to be largely buried in the lipid bilayer: more than 80% of it has become resistant to proteolysis. Apparently only short regions of 2.5 and 1.5 kD, from the N- and C-termini, are exposed to the lumenal and cytoplasmic compartments,

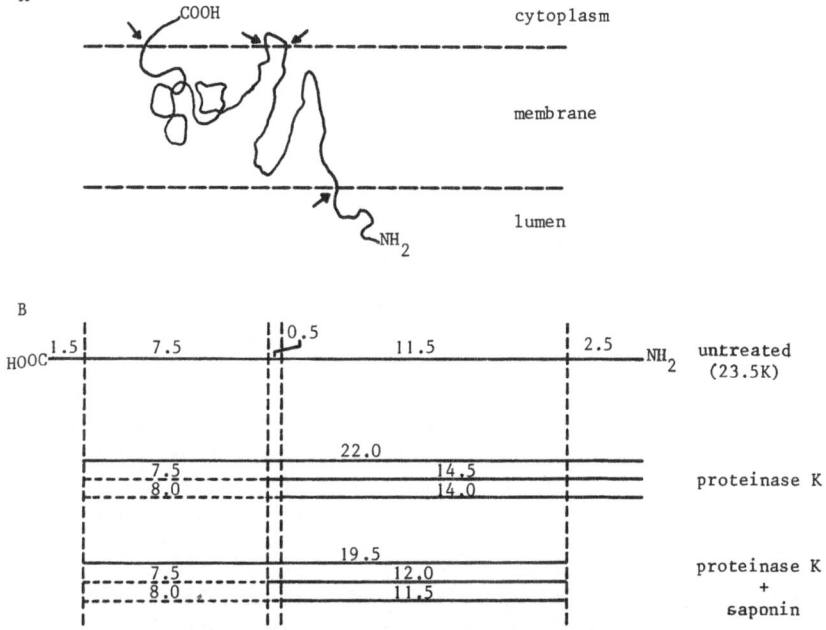

Fig.6. Schematic view of the topology of the E1 protein in the microsomal membrane. (A) summarizes the data presented in this paper. (B) represents the postulated cleavages observed using proteinase K as indicated by arrows in (A).

respectively. The remainder is sufficiently large to span the membrane several times, as shown schematically in Fig.6. This would be a novel feature for a viral glycoprotein, although several non-viral proteins are known which apparently cross the membrane more than once (25-28). Only bacteriorhodopsin is comparable, however, in appearing to lack substantial domains on either side of the membrane (29), but this protein is found in the unusual membrane of an Archaebacterium.

Insertion of E1 into membranes does not lead to the cleavage of an N-terminal leader peptide (Figs.1 and 4) as does usually occur with membrane glycoproteins. Other examples of spanning membrane proteins without a cleavable signal sequence are rhodopsin (30) and Band III protein (31); the same phenomenon has been found for a secreted protein, ovalbumin (32). No N-terminal peptide being cleaved off, the signal for insertion of E1 into membranes might well be located elsewhere in the molecule. Studying therefore the kinetics of its insertion, we found that the molecule can penetrate the membrane even after a large proportion of it, approximately 140-150 amino acids, has been synthesized (Fig.5). Thus the insertion signal could in principle be located anywhere within this region. A further comparison with ovalbumin and Band III protein can be made. It has been proposed that the signal sequence for these proteins is internal rather than N-terminal (31,33), although the precise location for ovalbumin remains controversial (34).

The E1 protein does not acquire its O-linked oligosaccharides in the rough ER, a result which confirms the cell fractionation data obtained by Niemann et al. (5). It is likely that these oligosaccharides are acquired as the completed virions pass through the Golgi complex (5,11). The attachment of the sugars to the 2.5 kD N-terminal domain seemed not to have altered the proteins' intramembranous configuration. In this respect a comparison between the E1 protein of murine and avian viruses will be valuable, since infectious bronchitis virus E1 is glycosylated only through N-linked oligosaccharides (35). O-linked sugars on animal virus structural proteins are rather rare. Their functions are still speculative. Glycoproteins bearing O-linked sugars have been described for vaccinia (36) and herpesvirus (11). It is interesting to note that these viruses also mature by budding from intracellular membranes.

The budding of MHV-A59 virions presumably involves the specific interaction between nucleocapsids present in the cytoplasm and E1 in ER membranes. Our results suggest that only the 1.5 kD C-terminal fragment of E1 is effectively available for such an interaction. It is probably this tiny portion of the molecule which is responsible for the high affinity of E1 for RNA (37).

Thus, the El glycoprotein of coronavirus has several features which distinguish it from the majority of membrane proteins. Some of these features should be clarified by analysis of the amino acid sequence of the protein (Armstrong et al., this volume).

ACKNOWLEDGEMENTS

We thank Bernard Dobberstein, Sharon Queally and Paul Quinn for critical reading of the manuscript; Maud Maas Geesteranus for typing; J.A. was supported by a European Fellowship from the Royal Society, and P.R. was supported at the EMBL by a short-term fellowship from the European Molecular Biology Organization.

REFERENCES

1. J.F. Smith and D.Y. Pifat, Virology 121:61 (1982).
2. A. Massalski, M.Coulter-Mackie and S.Dales, in: "Biochemistry and Biology of Coronaviruses", V. ter Meulen, S. Siddell and H. Wege, eds., Plenum Press, New York and London, pp. 111-118 (1981).
3. K.V.Holmes, E.W. Doller and L.S.Sturman, Virology 115:334 (1981).
4. M.E. Dubois-Dalcq, E.W. Doller, M.V. Haspel and K.V. Holmes, Virology 119:317 (1982).
5. H.Niemann, B. Boschek, D. Evans, M. Rosing, T. Tamura and H.-D. Klenk, EMBO J. 1:1499 (1982).
6. D.Chasey and D.J.Alexander, Arch.Virol. 52:101 (1976).
7. R.Ducatelle, W.Coussement, M.B. Pensaert, P. DeBouck and J.Hoorens, Arch.Virol. 68:35 (1981).
8. K.V.Holmes and J.N.Behnke, in: "Biochemistry and Biology of Coronaviruses", V. ter Meulen, S. Siddell and H. Wege, eds., Plenum Press, New York and London, pp. 287-299 (1981).
9. P.J.M.Rottier, M.C.Horzinek and B.A.M.van der Zeijst, J.Virol. 40:350 (1981).
10. H.Niemann, and H.-D. Klenk, J.Mol.Biol. 153:993 (1981).
11. D.C. Johnson and P.G. Spear, Cell 32:987 (1983).
12. W.J.M.Spaan, P.J.M.Rottier, M.C. Horzinek and B.A.M.van der Zeijst, Virology 108:424 (1981).
13. P.J.M.Rottier, W.J.M.Spaan, M.C.Horzinek and B.A.M.van der Zeijst, J.Virol. 38:20 (1981).
14. B.A.M. van der Zeijst, B.E. Noyes, M.-E. Mirault, B. Parker, A.D.M.E. Osterhaus, F.A. Swyryd, N. Bleumink, M.C. Horzinek and G.R. Stark, J.Virol., in press (1983).
15. F.H.Wilt, Cell 11:673 (1977).
16. H.R.B. Pelham and R.J.Jackson, Eur.J.Biochem. 67:247 (1976).
17. G. Blobel and B. Bobberstein, J.Cell Biol. 67:852 (1975).
18. H. Garoff, K. Simons and B.Bobberstein, J.Mol.Biol. 124:587 (1978).

19. W.M. Stanley, Anal.Biochem. 48:202 (1972).
20. J. Green, G. Griffiths, D. Louvard, P. Quinn and G. Warren, J.Mol.Biol. 152:663 (1981).
21. C. Bordier, J.Biol.Chem. 256:1604 (1981).
22. L.S. Sturman, Virology 77:637 (1977).
23. D.D. Sabatini and G. Blobel, J.Cell Biol. 45:146 (1970).
24. T.Obrig, J. Irvin, W. Culp and B. Hardesty, Eur.J.Biochem. 21:31 (1971).
25. R.Henderson and P.N.T.Unwin, Nature 257:28 (1975).
26. F.A.Dratz and P.A.Hargrave, Trends in Biochem.Sci. 8:128 (1983).
27. T.L. Steck, J.Supramol.Struc. 8:311 (1978).
28. M. Noda, H. Takahashi, T. Tanabe, M. Toyosato, S. Kikyotani, Y. Furutani, T. Hirose, H. Takashima, S. Inayama, T. Miyata and S. Numa, Nature 302:528 (1983).
29. Yu.A. Ovchinnikov, N.G. Abdulaev, M.Yu. Feigina, A.V. Kiselev, N.A. Lobanov, FEBS Lett. 100: 219 (1979).
30. I. Schechter, Y. Burstein, R. Zemell, E. Ziv, F. Kantor and D.S. Papermaster, Proc.Natl.Acad.Sci. USA 76:2654 (1979).
31. W.A. Braell and H.F. Lodish, Cell 28:23 (1982).
32. R.D. Palmiter, J.Gagnon and K.A. Walsh, Proc.Natl.Acad.Sci. USA 75:94 (1978).
33. V.R. Lingappa, J.R. Lingappa and G. Blobel, Nature 281:117 (1979).
34. R.D. Meek, K.A. Walsh and R.D. Palmiter, J.Biol.Chem. 257:12245 (1982).
35. D.F. Stern and B.M. Sefton, J.Virol. 44:804 (1982).
36. H. Shida and S. Dales, Virology 111:56 (1981).
37. L.S. Sturman, K.V. Holmes and J. Behnke, J.Virol. 33:449 (1980).

CHARACTERIZATION OF VIRAL PROTEINS SYNTHESIZED IN 229E INFECTED
CELLS AND EFFECT(S) OF INHIBITION OF GLYCOSYLATION AND GLYCO-
PROTEIN TRANSPORT.

M.C. Kemp[1,2,3], J.C. Hierholzer[4], A. Harrison[4] and
J.S. Burks[1,2,3]

[1]Center for Neurological Diseases/Rocky Mountain Multiple
Sclerosis Center, [2]Veterans Administration Medical Center
[3]University of Colorado School of Medicine, Denver
Colorado. [4]Division of Viral Diseases, Centers for
Disease Control, Atlanta, Georgia, U.S.A.

Coronaviruses were classified as a distinct group of viruses
in 1968 (1) and four members of this group are recognized as human
respiratory pathogens: These include B814 (2), the first human
coronavirus (HCV) isolated 229E (3), OC-43 (4) and 692 (5), identified by immunoelectromicroscopy only. In addition to the respiratory
pathogens, two coronaviruses have been isolated while working with
brain tissue from multiple sclerosis patients (6). These viruses
cross-react antigenically with OC-43 but neither of these viruses
have been implicated in respiratory disease.

The HCVs 229E and OC-43 together may account for 5-35% of the
upper respiratory infections of Americans (7). These viruses have
distinct biologic and biochemical properties. Antigenically, OC-43
is more related to the murine hepatitis virus (MHV) group, while
229E does not cross-react with this group (8). The HCV 229E is
readily adapted to grow in tissue culture, while OC-43 is difficult to grow except in the brain of newborn mice. Therefore, the
host range limitations of OC-43 preclude many biochemical studies.

Biochemical studies have shown that OC-43 and 229E both
have genomes with molecular weights of approximately 6×10^6 daltons
(9,10). The genome is of positive polarity, i.e. it acts as a mRNA,
and six additional intracellular mRNAs have been detected (10).
Previous studies have shown that OC-43 and 229E code for at least
six polypeptides with large variations in molecular weight (MW)
for these polypeptides being reported (11). The structural

composition of the HCV 229E was therefore debatable and little
information regarding the synthesis and processing of viral
specific peptides was available.

The object of the studies described herein was to determine:
1) The kinetics of synthesis of 229E polypeptides; 2) Whether
229E polypeptides are processed; and 3) The effects of tunicamycin,
an inhibitor of glycosylation, and monensin, an inhibitor of intracellular transport, on the synthesis of viral proteins.

Structural Proteins of HCV 229E

Analysis of purified HCV 229E proteins labeled with
^{35}S-methionine showed that the virus is comprised of three major
polypeptides. The largest polypeptide has a molecular weight of
180K and labeling studies with sugar precursors have shown that
this protein is glycosylated. The next largest polypeptide associated with the virion is a 50K phosphorylated protein, which has
been shown to be associated with the RNA genome. The third major
protein associated with the virion consists of a family of polypeptides having molecular weights of 25K, 23K and 21K, respectively.
Some variation in the amount of each of these respective proteins
was noted depending upon the viral preparations. With other coronaviruses differences in the molecular weights of these proteins
have been correlated with the level of glycosylation (12,13). We
have been unable to demonstrate glycosylation of the 25K, 23K or
21K proteins, respectively, using labeled sugar precursors. Glycosylation of the 25K protein is inferred from inhibitor studies
(see tunicamycin studies).

In addition to the three major polypeptides minor polypeptides having molecular weights of 107K, 92K and 39K, respectively,
have been detected.

Synthesis of Intracellular 229E Proteins

The kinetics of synthesis of intracellular 229E proteins
was investigated by pulse labelling infected cells for 15 min. at
different times post-infection (PI). The results presented in
Fig. 1, show that synthesis of proteins having molecular weights
equivalent to the structural proteins of the virion, i.e. 180K,
50K and 23K, respectively, are first detected at 6hr post-infection
(Fig. 1). Moreover, by 11hr PI, host protein synthesis is almost
completely shut-off as illustrated by the inhibition of actin
synthesis (46K dalton protein).

To investigate further the relationship of the proteins
detected in infected cellular extracts and improve our ability to

distinguish the viral related proteins, antiserum prepared against purified 229E virions was used to immunoprecipitate pulse labelled proteins. Infected cells were pulsed at different times PI for 15 min with ^{35}S-methionine or pulsed for 15 min and chased for 60 min.

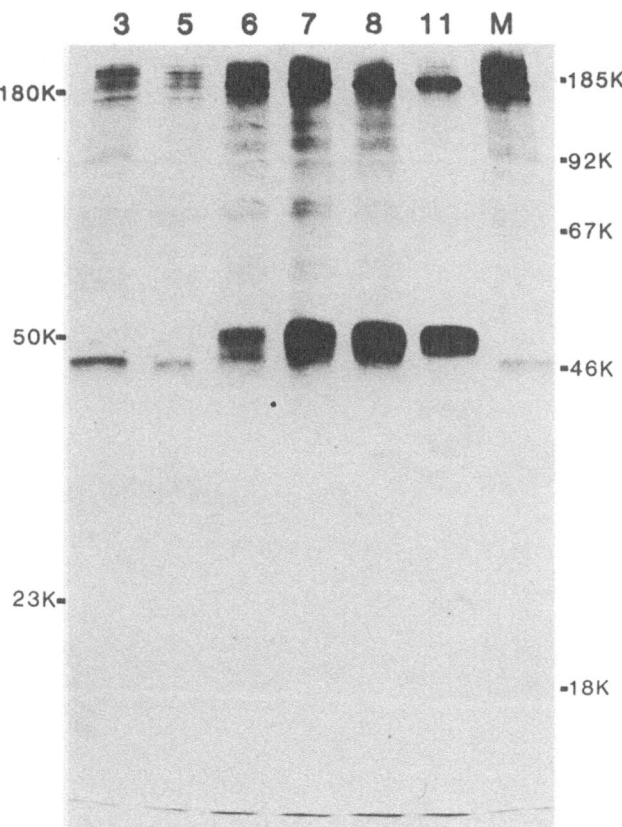

Figure 1: SDS-PAGE analysis of pulse-chase labeled polypeptides synthesized by 229E infected MRC$_5$ cells. Cells were infected at an M.O.I. of 10 TCID$_{50}$/cell and incubated with methionine-deficient medium for 30 min prior to pulse-labelling for 15 min with ^{35}S-methionine (400uCi/ml) in methionine-deficient medium. Cell extracts were prepared by scraping labelled cells into dissociation buffer containing SDS and 2-mercaptoethanol followed by boiling. Nucleic acid was removed from each extract by centrifugation and 100,000 trichloroacetic acid precipitable counts from each cell extract were applied to the gel. Electrophoresis was carried out as previously described (14). M, mock-infected extract prepared at 11hr PI.

As may be seen from Fig. 2, synthesis of pulse-labeled viral
related proteins can not be detected until 5hr PI at which time
minor amounts of the nucleocapsid protein (NP) are detected. At
6hr PI the 50K NP protein continues to be made but in vastly increased quantities and three additional proteins having molecular
weights of 180K, 23K and 21K were seen for the first time. At 7hrs
PI the amount of the 23K protein synthesized was increased and
a new protein having a MW of 39K was detected. At 8hr PI three
additional proteins having MW of 107K, 25K, and 18K (barely
visible), respecitvely, were observed. Additional viral specific
polypeptides were not detected beyond 8hr PI.

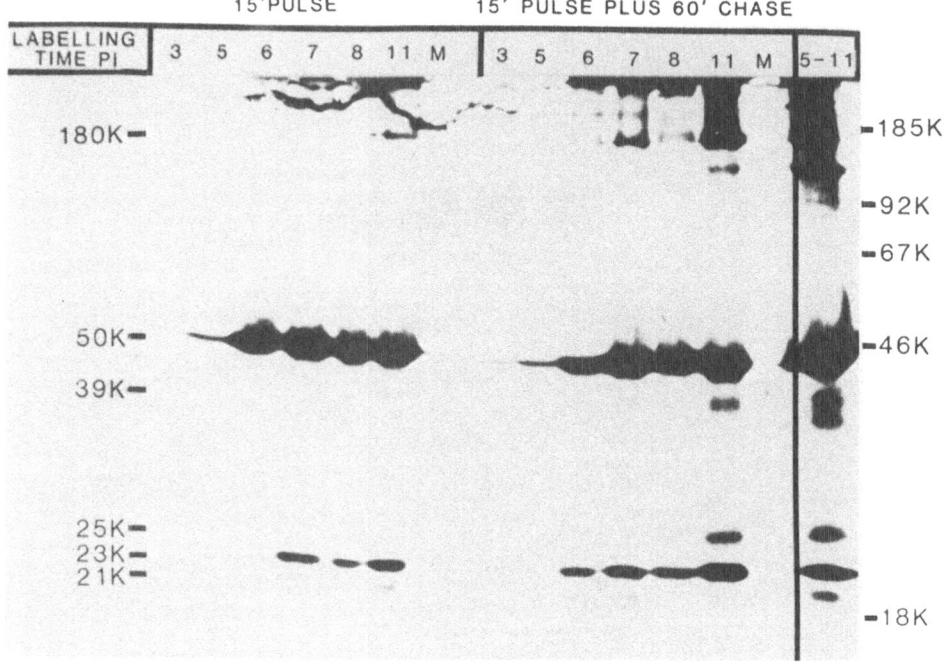

Figure 2: SDS-PAGE analysis of immunoprecipitates of labeled
229E proteins. Infected cells were pulsed for 15 min, pulsed for
15 min and chased for 60 min, or labeled from 5 to 11hr post-
infection. Cellular extracts were prepared from cultures labeled
with ^{35}S-methionine and 229E proteins were immunoprecipitated
with rabbit anti-229E serum using the procedure described by
Famulari and Jelalian (16). M=mock-infected immunoprecipitate prepared at 11hr PI.

To determine if the viral proteins synthesized during a 15
min pulse underwent post-translational cleavage or modification,
infected cells were pulsed for 15 min with ^{35}S-methionine and
chased for 60 min with an excess of unlabelled methionine. We were
unable to demonstrate the synthesis of additional viral proteins

during a 60 min chase (Fig. 2), but synthesis of some of the viral polypeptides could be detected earlier in the infectious cycle. At 6hr PI following a pulse-chase, all viral proteins were detectable that could not be seen until 8hr PI following a 15 min pulse (Fig. 2). The amount of each protein synthesized at different times varied considerably. Synthesis of the 50K, 23K and 18K polypeptides remained relatively constant from 6 to 11hr. PI. Formation of the 180K, 107K, 39K and 25K viral proteins, respectively, increased during the infectious cycle, until maximal synthesis was reached at 11hr PI.

Sturman (15) showed that the 180K glycoprotein of A59 is susceptible to proteases resulting in the formation of a 90K protein. To determine if longer labeling resulted in the accumulation of smaller glycoproteins, cells were labeled from 5 to 11 hour PI and the immunoprecipitable proteins were analyzed (Fig. 2). The amount of the 107K glycoprotein was increased significantly during a longer labelling period and a minor glycoprotein having a molecular weight of 92K was observed (Fig. 2).

These results suggested that precursors to the 180K and 25K proteins may undergo post-translational processing. In addition, it may be noted that significant quantities of labeled material did not penetrate the gel (Fig. 2), especially pulse-chase labeled proteins. Labeled proteins observed at the top of the gel could have represented aggregated glycoprotein since the samples were disrupted for electrophoresis by boiling in the presence of SDS and 2-mercaptoethanol. This procedure has been shown to cause virus glycoproteins to aggregate (22). These conditions may have led to the formation of the 39K and 18K proteins as well.

During a short 15 min pulse, detection of a glycosylated or partially glycosylated precursor to the 180K protein was expected, but a protein of this nature was not observed (Fig. 2). The possibility remained that the precursor aggregated and did not penetrate the gel, therefore, conditions of dissociation were altered. At 11hr PI, infected cells were pulsed for 15 min and chased from 15 to 105 min with excess unlabelled methionine. Samples were taken at 15 min intervals. Viral related proteins were immunoprecipitated and dissociated at 37°C for 30 min in the presence of SDS and 2-mercaptoethanol. Following electrophoresis the only proteins detectable were the 180K, 50K, 25K, 23K and 21K proteins, respectively. During the chase, the amount of the 25K protein increased whereas the amount of the 23K and 21K protein decreased suggesting that the 23K and 21K proteins are processed to yield the 25K protein. A precursor to the 180K protein was not observed but slight increases in the amount of the 180K protein were noted during the chase. When the conditions of dissociation were altered, the 107K, 92K, 39K and 18K proteins, respectively, were not observed, suggesting further, that these proteins are formed by aggregation or contain heat labile bonds.

Synthesis of Intracellular 229E Proteins in Tunicamycin Treated Cells

To further define the processing events that 229E proteins appeared to undergo, we analyzed the effect(s) of tunicamycin on viral protein synthesis. Tunicamycin is an antibiotic analogue of UDP-N-acetylglucosamine which blocks the synthesis of dolicholpyro-phosphate-N-acetylglucosamine (17,18). The result of this inhibition is the prevention of the en bloc transfer of core oligosaccharides to asparagine residues of nascent glycoprotein precursor molecules. Thus, glycoproteins synthesized in tunicamycin treated cells do not acquire N-glycosidically linked oligosaccharides.

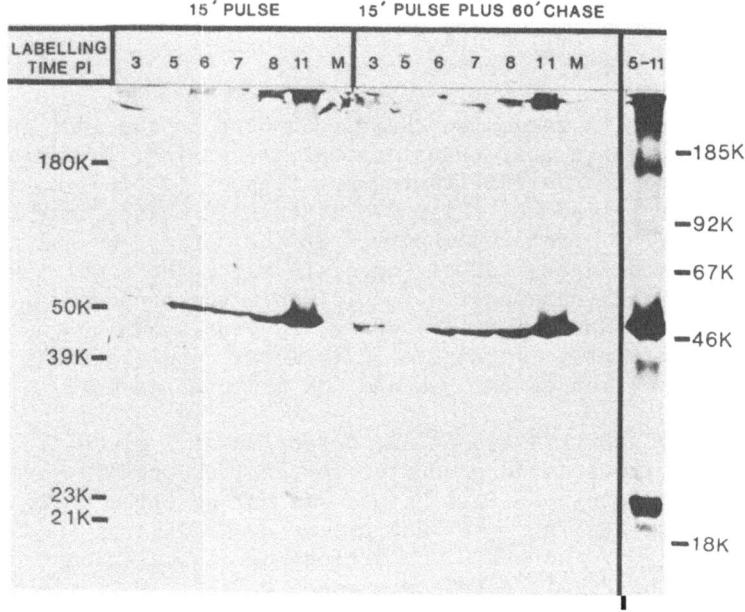

Figure 3: SDS-PAGE analysis of immunoprecipitates of labeled 229E proteins synthesized by tunicamycin treated cells. Infected cells were treated with 2 μg/ml of tunicamycin starting at 1hr post-infection. Labeling procedures were the same as described in Fig. 1 and 2. M=mock-infected immunoprecipitate prepared at 11hr PI.

Infected cells were treated with tunicamycin (2 μg/ml) starting at 1hr PI and infected cells were pulse labeled or pulse chased as in the above experiment. Viral proteins labeled for 15 min in tunicamycin treated cells at designated time periods are shown in Fig. 3. Synthesis of the 50K NP protein began at

approximately 6 hours PI in tunicamycin treated (Fig. 3) and untreated cells (Fig. 1 and 2). At 7hr PI, trace amounts of the 23K
protein were detected in tunicamycin treated cells and by 11hr PI
(Fig. 3) the 50K, 23K and 21K proteins, respectively, were clearly
visible. Noticeably absent were the 180K, major glycoprotein, and
the 25K protein. The results obtained following a 15 min pulse
and 60 min chase (Fig. 3) did not differ appreciably from the 15
min pulse studies. But, when tunicamycin treated cells were labeled
with ^{35}S-methionine from 5 to 11 hours PI (Fig. 3), small amounts
of the 180K and the 25K protein were detected compared to untreated cells (Fig. 2). More notable was the large amount of 23K
protein that accumulated in tunicamycin treated cells during the
labelling period from 5 to 11 hours PI.

These studies suggested that: 1) The 180K and 25K proteins
are N-glycosylated; 2) the 23K and 21K proteins may be precursors
to the 25K protein and 3) a non-N-glycosylated precursor to the
180K protein can not be demonstrated in tunicamycin treated infected cells. But as previously noted, when samples were incubated
at 100°C prior to electrophoresis, labeled material remained at
the gel origin and similarly labeled material can be seen at the
top of Fig. 3. To rule out the possibility that the precursor
remained at the origin, the dissociation conditions were altered.
The immunoprecipitated proteins were heated at 37°C as opposed
to the previous dissociation by boiling and then analyzed by SDS-
PAGE. Only the 50K, 23K and 21K proteins, respectively, were
synthesized during a 15 minute pulse. Following a 30 minute chase,
the amount of the 50K and 23K proteins synthesized was unchanged,
i.e. the 23K protein did not appear to chase. After altering the
dissociation conditions, a precursor to 180K was not noted and
label at the top of the gel dissappeared. The 25K protein was
totally absent. Therefore, it was concluded that the 180K and 25K
proteins, respectively, are N-glycosylated.

Synthesis of Intracellular 229E Proteins in Monensin Treated Cells

Based on the studies described above the 180K and 25K proteins undergo post-translational modification by the addition of
N-glycosidically linked oligosaccharides, and the electrophoretic
properties of a number of the viral proteins are altered by the
conditions of dissociation prior to electrophoresis. We were
interested in determining what effect(s) inhibition of transport
of nascent glycoprotein precursors might have on processing of
the viral proteins, because coronaviruses are assembled at membrane sites within the cytoplasm. Monensin, a monovalent ionophore
that inhibits the transport and plasma membrane expression of
membrane associated glycoproteins (19,20,21) was chosen as an
inhibitor. Monensin (10^{-6}M) was added to infected cells at 1hr

PI and treated cells were pulse labeled for 15 min or pulsed
for 15 min and chased for 60 min at different times PI. As may be
seen from Fig. 4, monensin did not alter the onset of viral protein
synthesis, i.e. at 5 - 6hr PI, compared to untreated infected cells
(Fig. 2). However, there was a noticeable difference in the
relative amount of viral proteins synthesized in monensin treated
cells. In treated cells only the 50K protein is detectable (Fig. 4)
at 6hr PI, whereas, in non-treated cells the 180K, 50K, 23K and
21K proteins, respectively, were synthesized during a 15 minute
pulse (Fig. 2) by 6hr PI. The amount of the 50K protein synthesized
in monensin treated cells was approximately the same as that
synthesized in untreated cells. By 7hrs PI trace amounts of the
39K and 23K proteins (Fig. 4) were observed. At 11hr PI synthesis
of the 180K, 50K, 39K and 23K protein, respectively, were evident,
but there appeared to be an increased accumulation of the 23K
protein (Fig. 4) compared to the amount synthesized in untreated
cells (Fig. 2).

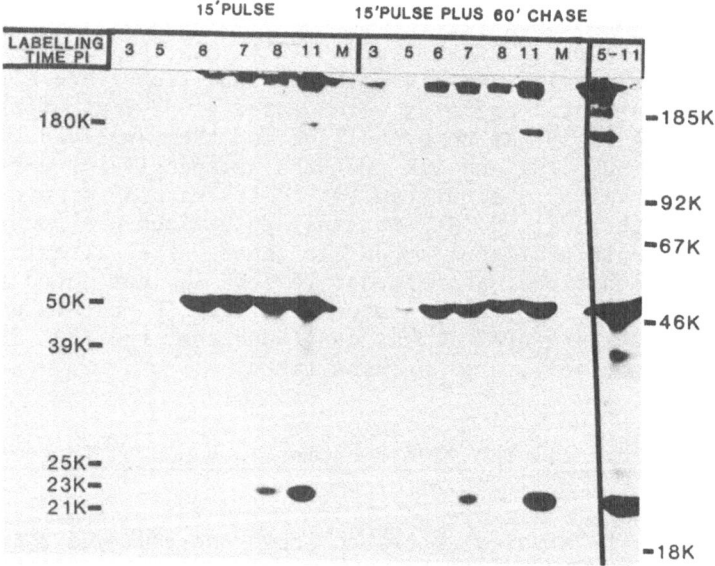

Figure 4: SDS-PAGE analysis of immunoprecipitates of labeled
229E proteins synthesized by monensin treated cells. Infected
cells were treated with 10^{-6}M monensin starting at 11hr PI. Labeling procedures were the same as described in Fig. 1 and 2. M=mock-
infected immunoprecipitate prepared at 11hr PI.

Synthesis of the 180K and 25K proteins was not observed
during a 15 min pulse until 11hr PI in monensin treated cells
(Fig. 4), whereas, the 180K protein was detectable during a 15 min
pulse at 6hr PI in untreated cells (Fig. 2). Following a pulse of

15 min and chase of 60 min, both the 180K and 23K proteins were noted at 7hr PI in monensin treated cells. At 11hr PI (Fig. 4) trace amounts of the 25K protein were visible and significant amounts of the 180K protein were detectable, but the amounts were substantially less than that seen in untreated cells (Fig. 2). The 107K and 92K proteins that may be derived from the 180K protein were not present in monensin treated cells. The effect of inhibition of glycoprotein transport was demonstrated further by long term labelling from 5-11hr PI. Small amounts of the 25K and 21K protein were detected during the long term labelling period but there appears to be an overall accumulation of the 23K protein. Moreover, only small amounts of the 180K protein (Fig. 4) were observed at 11hr PI in monensin treated cells, whereas in pulse-chase experiments, large amounts of the 180K protein were observed at 7hr PI in untreated cells (Fig. 2).

Proteins isolated from monensin treated cells and prepared for electrophoresis by boiling accumulated at the top of the gel like those synthesized in untreated and tunicamycin treated cells. Therefore, the conditions of dissociation were altered as described for proteins synthesized in untreated cells. At 11hr PI, monensin treated cells were pulsed for 15 minutes and chased from 15 to 105 minutes with excess unlabelled methionine. Proteins were immunoprecipitated from cell extracts at 15 minute intervals and separated by gel electrophoresis. Under these conditions the 180K, 50K, 25K, 23K and 21K proteins, respectively, are detectable but the amount of the 180K and 25K proteins synthesized are substantially less than in untreated cells. These results suggest that the addition of N-glycosidically linked oligosacharides to the 180K and 25K proteins is significantly reduced in monensin treated cells, which may lead to an accumulation of the 23K protein and possibility to the catabolism of the 180K unglycosylated precursor.

Discussion

The structural protein composition of the HCV 229E differs little from that reported for other coronaviruses (13,15,22-25). It is comprised of three major polypeptides, a high molecular weight glycoprotein, 180K, a phosphorylated nucleoprotein, 50K, and a family of proteins having molecular weights of 25K, 23K and 21K, respectively. In addition to these major proteins, minor polypeptides having molecular weights of 107K, 92K and 39K, have been shown to be associated with virions.

One of the objectives of the study presented herein was to determine if 229E proteins undergo post-translational processing. This study indicates that at least two proteins, the 180K and 25K proteins, respectively, undergo glycosylation, a post-translational event. Variation in molecular weight(s) of the small viral pro-

tein(s), i.e. the 25K, 23K and 21K proteins, respectively, has
been attributed to differences in the glycosylation pattern of
these proteins (12,13). Using labeled sugar precursors we have
been unable to demonstrate the glycosylation of the 25K, 23K or
21K proteins, respectively, but it is likely that the 25K protein
is N-glycosylated. Evidence for N-glycosylation of the 25K protein
is based on two studies: (1) When pulse-chase labeled proteins
were immunoprecipitated from tunicamycin-treated cells the 25K
protein could not be detected, whereas an accumulation of the
23K protein was observed; and 2) treatment of the infected cells
with monensin delayed and substantially decreased the synthesis
of the 25K protein. The effect of tunicamycin is to block
N-glycosylation and monensin alters transport of glycoproteins
through the golgi complex, where N-glycosidically linked oligosaccharides are processed. The net effect is inhibition or slowing
of glycosylation of the 25K protein and this was the phenomenon
which was observed. Therefore, the 25K protein is probably
N-glycosylated.

Other investigators (12, 26) have reported evidence for the
addition of O-linked oligosaccharides to a polypeptide having a
molecular weight of 23K in A59 infected cells. Monensin has been
reported to inhibit the addition of O-linked oligosaccharides
to herpesvirus glycoproteins (27), but an accumulation of the
presumed unglycosylated precursor 21K protein in monensin treated
229E infected cells was not noted. Moreover, in herpesvirus infected cells post-translational modification by the addition of
O-linked oligosaccharides appears to be a late event in the golgi
apparatus. In MRC$_5$ cells, the addition of O-linked oligosaccharides
must occur very rapidly since the 21K and 23K proteins appear
simultaneously at 6hr PI and the 23K protein is more readily
detected than the 21K protein. If O-glycosylation of the 21K
protein does not occur, then we do not have an explanation for
event(s) leading to the synthesis of the 23K protein.

The 180K protein in addition to being glycosylated, may be
further modified by cellular proteases. A 107K protein was detected
in cells pulsed for 15 min at 8hr PI but when cells were pulsed
for 15 min and chased for 60 min, the 107K protein was detected
at 6hr PI. The 92K protein was only detected when cells were
labeled from 5 - 11hr PI. The relationship between the 107K and
92K proteins has not been established but they are glycosylated
and are immunoprecipitated by rabbit anti-229E serum. Sturman
(15) showed that the 180K protein of A59 is cleaved by proteases
to yield two proteins, both having a molecular weight of 90K.
Whether the 107K and 92K together equal the 180K protein or
whether the 107K is processed further to yield the 92K protein
has not been determined. It is noteable that the 107K and 92K
proteins were absent from immunoprecipitates that were prepared for
electrophoresis by incubation at 37°C. This result suggests that

proteins were absent from immunoprecipitates that were prepared for electrophoresis by incubation at 37°C. This result suggests that breakdown of the 180K protein may occur because of heat-labile bonds rather than by the action of proteases.

Siddell et al (25) observed processing of a precursor 150K protein in JHM infected cells to a glycosylated 170K protein that appeared to undergo further processing to yield a glycosylated 98K molecule. A precursor to the glycosylated 180K protein of 229E could not be detected. But the inability to detect non-glycosylated precursors is not restricted to our system. The hemagglutinin (HA) glycoprotein of fowl plaque virus an influenza virus is degraded when it is not glycosylated (28,29), whereas the HA protein of WSN, another influenza virus, can be detected in an unglycosylated form designated HA_0 (30) and it is incorporated into virions. Thus, processing of precursor proteins depends to a certain extent on the virus-cell system.

Two other proteins having molecular weights of 39K and 18K, respectively, were consistently detected when immunoprecipitated proteins from infected cells were boiled before electrophoresis. However, if samples were prepared for electrophoresis by dissociation at 37°C these proteins could not be detected. It is therefore probable that these proteins form as a result of the dissociation conditions as previously shown for A59 (22).

REFERENCES:

1. D.A.J. Tyrrell, J.D. Almeida, D.M. Berry, C.H. Cunningham, D. Hamre, M.S. Hofstad, L. Mallucci, and K. McIntosh, Corona-viruses, Nature 220:650(1971).
2. D.A.J. Tyrrell and M.L. Bynoe, Cultivation of a Novel Type of Common-Cold Virus in Organ Cultures, Brit. Med. J. 1:1467(1965).
3. D. Hamre and J.T. Procknow, A. New Virus Isolated from the Human Respiratory Tract, Proc. Soc. Exp. Biol. Med. 121:190(1966).
4. K. McIntosh, J.H. Dees, W.B. Becker, A.Z. Kapikian, and R.M. Chanock, Recovery in Tracheal Organ Cultures of Novel Viruses from Patients with Respiratory Disease, Proc. Natl. Acad Sci. U.S.A. 57:933(1967).
5. A.Z. Kapikian, H.D. James, S.J. Kelly, and A.L. Vaughn, Detection of Coronavirus Strain 692 by Immune Electron Microscopy, Immun. 7:11(1973).
6. J.S. Burks, B.L. DeVald, L.D. Jankovsky, and J.C. Gerdes, Two Coronaviruses Isolated from Central Nervous System Tissue of Two Multiple Sclerosis Patients, Science 209:933(1980).
7. L.J. Anderson, P.A. Patriarca, J.C. Hierholzer, and G.R. Noble, Viral Respiratory Illnesses, Med. Clinics, In Press.

8. M.R. Macnaughton, Structural and Antigenic Relationships Between Human, Murine and Avian Coronaviruses, Adv. Exp. Med. Biol. 142:19(1980).

9. G.A. Tannock, and J.C. Hierholzer, The RNA of Human Coronavirus OC-43, Virology 78:500(1977).

10. S.R. Weiss, and J.L. Leibowitz, Comparison of the RNAs of Murine and Human Coronaviruses, Adv. Exp. Med. Biol. 142:245(1980).

11. J.C. Hierholzer, Purification and Biophysical Properties of Human Coronavirus 229E, Virology 75:155.(1976)

12. K.V. Holmes, E.W. Doller, and L.S. Sturman, Tunicamycin Resistant Glycosylation of a Coronavirus Glycoprotein: Demonstration of a Novel Type of Viral Glycoprotein, Virology 115:334(1981).

13. D.F. Stern, and B.M. Sefton, Coronavirus Proteins: Structure and Function of the Oligosaccharides of the Avian Infectious Bronchitis Virus Glycoproteins, J. Virol. 44:804(1982).

14. M.C. Kemp, M.L. Perdue, H.W. Rogers, D.J. O'Callaghan, and C.C. Randall, Structural Polypeptides of the Hamster Strain of Equine Herpes Virus Type 1: Products Associated with Purification. Virology 61:361(1974).

15. L.S. Sturman, The Structure and Behavior of Coronavirus A59 Glycoproteins, Adv. Exp. Med. Biol. 142:1(1980).

16. N.G. Famulari, and K. Jalalian, Cell Surface Expression of the env gene polyprotein of dual tropic mink cell focus-forming murine leukemic virus, J. Virol. 30, 720(1979).

17. A.K. Takatsuki, K. Kohno, and G. Tamura, inhibition of biosynthesis of polyisoprenol sugars in chick embryo microsomes by tunicamycin, Agr. Biol. Chem. 39:2089(1975).

18. D.K. Struck, and W.J. Lennarz, Evidence for the Participation of Saccharide-Lipids in the Synthesis of the Oligosaccharide Chain of Ovalbumin, J. Biol. Chem. 252:1007(1977).

19. A.M. Tartakoff, and P. Vaggali, Plasma Cell Immunoglobulin Secretion Arrest is accompained by Alterations of Golgi Complex, J. Exp. Med. 146:1332(1977).

20. N.H. Uchida, H. Smilowitz, and M.L. Tanzer, Monovalent Ionophores Inhibit Secretion of Procollagon and Fibronectin from Cultured Fibroblasts, Proc. Natl. Acad. Sci. U.S.A. 76:1868(1979).

21. D.C. Johnson, and M.J. Schlesinger, Vesicular Stomatitis Virus and Sindbis Virus Glycoprotein Transport to the Cell Surface in Inhibited by Ionophores, Virology 103:407(1980).

22. L.S. Sturman, Characterization of a coronavirus. I. Structural Proteins: Effect of Preparative Conditions on the Migration of Protein in Polyacrylamide Gels, Virology 77:637(1977).

23. L.S. Sturman, and K.V. Holmes, Characterization of a Coronavirus. II. Glycoproteins of the Viral Envelope; Tryptic Peptide Analysis, Virology 77:650(1977).

24. H. Wege, Wege, K. Nagashima, and V. ter Meulen, Structural

Polypeptides of the Murine Coronavirus JHM, J. Gen. Virol. 42:37(1979).

25. S. Siddell, H. Wege, A. Barthel, and V. ter Meulen, Coronavirus JHM: Intracellular Protein Synthesis, J. Gen. Virol. 53:145(1981).

26. H. Niemann, and H. D. Klenk, Coronavirus Glycoprotein E1, A New Type of Viral Glycoprotein, J. Mol. Biol. 153:983(1981).

27. D.C. Johnson, and P.G. Spear, O - Linked Oligosaccharides are Acquired by Herpes Simplex Virus Glycoproteins in the Golgi Apparatus, Cell 32:987(1983).

28. H. D. Klenk, W. Hollert, R. Rott and C. Scholtissek, Association of Influenza Virus Proteins with Cytoplasmic Fractions, Virology, 57:28(1974).

29. R. T. Schwartz, T.M. Rohrschneider, and M.F.G. Schmidt, Suppression of Glycoprotein Formation of Semliki Forest Virus, Influenza and Avian Sarcoma Virus by Tunicamycin, J. Virol. 17:782(1976).

30. K. Nakamura, and R.W. Compans, Effects of Inhibitors on Glycosylation, Sulfation, and Assembly of Influenza Virus glycoproteins, Virology 84:303(1978).

DEFECTIVE REPLICATION OF PORCINE TRANSMISSIBLE GASTROENTERITIS VIRUS IN A CONTINUOUS CELL LINE

D.J. Garwes, Lynne Bountiff, G.C. Millson and
Carole J. Elleman

A.R.C. Institute for Research on Animal Diseases
Compton, Newbury, Berkshire RG16 0NN, U.K.

ABSTRACT

During a search for established cell lines to produce large quantities of porcine transmissible gastroenteritis virus (TGEV), we observed bright immunofluorescent staining 6-12h after infection of pig kidney derived LLC-PK1 line. Infectious virus yield was, however, 2 $\log_{10}$ lower than that from secondary adult pig thyroid (APT/2) cell cultures, although small plaques were visible by three days in cultures maintained under agarose, suggesting limited replication. Attempts to adapt TGEV to the LLC-PK1 cell line by 10 serial 20h passes were unsuccessful.

Procedures to purify virions from infected LLC-PK1 cells produced less than 1% of the particles isolated from parallel APT/2 cultures. Examination of intracellular viral RNA in actinomycin-D treated cells revealed similar amounts of genomic RNA and the 4 major subgenomic species in both cell types, suggesting that there was no defect in viral RNA replication. In vitro translation of polyadenylated RNA from infected APT/2 and LLC-PK1 cells, followed by immune precipitation of the products, showed similar profiles of precursors to structural polypeptides, confirming the functional integrity of the viral messengers in the restrictive cell.

Comparison of the viral polypeptides synthesised following infection of the two cell types showed that similar species were synthesised in both, corresponding to a group of 28-30,000 mol. wt. envelope glycopolypeptides, a 47,000 mol. wt. nucleoprotein and peplomer glycopolypeptides of about 200,000 mol. wt. The rate of viral polypeptide synthesis in LLC-PK1 cells was reproducibly

higher than in APT/2, resulting in the earlier detection of bands
and greater incorporation of isotope.   Tunicamycin at 1 µg/ml had
a similar effect in both cells, preventing glycosylation of the
26,000 mol. wt. precursor of the envelope glycopolypeptides and
synthesis of the 200,000 peplomer glycoprotein.   Degradation of
the nucleoprotein from 47,000 to 42,000 mol. wt. although detectable
in both cells was more marked in the LLC-PK1 cultures.
Phosphorylation of these proteins was readily demonstrated in both
cells, although phosphorylation of host proteins and, to some
extent, viral envelope proteins was considerably greater in the
LLC-PK1.   The significance of this finding with respect to virus
maturation is being investigated.

INTRODUCTION

     Our previous attempts to grow TGEV, FS772/70, in a continuous
line of cells had been unsuccessful.   We required a culture system
that could be scaled up beyond that possible with secondary adult
pig thyroid cells (APT/2) to produce sufficient viral components
for chemistry and serology.   Accordingly, we tested several
recently derived cell lines of pig origin for their ability to
support the replication of TGEV.   The pig kidney cell line
LLC-PK1[1] gave bright immunofluorescence after infection, although
little or no infectious virus was produced.   This appeared to be
a common feature of our viral isolate in continuous cultures, since
it was true for several other well established lines, including
swine testis (ST). Another isolate of TGEV, for example the Purdue
and Miller strains, that would grow in lines such as ST, could be
chosen but the present isolate had been studied   extensively
already.   It was originally isolated from an outbreak in the U.K.
and might be more typical of newly isolated strains from field
outbreaks.   This paper describes data from an investigation into
the cause of defective replication in LLC-PK1 cells infected with
TGEV (FS772/70).

MATERIALS AND METHODS

     Virus and cells.   The FS772/70 isolate of TGEV and its
cultivation in APT/2 cells has been described[2].   LLC-PK1 cells
were obtained from Flow Laboratories Ltd., Scotland, and were
maintained as stationary cultures in Eagles minimal essential
medium (EMEM) supplemented with antibiotics and 5% foetal calf
serum and buffered with 0.14% sodium bicarbonate.   For virus
growth, the media were used without serum and buffered at pH 6.8
with 50 mM HEPES, 0.14% sodium bicarbonate.

Plaque assay. As previously described[2], petri dish cultures were incubated for 1h at 37°C with serial dilutions of virus then overlaid with either medium 199/2.5% calf serum (APT/2) or EMEM/2.5% foetal calf serum (LLC-PK1) supplemented with 50 mM HEPES/0.14% sodium bicarbonate/antibiotics and 0.6% agarose. Plaques were visualised after 3d at 37°C by staining with crystal violet.

Immunofluorescence. Cultures were grown as monolayers in 96-well flat bottom plates and sufficient TGEV added to infect 30-50% of the cells. At appropriate times after infection, the medium was removed and the cell sheets fixed with 80% acetone for 10 mins at room temperature. During the study, a variety of antibody preparations were tested including porcine, feline and murine antisera, monoclonal hybridoma supernatant fluids and ascitic fluids. FITC-conjugated rabbit anti-species antibodies were obtained from Nordic Laboratories, London.

Virus purification. Frozen/thawed cultures were clarified at 15,000 xg for 20 mins then centrifuged through a stepped 10%/60% sucrose gradient at 70,000 xg for 90 mins, followed by a linear 20%-45% sucrose gradient at 70,000 xg for 90 mins. The radioactive viral band was located by scintillation counting and pelleted at 150,000 xg for 2 hours[3].

Incorporation of radioisotopes. For most of the experiments described in which isotopically labelled precursors were incorporated, cells were grown in plastic flasks, 25 cm^2 (Nunc, Gibco Europe Ltd.) and either infected with TGEV at an input multiplicity of 50-200 pfu/cell for 1-2h at 37°C or treated with a corresponding volume of uninfected culture medium. The inoculum was removed, the cells were rinsed with isotonic saline and 2ml of medium was added, to be replaced by a further 2ml of medium containing isotope for the appropriate time period. For incorporation of [^{3}H]-leucine or [^{35}S]-methionine EMEM lacking leucine or methionine was used, medium 199 lacking orthophosphate for ^{32}P -orthophosphate incorporation and complete medium 199 or EMEM for experiments involving [^{3}H]-uridine or [^{3}H]-glucosamine. All medium was serum-free and was buffered at pH 6.8 with 50 mM HEPES/0.14% sodium bicarbonate. Actinomycin-D (Calbiochem) was incorporated at 1µg/ml where indicated. Radioisotopes were obtained from Amersham International plc, England.

Electrophoresis: Polypeptide samples. At the times indicated in the text, the medium was removed from the cultures and the cell sheets were solubilised in 0.5ml of 2% sodium dodecyl sulphate, 5% β-mercaptoethanol, 20% (vol/vol) glycerol and 0.0625M TRIS pH 6.8. After heating at 100°C for 2 min, samples were electrophoresed in 8.75% polyacrylamide gels by the method of Laemmli[4]. Gels were fixed in trichloroacetic acid, 10% (w/v); glacial acetic

acid, 10% (v/v); methanol, 30% (v/v) and dried down directly
(^{32}P samples) or treated with ENhance (NEN GmbH, Drieichenheim;
all other isotopes) prior to drying and autoradiography.

   RNA samples.   Cultures labelled with [^{3}H]-uridine were
solubilised in 2% sodium dodecyl sulphate, 5% mercaptoethanol, 20%
glycerol, 1 x Loening buffer and electrophoresed in agarose as
previously described for TGEV[5] but with a horizontal 1% agarose
slab gel in place of the rod gels used previously.   For
autoradiography, gels were compressed under filter paper to reduce
their volume then enhanced overnight (NEN GmbH, Dreieichenheim) and
dried under vacuum.

   In vitro translation.   Polyadenylated RNA was extracted from
uninfected and infected cells with guanidinium thiocyanate[6] and
eluted from an oligo(dT)-cellulose column[7].   In vitro translation
was carried out with a rabbit reticulocyte lysate (Amersham
International plc, England) and monitored by the incorporation of
[^{35}S]-methionine.   The products were reacted with hyperimmune
serum raised in TGEV-infected cats and the immune precipitates
were collected on Staphylococcus aureus cells prior to electrophoresis as described above[8].

RESULTS

   Immunofluorescence.   Fluorescent cells could be visualised
by 6h after infection of LLC-PK1 and APT/2 cultures and the staining
increased in intensity to approximately 10h.   After this time the
number of infected cells in the APT/2 cultures increased whereas
the LLC-PK1 cultures showed little or no evidence of viral spread.
The numbers of initially infected cells were consistent with the
dilution of virus used, however, and were similar between the two
cell types, indicating that the susceptibility of the cells to
infection was not different.

   Plaque formation.   A similar conclusion could be drawn from
the results of plaque assay (Fig. 1).   The numbers of plaques
developing on the two cultures were approximately similar but the
size of the plaques after 3 days clearly indicated that the several
cycles of replication undergone in APT/2 cells had not occurred in
LLC-PK1.

   Infectious virus yield.   Whereas the infectivity yield from
a single cycle of virus replication in APT/2 cells was equivalent
to 30-50 pfu per cell, the infected LLC-PK1 produced only 1 pfu
per 2-10 cells.   An attempt was made to adapt the virus or select
a subpopulation capable of growing on LLC-PK1 cells.   Ten serial
passes through LLC-PK1 cultures, involving 20h of culture with

APT/2   LLC-PK1

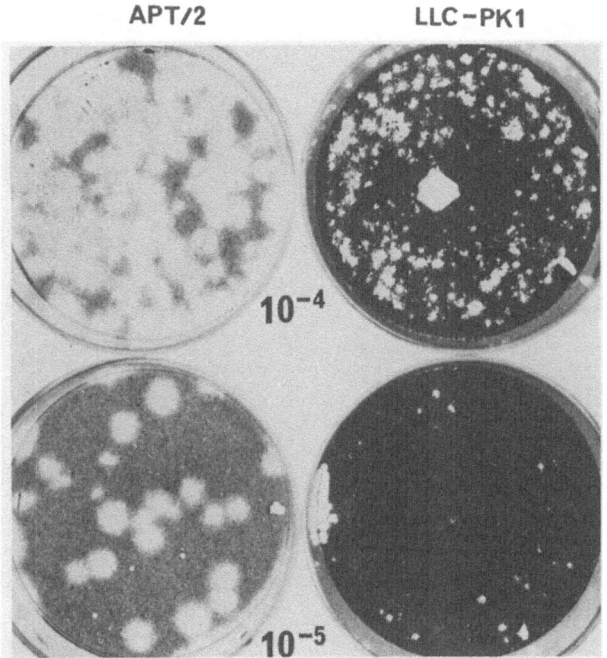

Fig. 1.   Plaque assay in monolayer cultures of APT/2 and LLC/PK1
           cells.   After 1h incubation with 0.1ml of TGEV at the
           dilution shown, the cultures were overlaid, incubated
           at 37°C for 3 days and stained with crystal violet.

virus, freeze-thawing and inoculating 10% of the culture into the
next flask, were assayed and the infectivity dropped by approximately 2 $\log_{10}$ during each of the first three passes.   No
infectivity was detectable from the fifth pass on.

    Virion purification.   To determine whether non-infectious
particles were produced by LLC-PK1 cells, parallel cultures of
APT/2 and LLC-PK1 were infected and incubated in the presence of
[^{3}H]-uridine or [^{3}H]-leucine.   Both cultures were then processed
to purify virus by gradient centrifugation and the radioactivity
monitored.   A clear band of radioactivity was detected in the
linear sucrose gradient of APT/2 material.   This was pelleted and
showed the expected profile of structural polypeptides after
electrophoresis (Fig. 2).   There was no corresponding peak of
radioactivity in the LLC-PK1 derived material and the small amount
of radioactivity that was recovered in the final pelleted
preparation did not correspond to any of the major structural
polypeptides.

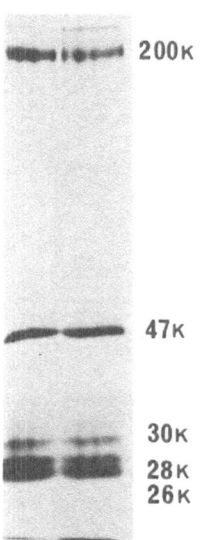

C 1 2 3 4 5 6 7 8

Fig. 2.   Electrophoresis of
TGEV structural polypeptides.
Two preparations of [^{3}H]-leucine
labelled virus, isolated from
APT/2 cultures, were purified
and electrophoresed as described.
Molecular weights were determined
by comparison with standard
proteins.

Fig. 3.   Agarose gel electrophoresis of [^{3}H]-uridine labelled
RNA from uninfected (track C) and
TGEV-infected (tracks 1-8) APT/2
cells incubated with actinomycin-
D.   Cultures were labelled for 3
hours before lysis: Tracks C &
no. 1, 0-3h; no. 2, 3-6h; no.
3, 6-9h; no. 4, 9-12h; no. 5,
12-15h; no. 6, 15-18h, no. 7,
18-21h; no. 8, 21-24h.

        Viral RNA synthesis.   Five major species of RNA were
synthesised in TGEV-infected APT/2 cells incubated with
actinomycin-D and [^{3}H]-uridine.   Fig. 3 shows the rates of
synthesis over 24h in cultures receiving an input multiplicity of
5-10 pfu/cell.   Although more of the largest species accumulated
during the ^{3}H labelling period, the relative proportions of the
bands stayed approximately the same during the growth cycle.   The
5 bands corresponded in size to genomic RNA and the 4 subgenomic
species described previously[9], shown in Fig. 4a.   Comparison of
the electrophoretic profiles obtained with RNA extracted from
infected, actinomycin-D treated APT/2 and LLC-PK1 cells (Fig. 4b)
showed that the number, molecular weights and relative proportions
of the bands is similar from the two cultures.

        RNA from uninfected and infected APT/2 and LLC-PK1 cultures
was extracted and the polyadenylated molecules purified on oligo
(dT)-cellulose.   This was then translated in a rabbit reticulocyte

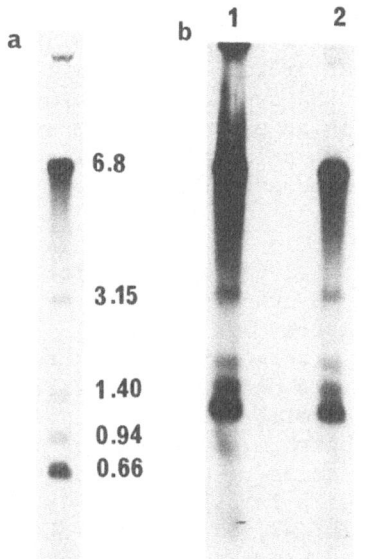

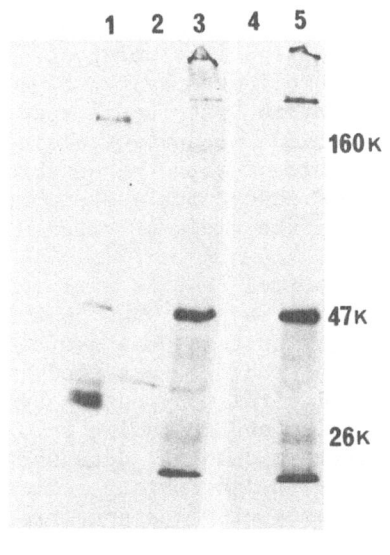

Fig. 4.   Agarose gel electrophoresis of TGEV-specific RNA.
a. APT/2-derived RNA with
molecular weights in megadaltons.
b. Comparison of APT/2-derived
(track 1) with LLC-PK1-derived
(track 2) viral intracellular
RNA.

Fig. 5.   Translation products
of viral mRNA.   Polyadenylated
RNA from uninfected (track 2) and
TGEV-infected (track 3) APT/2
cells and from uninfected (track
4) and TGEV-infected (track 5)
LLC-PK1 cells was translated in
a rabbit reticulocyte system in
the presence of [^{35}S]-methionine.
The products were precipitated
with immune feline antiserum and
compared by polyacrylamide gel
electrophoresis with purified
virus (track 1).

lysate and the products immune precipitated and electrophoresed in
polyacrylamide gel.   The autoradiographs shown in Fig. 5
demonstrate that proteins made by APT/2 and LLC-PK1 derived RNA
are very similar and correspond to the precursor molecules of
envelope polypeptides (26,000 mol. wt.) and peplomer (160,000 mol.
wt.) and the nucleoprotein (47,000 mol. wt.).   Other bands,
particularly those between 26,000 and 47,000 mol. wt. may correspond
to incomplete forms of the nucleoprotein or to non-structural
proteins.   The track of purified viral polypeptides shows some
evidence of nonglycosylated precursor to envelope protein (26,000
mol. wt.) but none of the peplomer precursor.   There does not
appear to be any defect, therefore, in the synthesis of viral RNA
in the LLC-PK1 cell nor in the coding ability of the RNA made.

Intracellular polypeptide synthesis.   Studies on the synthesis
of viral specific polypeptides by TGEV FS 772/70-infected cells
were complicated by the high level of host protein synthesis.
Actinomycin-D at 1μg/ml reduced cellular RNA synthesis by more than
98% but had no appreciable effect on cellular protein synthesis.
Pretreatment with the antibiotic for 12-18h prior to infection
reduced endogenous protein synthesis to some extent but also
reduced the yield of virus.

Optimal results were achieved by using input multiplicities of
infection in the range 50-200 pfu/cell.   Synthesis of most of the
cellular proteins was reduced to approximately 50% and viral
proteins could be detected by comparison with uninfected controls.
Maximum viral polypeptide synthesis occurred between 8-12h after
infection and following this the infected cells showed marked
cytopathic changes, detached from the substrate and lost their
ability to incorporate radioactive amino acids.   Fig. 6 shows the
appearance of virus specific bands during 2h labelling periods up
to 8h after infection.   The nucleoprotein (47,000 mol. wt.) is
the most apparent of the newly synthesised bands;   that it
comigrates in the gel with a host protein of similar size is

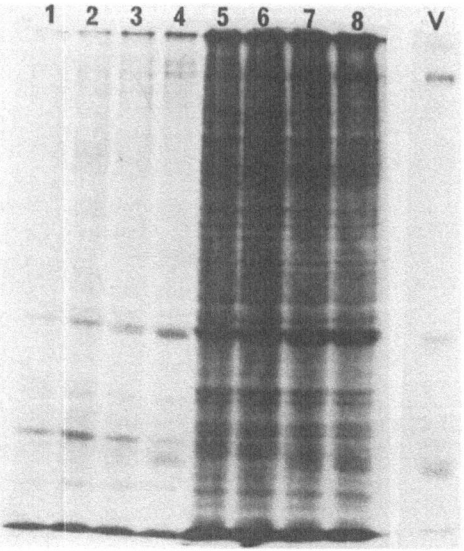

Fig. 6.   Synthesis of TGEV polypeptides.   APT/2 cells (tracks
           1-4) and LLC-PK1 cells (tracks 5-8) were infected with
           TGEV and labelled with [^{35}S]-methionine for 2h between
           0-2h (tracks 1 & 5), 2-4h (tracks 2 & 6), 4-6h (tracks
           3 & 7) and 6-8h (tracks 4 & 8).   The polypeptides from
           purified virions are shown in track V for comparison.

unfortunate, but its identity has been confirmed by electroblotting
onto nitrocellulose followed by reaction with TGEV antiserum, by
comparison of the bands from uninfected and infected cells by
oligopeptide mapping and, as discussed below, by the phosphorylation
of the nucleoprotein. A heterogeneous group of bands in the
28-30,000 mol. wt. region corresponds to the set of envelope
proteins seen in the purified virion but any small amount of
precursor to this species is masked by the presence of host proteins.
Similarly, there is little evidence of peplomer polypeptide or its
precursor in these gels, in part due to the relatively low amounts
synthesised and the presence of host proteins at the same location
but serological detection of electroblots has confirmed their
presence as a double band at 200,000 and 220,000 mol. wt. and a
small amount of material at 160,000 (data not shown).   The
patterns are clearer in Fig. 7 in which uninfected and infected
APT/2 and LLC-PK1 cells were labelled with [^{3}H]-leucine, [^{35}S]-
methionine or [^{3}H]-glucosamine between 6 and 12h after infection.
The peplomer proteins can be seen as a double band near the top of
the glucosamine tracks, but there was insufficient incorporation
of label into the 28-30,000 mol. wt. envelope proteins to detect

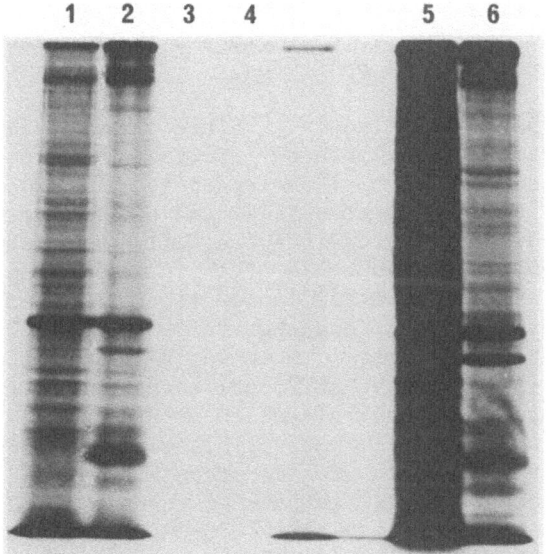

Fig. 7.   Intracellular polypeptides from uninfected (tracks 1 & 3)
           and TGEV-infected (tracks 2 & 4) APT/2 cells and from
           uninfected (track 5) and infected (track 6) LLC-PK1
           cells.   Tracks 1, 2, 5 & 6 received samples from cells
           labelled 4-8h after infection with [^{35}S]-methionine,
           while tracks 3 & 4 received samples from [^{3}H]-glucosamine-
           labelled cells.

them in this experiment.   It should be noted that there are no
major differences in the numbers or molecular weights of the viral
polypeptides seen in the APT/2 and LLC-PK1 cells and that all
except one of the bands identified can be found in purified virions.
The exception is the strongly labelled band with an apparent
molecular weight of 42,000.   This protein is produced late on in
the replication cycle and is more pronounced in LLC-PK1 cells than
in APT/2 cells.   Preliminary data from oligopeptide mapping
suggests that this protein has sequences common to the 47,000
mol. wt. nucleoprotein, thus it seems very likely that the 42,000
mol. wt. band represents a specific degradation product of the
nucleoprotein.   The 42,000 protein is found in neither purified
virions nor in vitro translation products but it is detected by
antiserum on electroblots.

The effect of tunicamycin, an inhibitor of N-linkage
glycosylation, on TGEV polypeptide synthesis is seen in Fig. 8.
There is a clear inhibition of envelope glycoprotein synthesis and
the accumulation of a band at 26,000 mol. wt., corresponding in
size to a major product from the in vitro translation and to a
minor component of the purified virion.   This non-glycosylated
precursor is detected with antibody after electroblotting but to
date the accumulation of isotopically labelled or antigenically
reactive precursor to the peplomer protein in the presence of
tunicamycin has not been demonstrated.

Phosphopolypeptide synthesis.   Since phosphorylation of the
viral nucleoprotein is likely to be important for its configuration
and the subsequent formation of nucleocapsid, the production of
phosphoproteins in TGEV-infected APT/2 and LLC-PK1 cells was
investigated.   Uninfected and infected cells were incubated with
[^{32}P]-orthophosphate between 6-12h after infection and were then
solubilised in SDS/mercaptoethanol and electrophoresed as described
above.   A representative autoradiograph is shown in Fig. 9 and
illustrates several features.   There was a low level of
phosphorylation in uninfected APT/2 cells whereas there were
several host proteins phosphorylated in uninfected LLC-PK1.   The
47,000 mol. wt. nucleoprotein was well labelled in both types of
infected cell but there were greater amounts of the 42,000 mol. wt.
product, also phosphorylated, in LLC-PK1 than in APT/2.   There
appeared to be phosphorylation of the 28-30,000 mol. wt. envelope
proteins in the LLC-PK1 cells.   Preliminary data from oligopeptide
analyses suggest that the phosphopeptide patterns of the 47,000
mol. wt. molecules from infected APT/2 and LLC are very similar,
if not identical, and that the phosphopeptides of the 42,000
mol. wt. species are contained in the 47,000 mol. wt. protein.
The phosphopeptides of the 28-30,000 mol. wt. group in the LLC-PK1
cultures, on the other hand, do not appear to be common to those
of 47,000 mol. wt. band, suggesting that the ^{32}P counts in the ·lower
area of the gel are not derived from degradation of the nucleoprotein.

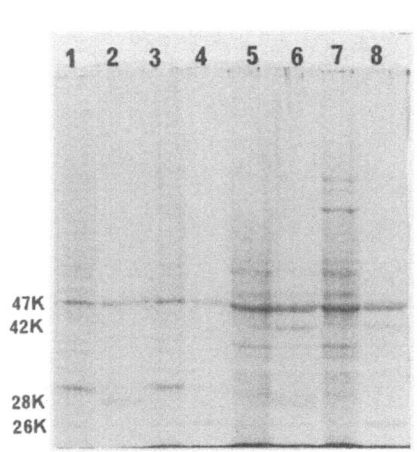

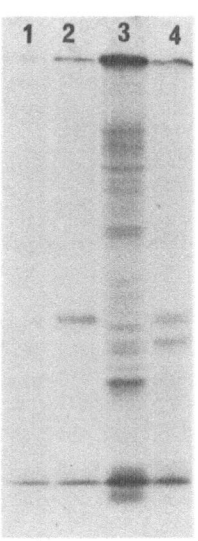

Fig. 8. The effect of tunicamycin on TGEV polypeptide synthesis. Uninfected (tracks 1 & 3) and infected (tracks 2 & 4) APT/2 cells and uninfected (tracks 5 & 7) and infected (tracks 6 & 8) LLC-PK1 cells were incubated in the absence (1, 2, 5, 6 & 7) or presence (3, 4, 7 & 8) of 1µg tunicamycin/ml and labelled with [^{35}S]-methione between 4-8h after infection.

Fig. 9. Intracellular phosphoproteins. Uninfected (tracks 1 & 3) and TGEV-infected (tracks 2 & 4) APT/2 and LLC-PK1 cells (respectively) were labelled with [^{32}P]-orthophosphate 6-12h after infection.

To establish whether the enhanced degradation of nucleoprotein to the lower molecular species in LLC-PK1 cells might account for their inability to produce virus, a time course of ^{32}P incorporation was carried out. Fig. 10 shows an autoradiograph of samples from 4h exposures to ^{32}P during 1-16h after infection and a pulse-chase sample labelled 4-8h then chased 8-12h after infection. The greater extent of phosphorylation was again apparent in the LLC-PK1 cell as was the faster synthesis of phosphorylated 47,000 and 42,000 mol. wt. species. The pulse-chase lanes show, however, that phosphonucleoprotein is lost from both cell types between 8-12h after infection. Whether this represents degradation of the protein concomitant with synthesis of new molecules, irreversible dephosphorylation or packaging and export out of the cell is not clear and is presently being investigated.

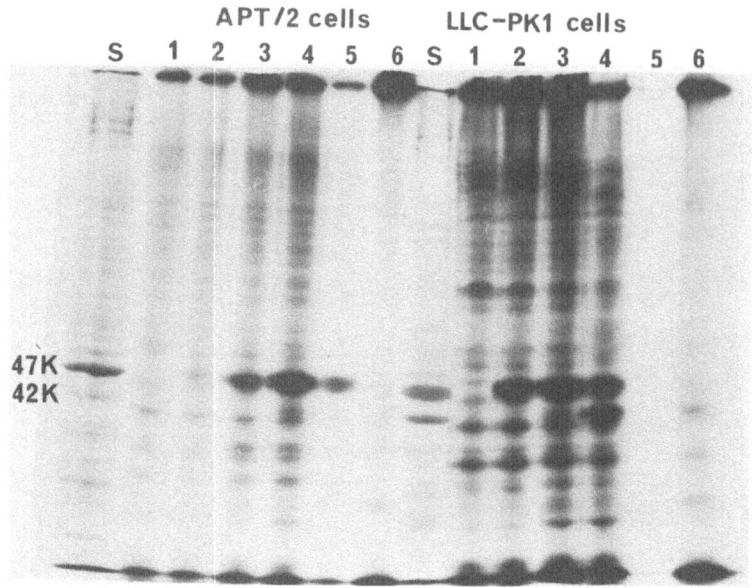

Fig. 10.   Rate of phosphoprotein synthesis. TGEV-infected cells
            were labelled with [³²P]-orthophosphate 1-4h after
            infection (track 2), 4-8h (track 3), 8-12h (track 4) and
            12-16h (track 5). Track 1 shows uninfected cells
            labelled 1-4h. The samples in track 6 were from
            infected cells labelled with [³²P]-orthophosphate 4-8h
            after infection and then incubated in fresh unlabelled
            medium between 8-12h after infection. The tracks
            marked 'S' contain samples from [³⁵S]-methionine
            labelled, infected cells for comparison.

DISCUSSION

     There are several points in the replication cycle of a
coronavirus that might be blocked in a non-permissive cell, from
viropexis and entry to maturation and release.   It is quite clear
from the experiments reported that the virus is capable of
initiating infection in LLC-PK1 cells as readily as in APT/2 cells,
giving the same number of infectious centres as measured by plaques
and fluorescent foci.   Having entered the LLC-PK1 cell, the virus
undergoes a phase of genomic RNA replication and formation of
subgenomic RNA species indistinguishable from that of infected
APT/2 cells as judged by amount, molecular weight and ability to
be translated in vitro.   That the messengers are equally functional
in the cell is indicated by the synthesis of viral antigens,
detected by immunofluorescence and radioimmune staining of
electroblots, and the precursors of the structural polypeptides.
The subsequent processing of these polypeptides by glycosylation

and phosphorylation appears to proceed as efficiently in the LLC–PK1 as in the APT/2 cell and cells show marked cytopathic changes at about the same time in both cultures.   Tunicamycin, an inhibitor of N–linked glycosylation, was shown to block the formation of both the envelope and peplomer glycopolypeptides in the two cell types.   The first reports of the effect of tunicamycin on coronaviruses had indicated that the polypeptide of mouse hepatitis virus envelope protein contained no N–linked carbohydrate[10,11,12] but was processed in the Golgi apparatus with O–linked glycosylation.   That this was not characteristic of coronaviruses generally was shown with infectious bronchitis virus[13] and the present study confirms the peculiarity of mouse hepatitis virus.

All the steps in the formation of the structural elements required for virion production appear, therefore, to be proceeding normally.   And yet, there are few or no demonstrable virus particles released from the cell even after freezing and thawing. This implies therefore that a maturation step in the infected LLC–PK1 cell is the location of the defect.

It is possible that the mechanism for assembling virus particles at the membrane of the endoplasmic reticulum is faulty in LLC–PK1 cells even though the organelle clearly functions adequately to support the cell.   Further studies involving electron microscopy of infected cells might throw light on this. Another possibility, and one that we are presently investigating, is that the maturation block resides in the nucleoprotein phosphorylation step.

Coronaviruses have been shown to contain a protein kinase capable of phosphorylating their nucleoprotein[14].   Thus, they would seem to have no requirement for a cellular protein kinase. Our data suggest, however, that while APT/2 cells appear to have little endogenous protein phosphorylation, LLC–PK1 cultures have an active protein kinase.   This may reflect the transformed state of the LLC–PK1 cell line; many transformed cells have been shown to carry oncornaviruses which code for an active protein kinase. Whereas the coronavirus protein kinase is active on serine residues[14,15] the oncornavirus enzyme has been shown to phosphorylate tyrosine[16].   We are presently studying the phospho-amino acids isolated from TGEV nucleoprotein produced in APT/2 and LLC–PK1 cells to determine whether there are differences.   It is not inconceivable that the presence of a phosphotyrosine residue at a site in the nucleoprotein essential for its secondary or tertiary structure might so alter the conformation of the molecule to make it unable to form nucleocapsids and so start the virus maturation process.   Different strains of TGEV might have small differences in the primary amino acid sequence of their nucleo-protein such that phosphorylation at sites other than serine could determine their ability to grow in transformed cell lines.

ACKNOWLEDGEMENTS

    We thank Miss Fiona Stewart for her technical assistance,
Mr. P.D. Luther for providing the cell cultures and
Dr. D.J. Reynolds for porcine and feline antisera to TGEV.

REFERENCES

1.   R.N. Hull, W.R. Cherry, and G.W. Weaver, The origin and
        characteristics of a pig kidney cell strain, LLC-PK1,
        In Vitro 12:670 (1976).
2.   D.H. Pocock, and D.J. Garwes, The influence of pH on the growth
        and stability of transmissible gastroenteritis virus
        in vitro, Arch. Virol. 49:239 (1975).
3.   D.J. Garwes, and D.H. Pocock, The polypeptide structure of
        transmissible gastroenteritis virus, J. gen. Virol. 29:25
        (1975).
4.   U.K. Laemmli, Cleavage of structural proteins during the
        assembly of the head of bacteriophage T4, Nature 29:680
        (1970).
5.   D.J. Garwes, D.H. Pocock, and T.M. Wijaszka, Identification of
        heat-dissociable RNA complexes in two porcine coronaviruses,
        Nature 257:508 (1975).
6.   T. Maniatis, E.F. Fritsch, and J. Sambrook, in· "Molecular
        Cloning: a laboratory manual," Cold Spring Harbor
        Laboratory (1982).
7.   H. Aviv, and P. Leder, Purification of biologically active
        globin messenger RNA by chromatography on oligothymidylic
        acid-cellulose, Proc. Nat. Acad. Sci. USA 69:1408 (1972).
8.   R.A. Lamb, P.R. Etkind, and P.W. Choppin, Evidence for a
        ninth influenza viral polypeptide, Virology 91:60 (1978).
9.   D.E. Dennis, and D.A. Brian, Coronavirus cell-associated
        RNA-dependent RNA polymerase, in "Biochemistry and Biology
        of Coronaviruses," V. ter Meulen, S. Siddell, and H. Wege,
        eds., Plenum Press, New York (1981).
10. K.V. Holmes, E.W. Doller, and L.S. Sturman, Tunicamycin
        resistant glycosylation of a coronavirus glycoprotein:
        demonstration of a novel type of viral glycoprotein,
        Virology 115:334 (1981).
11. H. Niemann, and H.-D. Klenk, Coronavirus glycoprotein E1, a
        new type of viral glycoprotein, J. Mol. Biol. 153:993
        (1981).
12. P.J.M. Rottier, M.C. Horzinek, and B.A.M. van der Zeijst,
        Viral protein synthesis in mouse hepatitis virus strain
        A59-infected cells: effect of tunicamycin, J. Virol.
        40:350 (1981).

13. D.F. Stern, and B.M. Sefton, Coronavirus proteins: structure and function of the oligosaccharides of the avian infectious bronchitis virus glycoproteins, J. Virol. 44:804 (1982).
14. S.G. Siddell, A. Barthel, and V. ter Meulen, Coronavirus JHM: a virion associated protein kinase, J. gen. Virol. 52:235 (1981).
15. S.A. Stohlman, and M.M.C. Lai, Phosphoproteins of murine hepatitis viruses, J. Virol. 32:672 (1979).
16. T. Hunter, and B.M. Sefton, Protein kinases and viral transformation, in "Molecular action of toxins and viruses." Cohen and van Heyningen, eds., Elsevier Medical Press, Amsterdam (1982).

STRUCTURAL CHARACTERIZATION OF IBV GLYCOPROTEINS

David Cavanagh

Houghton Poultry Research Station
Houghton, Huntingdon
Cambs. PE17 2DA.   U.K.

INTRODUCTION

Avian infectious bronchitis virus (IBV) causes economically important disease in chickens, affecting both respiratory and non-respiratory tissues. Like other coronaviruses IBV virions contain three virus-coded protein structures, the spike (S; surface projection, peplomer), nucleocapsid (N) and matrix (M) proteins[1]. The polypeptides of M and N proteins have been identified. The M protein comprises a polypeptide of mol.wt. 23 000 (23K) which is glycosylated to different extents, the major glycopolypeptide being about 30K[2,3,4]. A polypeptide of about 50K forms the N protein[5]. However, although many papers have been published on the composition of IBV, there has been a distinct lack of agreement on the number and mol.wt. of the polypeptides which form the spikes (for references see[1,6].

Our initial work indicated that S comprised two glycopoly-peptides S1 (90K) and S2 (84K)[7]. As will be shown, part of the confusion is because of the variable presence in virus preparations of contaminating host polypeptides which are sometimes present in quantities greater than the spike polypeptides. Also, SDS-poly-acrylamide gel electrophoresis (SDS-PAGE) has shown that one of the S polypeptides (S2) stains poorly with Coomassie Brilliant Blue and has a tendency to aggregate.

Stern & Sefton[8] have recently shown, using tryptic peptide analysis, that S1 and S2 are derived from a common precursor molecule, showing that both S1 and S2 are virus-coded polypeptides. We show that purified S, from both radiolabelled and non-labelled virus, comprises both S1 and S2 and report on how these two glyco-

polypeptides associate with each other to form S. In addition we have
examined the nature of the oligosaccharides of S1, S2 and M.

METHODS

    Radiolabelled and non-labelled IBV, strains M41 and D41, was pre-
pared and analysed by SDS-polyacrylamide gel electrophoresis (SDS-
PAGE) as described by Cavanagh[4,6,7]. The preparation of IBV S protein has been described[6]. Briefly, IBV-Mr1 was dissociated with Non-
idet P40 (NP40) and centrifuged at 85B g_{av} for 16h at 4°C in a 10-55%
(w/w) sucrose gradient in NET buffer (100 mM NaCl, 1 mM EDTA, 10 mM
tris-HCl, pH 7.4) containing 0.1% NP40 and 1M NaCl or KCl until S had
travelled about one third of the length of the tube. For the estimation of the mol. wt. of S the protein was used straight from preparative gradient. 25 ul containing S protein was diluted with 75 ul of
NET buffer containing 0.1% NP40 and 5 ug of bovine catalase. This was
layered on top of a 6 ml 5/20% (w/v) sucrose gradient in NET buffer
containing 0.1% NP40 and centrifuged in a 3 x 6.5 ml MSE swing-out
rotor at 4°C for 16h at 70K g_{av}. Fractions of 100 ul were collected
and the constituent polypeptides detected by SDS-PAGE. The gels were
stained with Coomassie Brilliant Blue, destained, and the S polypeptides visualised by silver staining[9]. Pre-staining with Coomassie
Brilliant Blue enhanced the sensitivity of the silver stain. The mol.
wt. of S was estimated using the formulae of Martin & Ames[10].

    For studies with urea and SDS volumes of 100 or 200 ul of 35_S-
methionine-labelled IBV-M41 in NET buffer containing sucrose (about
40% w/w) and 50 ug/ml of BSA were mixed with an equal volume of urea,
in 5 mM tris-acetate pH 7.4 contining 50 ug/ml of BSA, or SDS, in NET
buffer without BSA, at twice the desired final concentration. Control
virus was mixed with buffer only. After 1h at 37°C (urea) or 30 min.
at 25°C (SDS) the suspensions were diluted to 750 ul with NET buffer
containing 50 ug/ml of BSA and loaded into 1 ml tubes and centrifuged
in an MSE 3 x 6.5 ml swing-out rotor with the appropriate adaptor at
80K g for 2 h at 25°C. Pellets were recovered using 2% SDS and 2%
2-mercaptoethanol. For DTT treatment ^{35}S-methionine-labelled virus
was incubated at 37°C for 1 h with an equal volume of buffer containing DTT at twice the desired final concentration. The virus was then
sedimented to equilibrium in 25-55% (w/w) sucrose gradient at 30K g_{av}
for 16 h at 4°C.

    Endo- and exoglycosidases were used as described by Cavanagh[4]
and in the legend to Fig. 1.

RESULTS

Glycosylation of IBV polypeptides

    Stern et al.[2] have shown theat several polypeptides of IBV-
Beaudette, analogous to polypeptides of 34K, 30K/28K, 26K and 23K

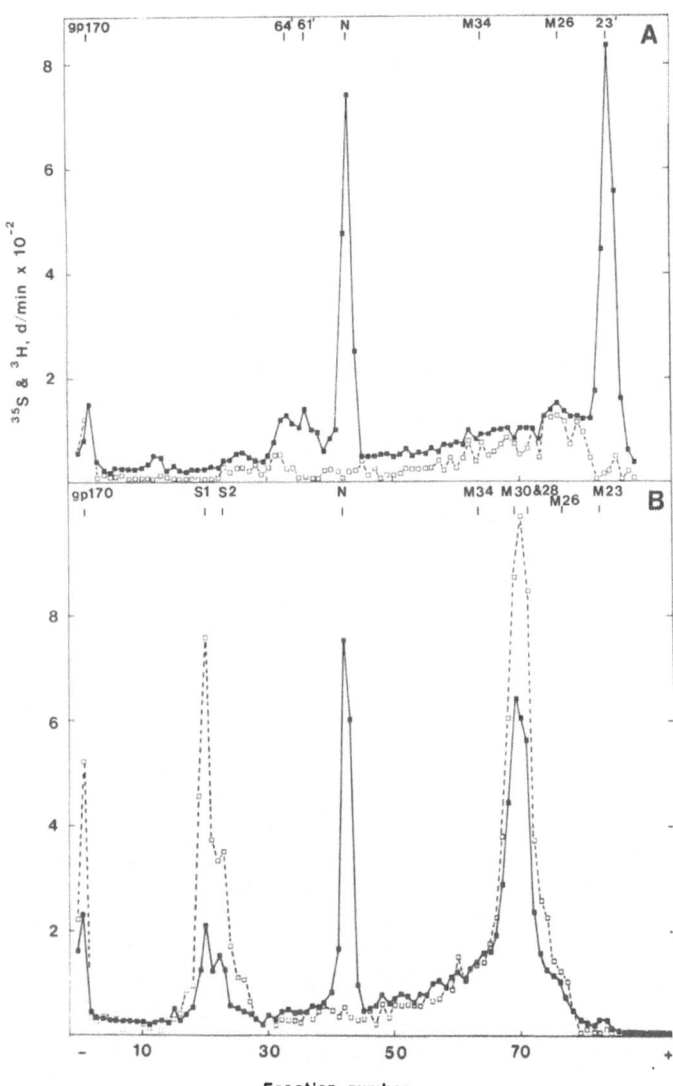

Fig. 1. SDS-PAGE of IBV-M41 labelled with ^{35}S-methionine (■) and ^{3}H-mannose (□) after incubation at 37°C for 40h at pH 6.0 with (A) a mixture of 25 mU/ml endoglycosidase H, 50 mU/ml endoglycosidase D, 50 mU/ml neuraminidase, 100 mU/ml b-N-acetylglucosaminidase and 100 mU/ml b-galactosidase, and (B) no enzyme. Both samples contained 1mM phenylmethylsulphonyl fluoride. 64', 61' and 23' refer to the mol. wt. (x10[-3]) of polypeptides which are the products of hydrolysis by endoglycosidase H.

(M34 to M23) in our studies with IBV-M41, all give the same peptide maps. With the exception of M23, which is normally present in very small amounts, the M polypeptides of IBV were glycosylated, as shown by the incorporation of 3H-mannose (Fig. 1) and 3H-glucosamine. Analysis in 5 polyacrylamide gels of IBV-D41 labelled with 15 3H-labelled amino acids and ^{35}S-methionine showed that the 3H/^{35}S d/min (disintegrations per min) ratios for M23, M26, M28, M30 and M34 were 1.9, 1.9, 1.8, 1.9 and 1.9 respectively. Similar analysis of IBV-D41 labelled with 3H-glucosamine and ^{35}S-methionine gave 3H/^{35}S d/min ratios for M23, M26, M28, M30 and M34 of 1.2, 2.2, 3.2, 4.1 and 6.3 respectively. These data support the view of Stern et al.[2] that M23-M34 have the same polypeptide moiety but differ in their degree of glycosylation, this increasing with increasing mol.wt.

In order to determine whether the oligosaccharides of the S1, S2 and M polypeptides were N- or O-glycosidically linked, whether they were of the high mannose or complex type, and the proportion of the glycopolypeptide mol.wt. accounted for by the oligosaccharides, radio-labelled IBV-M41 was treated with endoglycosidase-H and -D. These enzymes remove high mannose and complex oligosaccharides respectively which are N-glycosidically linked to polypeptides.[11-13] The specificity of endoglycosidase H is such that if a polypeptide had only high-mannose oligosaccharides, endoglycosidase H would be expected to yield a polypeptide with some residual N-acetylgluco-samine but no mannose. Such polypeptides were generated from S1, S2, M30 and M28. Endoglycosidase H removed oligosaccharides from both S1 and S2 of virus doubly labelled with ^{35}S-methionine and 3H-mannose (Fig. 1) or 3H-glucosamine. The products of hydrolysis were generally heterogenous and their mol.wt. varied among experiments. Mean mol.wt. values of 71K + 7K and 64K + 3K were obtained from 8 experiments. The smallest products, with mol.wt. of 64K and 61K, were obtained in the experiment shown in Fig. 1. Enzyme concen-trations of up to 125 mU/ml did not decrease the size of S1 and S2 to less than in Fig. 1. Endoglycosidase D had no detectable effect on the S polypeptides by itself or with the exoglycosidases neuraminase, b-galactosidase and N-acetylglucosaminidase[13] without or with (Fig. 1.) endoglycosidase H. These results indicate that the oligosaccharides of S1 and S2 are N-glycosidically linked and are probably of the high-mannose type.

In all experiments the effect of endoglycosidase H on the M glycopolypeptides of IBV-M41 was the same: most of M30 and M28 were converted to a polypeptide of 23K with no mannose (Fig. 1.) and little glucosamine. Endoglycosidase D had no detectable effect on any of the M polypeptides. These results indicate that the oligo-saccharides of M30 and M28 are N-glycosidically linked, high mannose side chains, and that the oligosaccharides of M34 and M26 are diff-erent from those of M30 and M28. This is in contrast to MHV and

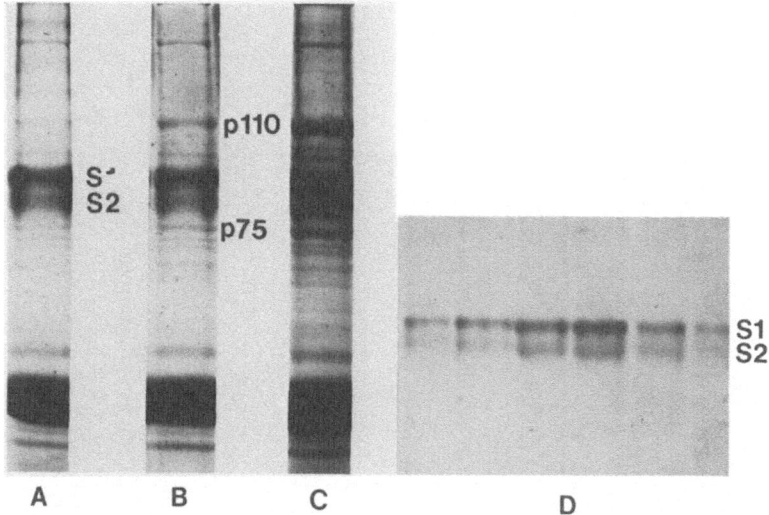

Fig. 2. SDS-PAGE of (a,b,c) 3 non-labelled preparations of IBV-M41;
(d) non-labelled purified S polypeptides. IBV-M41 (2-4 mg of protein) was dissociated with 2% NP40 in 1M KCl in NET and sedimented in
a 10-55% (w/w) sucrose gradient containing 0.1% NP40 and 1M KCl in
NET. Only the S-containing fractions are shown in (d). Gels were
stained with Coomassie Brilliant Blue. Only the half of the 10%
acrylamide gel is shown.

bovine coronavirus L9 in which the matrix glycopolypeptide has
exclusively O-linked oligosaccharides and lacks mannose[14]. The
results above also indicate that the polypeptide moieties of S1 and
S2 are about 60K, and that of M 23K.

Polypeptide of IBV Spikes

Analysis of non-labelled IBV-M41 polypeptides by SDS-PAGE and
staining showed that all preparations contained S1 and S2, although
S2 was less readily detectable than S1 unless the gel was heavily
over-loaded with respect to N (Fig. 2A-C). In 75% of preparations
S1 was the major polypeptide of > 54K, while in the remainder polypeptides of 110K (p110) and 75K (p75) were present in similar amounts
to S1. In some preparations p110 and 75 were barely detectable. S
prepared from non-labelled virus contained S1 and S2 but no other
high mol.wt. polypeptides (Fig. 2D). The S of Fig. 2D was derived
from a virus preparation which had a greater than usual amount of
p110 and p75. However, these polypeptides remained near the top of
the gradient, away from the S-containing fractions.

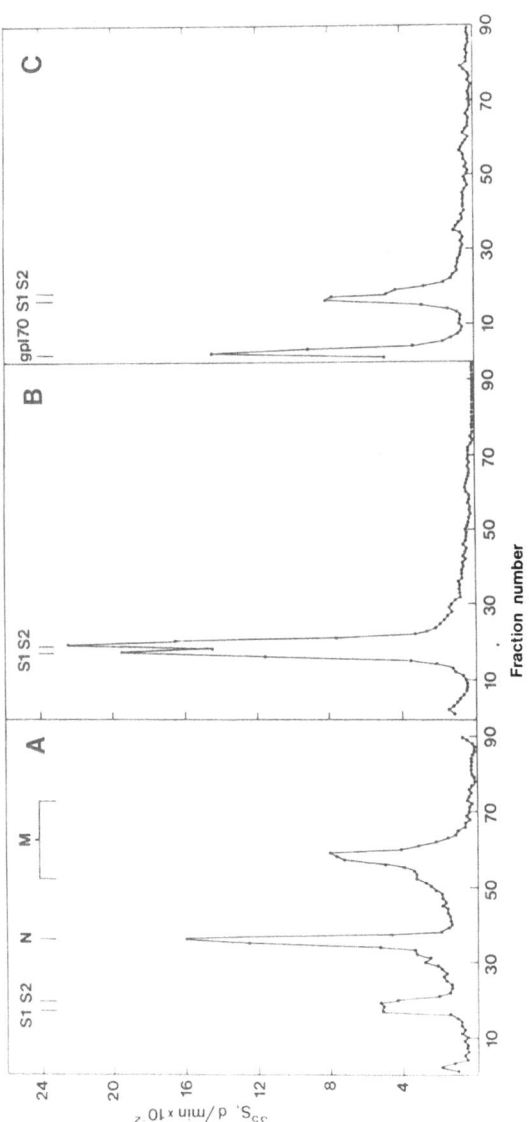

Fig. 3.   SDS-PAGE of ^{35}S-methionine-labelled IBV-M41 polypeptides. Virus (a) was
dissociated with 1% NP40 or 5% octyglucoside (OG) and sedimented in
10–55% (w/w) sucrose gradients containing 0.1% NP40 or 1% OG respectively.
Three peaks of radio-label were obtained: (b) and (c) show the polypeptides
present in the middle peak of the (b) NP40– and (c) OG-containing gradients
respectively.

S1 and S2 were clearly present in the majority of radiolabelled IBV-M41 preparations (Fig. 6) and in the S isolated from
them (Fig. 3). As can be seen in Fig. 3D, S2, and to a lesser extent
S1, has a tendency to form aggregates with an apparent mol.wt. of
170K. We have observed that with IBV-Beaudette and other strains
the aggregation of S2 is often greater than with IBV-M41. Dissociation of virus at 100°C did not consistently prevent this aggregation.

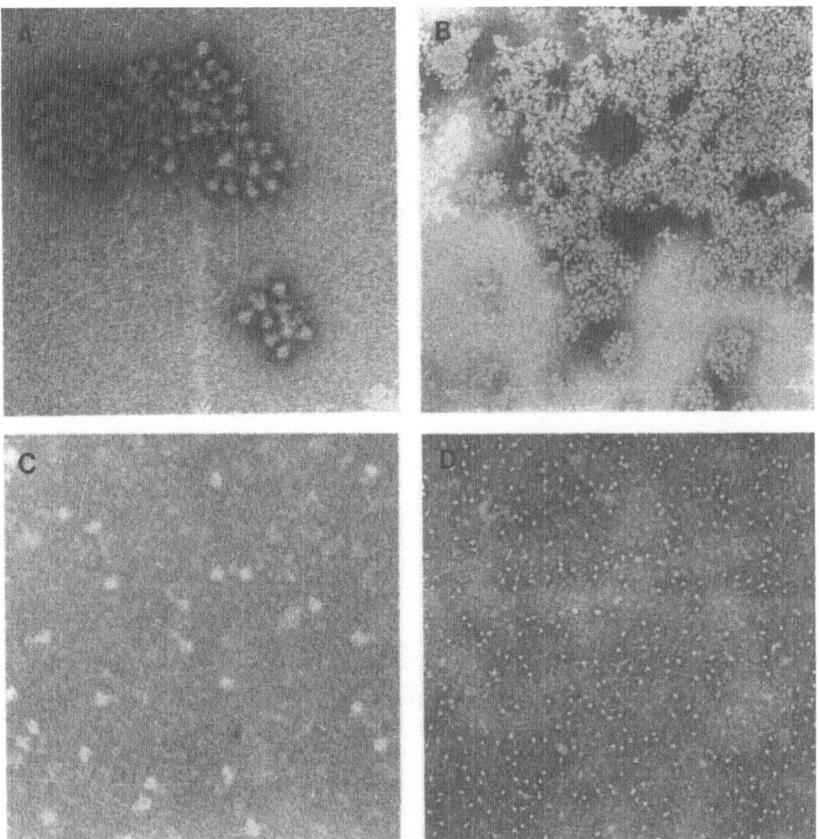

Fig. 4. Electron microscopy of purified spikes from IBV-M41. Spikes
were separated from M and N protein by disruption of the virus with
2% NP40 and sedimentation in a 10-55% (w/w) sucrose gradient containing 0.1% NP40 and 1M NaCl. The spike containing fractions of one
preparation were dialysed against water containing 0.1% NP40 lyophilized and resuspended to give a 10-fold concentration (a,b). Another
preparation of spikes was examined without prior dialysis or lyophilization (c,d). Magnification (a,c) x 178000, (b,d) x 55000.

SDS-PAGE of IBV-M41 radiolabelled with a mixture of 15 3H-labelled
amino acids and ^{35}S-methionine indicated that S contains S1 and S2 in a
1:1 molar ratio[6]. Radioimmunprecipitation with an anti-S monoclonal
antibody precipitated equal amounts of S1 and S2 after dissociation
of virus with NP40, a further indication that S1 and S2 are associated with each other (Mockett, A.P.A., Cavanagh, D. and Brown T.D.K.
unpublished observation).

Molecular weight of S protein

The mol.wt. of S was estimated by co-sedimenting S with catalase
in 5-20% (w/v) sucrose gradients containing NP40. Electron microscopy of non-labelled S which had been concentrated by dialysis and
lyophilization showed that S had formed rosettes by aggregation at
their narrow hydrophobic ends, and also larger aggregates by their
bulbous hydrophilic ends (Fig. 4A,B). Such aggregates were obviously
unsuitable for mol.wt. estimations. However, electron microscopy
showed that S which had been neither dialysed nor concentrated had
not aggregated (Fig. 4C, D) Consequently, S was used direct from
preparative sucrose gradients. S sedimented in one band ahead
of catalase (mol.wt. 250K) (Fig. 5) . A mol.wt. estimate for S
of 354K $\pm$ 17K was obtained from three experiments. Ziemiecki &
Garoff[15] have shown that the spikes of Semliki Forest virus, mol.wt.

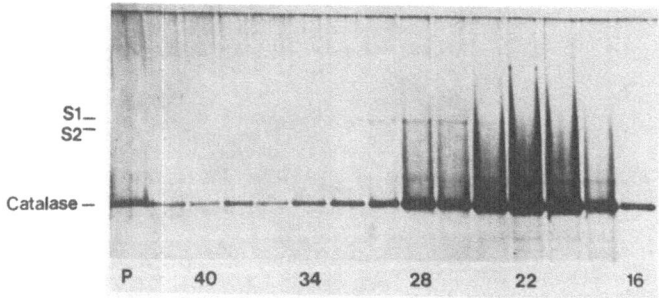

Fraction no.

Fig. 5. Mol.wt. estimation of S from IBV-M41. Spikes were obtained
as described for Fig. 5. and were not dialysed or lyophilized. S was
co-sedimented with 5 ug of catalase in a 5-20% (w/v) sucrose gradient
containing 0.1% NP40. Fractions of 100 ul were collected and 40 ul
of alternate fractions analysed by SDS-PAGE followed by silver staining. Only the top part of the gel is shown. The right hand side of
the gel corresponds to the upper part of the sucrose gradient.
Pelleted material was resuspended in 140 ul of 2% SDS and 2% 2-mer-
captoethanol and 40 ul (P) analysed in the gel.

111K, bound 0.21 mg of non-ionic detergent per 1.0 mg of protein.
IBV S protein undoubtedly bound NP40 which would have led to an over-
estimate of the mol.wt. of S. The formulae used to calculate the
mol.wt. of S apply most accurately to proteins which are essentially
spherical molecules. The elongated shape of S would have reduced
the sedimentation rate compared with a spheric molecule and would
have resulted in an underestimate of the mol.wt.[16]. While these
errors have not been quantified we know that the mol.wt. of S has to
be multiples of 174K, since S comprises equimolar amounts of S1 and
S2 [6]. Thus the mol.wt. estimate for S from sucrose gradient analysis
of 354K $\pm$ 17K indicates strongly that S is a tetramer. Experiments
with radiolabelled S which had been concentrated gave a major peak
equivalent to that obtained with non-labelled S. In addition some
S1 and S2 was present near the top of the gradient. In some preparations the amount of material in this peak was the same as in the
354K peak, indicating extensive breakdown of some spikes.

Nature of association of S1 and S2.

     After incubation of IBV-M41 at 37°C with 2M urea and pelleting
of the virus, most of S1 had been removed from the virus (Fig. 6).
Analysis of the supernatant by electrophoresis in tube gels showed
that S1 was intact and was the predominant polypeptide present. The
amount of S2, N and M present in the supernatants was very similar
to that from the control virus. Essentially the same result was
achieved with 6M urea.

     Similar results were obtained with SDS (Fig. 7) as had been
obtained with urea. The concentration of SDS that caused selective
removal of S1 varied among experiments and was critical within each
experiment. Thus in the experiment illustrated in Fig. 7. 0.01%
SDS removed most of S1 (Fig. 7B), 0.015% removed even more (Fig. 7C)
while 0.022% SDS disrupted more than 50% of the virus particles.
Inspection of Fig. 7, confirmed by quantitative analysis of the polypeptides in the supernatants by tube gel SDS-PAGE, shows that 0.010%
SDS caused the release of some N but not M polypeptide while even
more N, but not M, was released by 0.015%.

     These results indicate that S2 is more strongly associated with
the virus membrane than S1. Indeed S1, may not be in contact with
the membrane.

     That S1 can be separated from S2 by urea or SDS alone indicates
that disulphide bonds are not responsible for the association of S1
and S2. This was emphasized by the observations that IBV-M41 spikes
were dissociated into their S1 and S2 components just as readily by
SDS alone as by SDS with 2-mercaptoethanol at 100°C (Fig. 8) or 25°C.
This also indicates that the two molecules of S1 per spike are not
linked by disulphide bonds, and likewise for S2. After incubation
of ^{35}S-methionine labelled IBV-M41 at 37°C for 1h with 100 mM

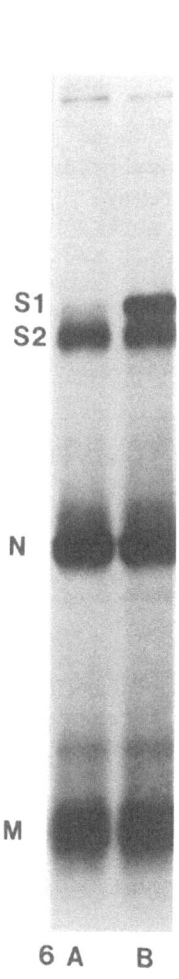

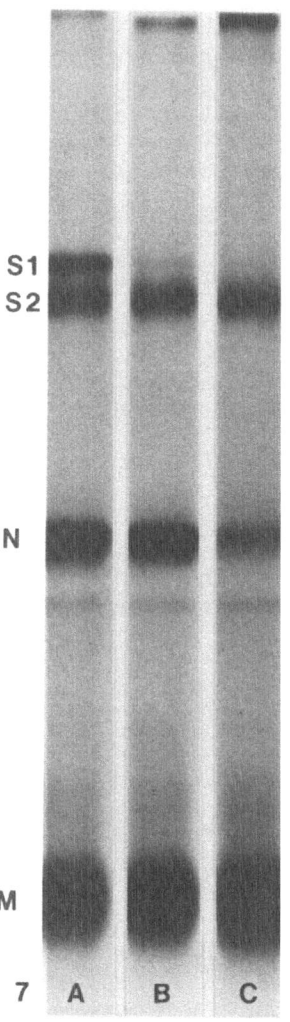

Fig. 6. Selective release of S1
by urea. ^{35}S-methionine-label-
led IBV-M41 was incubated with
or without (control) 2M urea for
1h at 37°C. The virus was pelleted and then analysed by SDS-
PAGE in a slab gel and radio-
label detected by fluorography:
(a) control, (b) urea-treated
virus.

Fig. 7. Selective release of S1
by SDS. ^{35}S-methionine-labelled
IBV-M41 was held at 25° for 30 min.
with or without (control) SDS.
The virus was pelleted and analysed
as described in Fig. 6: (a) control;
(b,c) virus after treatment with
(b) 0.010% SDS and (c) 0.015% SDS.

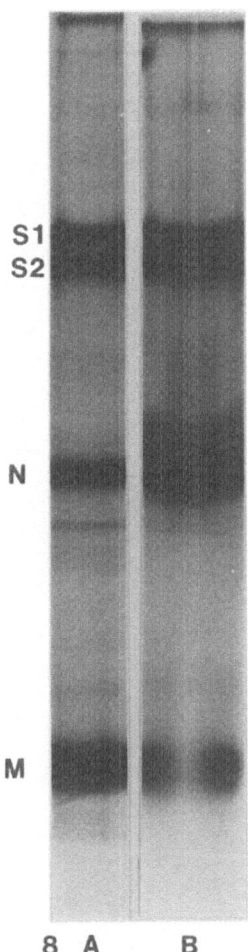

Fig. 8. ^{35}S-methionine-labelled IBV-M41 was heated at 100°C for
1 min with (a) 2% SDS and 2% 2-mercaptoethanol or (b) 2% SDS alone
and then analysed as in Fig. 6.

dithiothreitol (DTT) the buoyant density of the virus in sucrose
gradients was decreased from 1.18 g/ml to 1.16 g/ml. However,
SDS-PAGE showed that no polypeptides had been removed. After
incubation at 37°C for 1h of purified non-labelled spikes with 1 M
DTT electron microscopy showed that the characteristic shape of the
spikes had gone and also that they had aggregated much more than in
the control. These results suggest that intrapeptide disulphide
bonds do occur in S1 or S2 or both.

CONCLUSIONS

Results obtained with glycosidases have shown that S1, S2 and
M30 and M28 of IBV have high mannose, N-linked oligosaccharides.
The mol.wt. of the polypeptide moiety of the IBV M glycopolypeptide
is very similar (23K) to that of murine hepatitis virus (MHV)[1] but
the degree of glycosylation is much greater. This is probably
related to the fact that the oligosaccharides of the M protein of
MHV are of a different type and are O-linked to the M polypeptide[14].
Our results indicate that IBV S is an oligomeric protein
comprising two molecules of each of the glycopolypeptides S1 and S2,
to give a mol.wt. of approximately 350K. Under certain conditions[7]
urea can remove both S1 and S2 from the virion, without disrupting
the membrane or releasing M, indicating that S is a peripheral protein. Our more recent findings indicate that S2 anchors S to the
membrane while S1 has little or no contact with the membrane.
The association of S1 and S2 is not a strong one and intrapeptide,
but not interpeptide, disulphide bonds exist in S. Fig. 9. is a
simplistic representation of IBV S protein. This "ice cream cone"
model is appropriate in that just as it is easy to lose ice cream
from a cone while still holding the cone, so S1 is easily displaced
from S2 while S2 remains in the membrane.

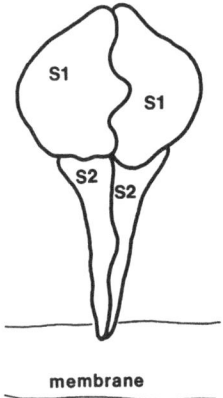

Fig. 9. A model for IBV S protein.

REFERENCES

1. S. G. Siddell, H. Wege and V. Ter Meulen. The structure and replication of coronaviruses. Curr. Top. Microbiol. Immunol. 99: 131 (1982).
2. D. F. Stern and B. M. Sefton. Structural analysis of virion proteins of the avian coronavirus infectious bronchitis virus. J. Virol. 42: 208 (1982).
3. D. F. Stern and B. M. Sefton. Coronavirus proteins : structure and function of the oligosaccharides of the avian infectious bronchitis virus glycoproteins. J. Virol. 44: 804 (1982).
4. D. Cavanagh. Coronavirus IBV glycopolypeptides : size of their polypeptide moieties and nature of their oligosaccharides. J. Gen. Virol. 64: 1187 (1983).
5. M. R. Macnaughton, M. H. Madge, H. A. Davies and R. R. Dourmashkin. Polypeptides of the surface projections and the ribonucleoprotein of avian infectious bronchitis virus. J. Virol. 24: 821 (1977).
6. D. Cavanagh. Coronavirus IBV : further evidence that the surface projections are associated with two glycopolypeptides. J. Gen. Virol. 64: in press (1983).
7. D. Cavanagh. Structural polypeptides of Coronavirus IBV. J. Gen. Virol. 53: 93 (1981).
8. D. F. Stern and B. M. Sefton. Coronavirus proteins : biogenesis of avian infectious bronchitis virus virion proteins. J. Virol. 44: 794 (1982).
9. J. Morrissey. Silver stain for proteins in polyacrylamide gels. A modified procedure with enhanced uniform sensitivity. Anal. Biochem. 117: 307 (1981)
10. R. G. Martin and B. N. Ames. A method for determining the sedimentation behavior of enzymes : application to protein mixtures. J. Biol. Chem. 236: 1372 (1961).
11. A. L. Tarentino and F. Maley. Purification and properties of an endo-B-N-acetylglucosaminidase from Streptomyces griseus. J. Biol. Chem. 249: 811 (1974).
12. A. L. Tarentino, F. H. Plummer and F. Maley. The release of intact oligosaccharides from specific glycoproteins by endo-B-N-acetylglucosaminidase H. J. Biol. Chem. 249: 818 (1974).
13. N. Koide and T. Muramatsu. Endo-B-N-acetylglucosaminidase acting on carbohydrate moieties of glycoproteins. J. Biol. Chem. 249: 4897 (1974).
14. H. Niemann and H-D. Klenk. Coronavirus glycoprotein E1, a new type of viral glycoprotein. J. Mol. Biol. 153: 993 (1981).
15. A. Ziemiecki and H. Garoff. Subunit composition of the membrane glycoprotein complex of Semliki Forest virus. J. Mol. Biol. 122: 259 (1978).

16. R. Eason and A. M. Campbell. Analytical centrifugation, in
     "Centrifugal Separation in Molecular Biology and Cell
     Biology" G. D. Birnie and D. Rickwood, eds., Butterworths,
     London. (1978).

USE OF MONOCLONAL ANTIBODIES TO ASSESS ANTIGENIC RELATIONSHIPS

OF AVIAN INFECTIOUS BRONCHITIS VIRUS SEROTYPES IN THE UNITED STATES

D. B. Snyder and W. W. Marquardt

Virginia-Maryland Regional College
  of Veterinary Medicine
University of Maryland
College Park, Maryland 20742

Avian infectious bronchitis virus (IBV), the etiology of a highly infectious and contagious respiratory disease of young chickens, has been under scrutiny for about 50 years. Since the early reports on the manifestations of the disease, a large number of apparently distinct serotypes of the virus have been identified in the United States. One classification scheme was derived in our laboratory by reciprocal virus neutralization tests carried out in tracheal organ culture[3]. However, there is some controversy as to the absolute number of IBV serotypes in existence and the groups into which they are assigned. Hopkins[2] obtained seven serotypes as determined by neutralization assays with cloned virus in cell culture.

All but a few designated serotypes, and new isolates appear to have a distribution peculiar to a given area. Control of the disease is attempted with modified-live virus vaccine administered to chicken flocks on the basis of prevalence of the disease causing serotype in that area. In the Delaware-Maryland-Virginia (Delmarva) area four serotypes are currently employed as vaccines. They are the Mass-41, Conn, JMK and ARK-99 serotypes.

Infectious bronchitis outbreaks in flocks which have been vaccinated for IBV do occur and there are several apparent causes for this. First, vaccines themselves may cause disease in stressed birds; second, non-indigenous viruses may be imported from other geographic areas of the U.S.; and third, the appearance of antigenic variants in the environment may also cause these breaks.

The poultry industry is interested in preventing disease, whereas virologists wish to know whether new serotypes are evolving. Therefore, both the poultry industry and virologists would like to define the antigenic repertoire of IBV. However, a rapid serotypic identification of IBV is not possible when using currently available isolation and identification procedures. Further, in vitro serotypic differences may have little practical significance in relation to what in vivo protection a serotype may or may not elicit. It is this parameter which is ultimately important, but one that has only in recent years begun to be defined. Results of in vivo cross-challenge studies by us and others, employing IBV serotypes defined as distinct by serum neutralization tests, both support and contradict in vitro results.

We have recently confirmed and extended the use of a tracheal ciliary activity test[5] first reported by Darbyshire[1], for use in the assessment of in vivo protection to various serotypes of IBV. Briefly, two-week-old specific pathogen free chickens are vaccinated with the serotypes of interest. The chickens are allowed to develop an immunity for three weeks and are then challenged with homotypic and heterotypic viruses. After three days, the chickens are sacrificed and their tracheas are removed and tracheal rings are examined for ciliary activity. Tracheal rings from protected birds show strong ciliary movement while those from unprotected birds show cessation of ciliary activity. This criterion may also be used to correlate in vivo resistance with enzyme-linked immunosorbent assay (ELISA) antibody titer to IBV[6].

Experimental results thus far from in vivo cross-challenge studies indicate that putative, distinct antigenic serotypes in vitro may actually be very closely related from a protection standpoint. Further, certain serotypes elicit protection against themselves and other serotypes, but others elicit only one-way protection. Thus, one-way crosses of protection may be obtained, which suggests further variation in antigenic complexity as recognized in vivo. Table 1 shows results of in vivo reciprocal JMK-Conn challenges which exemplify one-way cross protection. This and similar work indicate the need for caution when extrapolating in vitro results for use in vivo, particularly when one is selecting potential vaccine candidates.

To facilitate rapid diagnostic methods, and in order to map the antigenic relationships of IBV at the epitope level, we have prepared batteries of monoclonal antibodies (mcabs) to three of four serotypes prevalent on the Delmarva Peninsula. They are the Mass-41, Conn and JMK serotypes. Two monoclonal antibodies, which are specific for the Mass-41 serotype and one monoclonal antibody apparently specific for the JMK serotype have been obtained.

Table 1. Results of Cross-Protection Tests in Chickens Immunized
          with the JMK and Conn Serotypes of Infectious Bronchitis
          Virus.

| | | Three days post challenge | |
Immunizing Virus	Challenge Virus	Ciliostasis	Virus Recovery
None	Conn	4/4[a]	4/4
Conn	Conn	0/6	0/6
Conn	JMK	4/4	6/6
None	JMK	4/4	4/4
JMK	JMK	0/6	0/6
JMK	Conn	0/6	0/6

[a] Number positive of number tested.

Specificities of the antibodies were determined by indirect ELISA
and fluorescent antibody tests. Monoclonal antibodies, specific
for the Mass-41 serotype, were observed by specific fluorescence
to be reacting in the cytoplasm of Mass-41 virus infected chorio-
allantoic membrane cells, but not in heterotypically infected cells,
or those from normal control membranes. Forty-four other mcabs have
been derived, eight of these have unique ELISA reactivity patterns
against the four serotypes and are under further study. All eight
antibodies have been tested for specificity against the four IBV
serotypes (Mass-41, Conn, JMK, ARK-99), purified Newcastle disease
virus, normal allantoic fluid preparations and actin. Actin was
included in these studies because of previous reports[4], which we
have confirmed, that it will co-purify with egg propagated IBV.
The ELISA reactivity patterns of these mcabs are reported in Table
2.

We conclude that mcabs to IBV will be useful in rapid diagnos-
tics and epidemiological studies as serotype specific antibodies
become available for serotypes present in a given geographic area.
They will also be useful as probes for dissecting the virion
structure and elucidating functional relationships.

At this time we are characterizing derived mcabs to these
three serotypes of IBV in order to map their polypeptide specificities and to study the functions of the viral proteins.

Table 2.   ELISA Reactivity Patterns of Monoclonal Antibodies
           Against Selected Antigen Preparations.

Solid phase antigen

Monoclonal Antibody	Mass-41	Conn	JMK	ARK-99	NDV[a]	NAF[b]	Actin
LAS I	++++[c]	-[d]	-	-	-	-	-
LAS II	+/-	-	++++	-	-	-	-
8.1	++	++	++	++	-	-	-
H	++++	+	++	ND[e]	-	-	-
C	++++	++++	+	ND	-	-	-
2	++	+	++++	ND	-	-	-
H.7	++++	++++	++++	ND	-	+/-	-
8b	++++	++++	++++	ND	++++	++++	-

[a] NDV is Newcastle disease virus.

[b] NAF is normal allantoic fluid.

[c] Normalized reaction strength, + is weak, ++++ is strong.

[d] Negative reaction.

[e] Not done.

ACKNOWLEDGMENTS

     We would like to thank Dr. Kathryn V. Holmes, Uniformed
Services University of the Health Sciences, Bethesda, Maryland
for presenting this information at the workshop on our behalf.

     This report was taken in part from a dissertation to be
submitted to the Graduate School, University of Maryland, by the
senior author in partial fulfillment of the requirements for the
Ph.D. degree in the Virginia-Maryland Regional College of
Veterinary Medicine.

     This research was supported in part, by Grant No. 59-2241-1-
2-070-0 from the Cooperative State Research Service (CSRS), Science
and Education, United States Department of Agriculture and by Avrum
R. Gudelsky Research Funds.

     Scientific Article No. A-3508 Contribution No. 6581   of the
Maryland Agricultural Experiment Station, College Park, Maryland.

REFERENCES

1. Darbyshire, J. H. Assessment of cross-immunity in chickens to strains of avian infectious bronchitis virus using tracheal organ culture. Avian Pathol. 9:179-184. 1980.

2. Hopkins, S. R. Serological comparisons of strains of infectious bronchitis using plaque purified isolants. Avian Dis. 18:231-239. 1974.

3. Johnson, R. B. and W. W. Marquardt. The neutralizing characteristics of strains of infectious bronchitis virus as measured by the constant-virus variable-serum method in chicken tracheal cultures. Avian Dis. 19:82-90. 1975.

4. Lomniczi, B. and J. Morser. Polypeptides of infectious bronchitis virus. I. Polypeptides of the virion. J. Gen. Virol. 55:155-164. 1981.

5. Marquardt, W. W., S. K. Kadavil and D. B. Snyder. Comparison of ciliary activity and virus recovery from tracheas of chickens and humoral immunity after inoculation with serotypes of avian infectious bronchitis virus. Avian Dis. 26:828-834. 1982.

6. Snyder, D. B., W. W. Marquardt and S. K. Kadavil. Ciliary activity: A criterion for associating resistance to infectious bronchitis virus infection with ELISA antibody titer. Avian Dis. 27:485-490. 1983.

MONOCLONAL ANTIBODIES TO THE THREE CLASSES OF MOUSE HEPATITIS VIRUS STRAIN A59 PROTEINS

Marck J.M. Koolen, Albert D.M.E. Osterhaus*, Kees H.J. Siebelink*, Marian C. Horzinek and Bernard A.M. van der Zeijst

Institute of Virology, Veterinary Faculty, State University of Utrecht, and *National Institute of Public Health, Bilthoven, The Netherlands

Hybridoma cell lines producing monoclonal antibodies to mouse hepatitis virus strain A59 (MHV-A59) have been established by fusion of spleen cells of immunized mice with P3X63Ag8.653 mouse plasmacytoma cells. Culture fluids were screened for their ability to immunoprecipitate virus-specific proteins from ^{35}S-methionine-labeled infected cells. Eleven clones were obtained which fell into three classes (Figure 1).

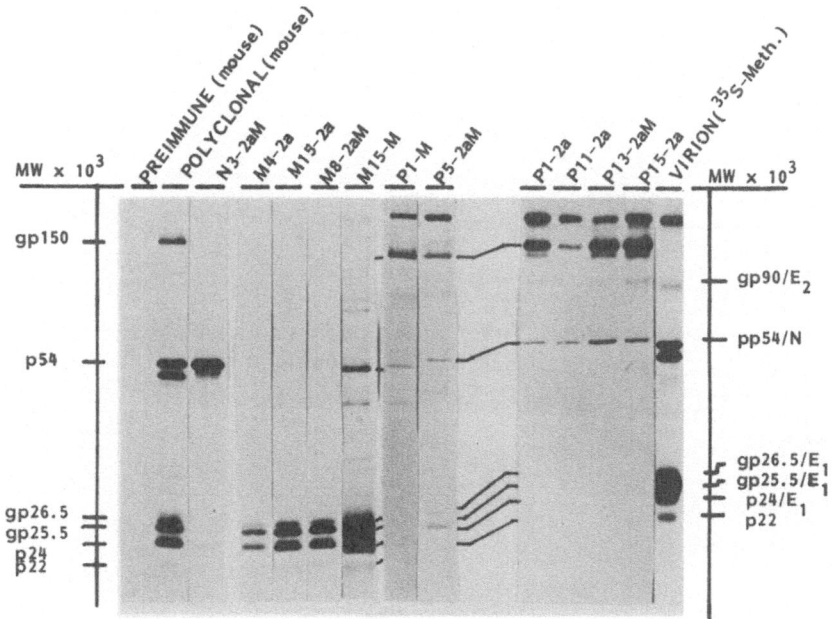

Figure 1

One clone reacted with the nucleocapsid protein (N). Four clones reacted with the matrix protein (E1) which is present, both in infected cells and in virions, as the unglycosylated form gp24/E1 and two glycosylated forms gp25.5/E1 and gp26.5/E1. All three modifications of E1 were precipitated which is in agreement with earlier fin;erprinting data for MHV strain JHM (1). The third class consisted of six clones specific for E2. The hybridomas produced IgG2a and/or IgM antibodies. The presence of two Ig species was not due to insufficient cloning, since the results remained the same after additional cloning. Possibly these cell lines carry out the IgM/IgG switch. Monoclonal antibodies against the viral glycoproteins, E1 and E2 recognized viral proteins on the surface of infected L929 cells but not on Sac(-) cells. Four out of six of the anti-E2 but none of the anti-E1 clones were able to neutralize the virus in the absence of complement. On the addition of complement a slight increase in neutralization by three anti-E1 clones was observed (Table).

Table 1. SUMMARY OF MONOCLONAL ANTIBODIES

HYBRIDOMA CELL LINES	POLYPEPTIDE SPECIFICITY	IMMUNOGLOBULIN ISOTYPE[*]	% NEUTRALIZATION AT ANTIBODY DILUTIONS[✰]					
			NO COMPLEMENT ADDED			COMPLEMENT ADDED		
			1/10	1/100	1/500	1/10	1/100	1/500
N3-2aM	N	IgG2a/IgM	12	5	10	1	1	7
P1-2a	E_2	IgG2a	100	83	49	100	79	54
P11-2a	E_2	IgG2a	42	7	7	44	11	-10
P13-2aM	E_2	IgG2a/IgM	4	12	12	31	8	-17
P15-2a	E_2	IgG2a	100	90	60	100	89	60
P1-M	E_2	IgM	17	2	10	17	8	-3
P5-2aM	E_2	IgG2a/IgM	99	97	90	100	97	30
M4-2a	E_1	IgG2a	2	-6	1	22	18	0
M15-2a	E_1	IgG2a	4	-6	-2	12	10	-4
M8-2aM	E_1	IgG2a/IgM	4	-1	4	8	-8	-2
M15-M	E_1	IgM	6	-8	-10	15	37	24

[*] As determined by Ouchterlony immuno diffusion test.

[✰] Monoclonal antibodies were adjusted to an initial concentration of 5 mg/ml of the active immuno-globulin isotype.

Further studies are in progress to elucidate the relationship between the various species of E2 with monoclonal antibodies directed against gp150.

REFERENCE

1. Siddell, S.G., J.gen.Virol. 62:259-269 (1982).

ANTIGENIC AND POLYPEPTIDE STRUCTURE OF BOVINE ENTERIC CORONAVIRUS

AS DEFINED BY MONOCLONAL ANTIBODIES

J.F. Vautherot[1], J. Laporte[1], M.F. Madelaine[1],
P. Bobulesco[1], and A. Roseto[2]

(1) INRA, Station de Recherches de Virologie et
     d'Immunologie, F-78850, Thiverval-Grignon

(2) Hôpital Saint-Louis, Unité INSERM U 107,
     12 bis rue de la Grange aux Belles F-75010-Paris

INTRODUCTION

Bovine enteric coronavirus (BECV), characterized by Stair
et al (1972), is now recognized as one of the viral agents that
cause acute diarrhoea in young calves (Stair *et al*, 1972). Virions
are large and pleomorphic (100 to 150 nm in diameter) and possess
a fringe of characteristically club-shaped peplomers, 20 nm long
(Sharpee *et al*, 1976). Polypeptide analysis revealed 3 major
proteins including glycoproteins of high (GP 65/125 - 65,000 and
125,000 daltons in molecular weight) and low (GP25) molecular
weight and a phosphorylated protein (VP 50) (King and Brian, 1982;
Laporte and Bobulesco, 1981). Two minor glycoproteins have also been
described, GP 105 and GP 100 (King and Brian, 1982 ; J. Laporte,
personal communication). Detergent treatment and limited proteolysis of purified virions enabled to localize the structural proteins (King and Brian, 1982 ; Bobulesco, 1983). The peplomers are
mainly constituted of GP 125, a glycoprotein which is reduced to
a GP 65 component by 2-Mercaptoethanol (2-ME), and of GP 105 and
GP 100. On these outer projections are located the structural sites
responsible for haemagglutination and virus to cell interactions.
GP 25 is more deeply embedded in the virion envelope and interacts
with the internal nucleoprotein (Bobulesco, 1983). VP 50 is an
internal phosphoprotein, closely associated with the viral genome
(King and Brian, 1982).
    Current evidence indicates that the coronaviruses which affect
mammals can be classified in two antigenically distinct groups
(Pedersen *et al*, 1978 ; Gerna *et al*, 1982) a) OC_{43} group to which

belong BECV, haemagglutinating encephalitis virus of swine (HEV),
murine hepatitis virus (MHV), diarrhoea virus of infant mice (DVIM),
rat sialodacryoadenitis virus (SDAV),   human enteric coronavirus
(HECV)   b) 229 E group comprising the viruses of transmissible
gastroenteritis of swine (TGEV), feline infectious peritonitis
(FIPV) and canine enteric coronavirus (CCV). Common antigenic
determinants were described on the three structural polypeptides
of TGEV, FIPV and CCV (Horzinek *et al*, 1982), but little is known
on the precise antigenic relationships at the molecular level
between the coronaviruses of the OC43 group.

This report describes the characterization of monoclonal antibodies to BECV, 8 of which reacted with GP 105. These monoclonal
antibodies helped to define two biological activities associated
with GP 105, haemagglutination and virus to cell interaction.
Antigenic relationships between BECV and other coronaviruses, as
well as within BECV isolates, were studied using monoclonal antibodies.

MATERIALS AND METHODS

Cell-lines and viruses

HRT 18 cell-line (a human rectal tumor cell-line isolated by
Tompkins *et al*, 1974) was grown as previously described (Laporte
et al, 1981) except that tylosine (10 µg/ml) and lincomycine
(200 µg/ml) were added to the medium instead of penicillin and
steptomycin. BECV G110 (Laporte *et al*, 1979 ; L'Haridon *et al*,
1981), F_{15} (Laporte *et al*, 1979 ; Laporte and Bobulesco, 1981),
NCDCV (Mebus *et al*, 1973), danish and british isolates (Bridger
et al, 1978), as well as HEV, OC_{43} (Weiss, 1983), and a bovine
respiratory coronavirus (Thomas *et al*, 1982) were serially passaged on HRT 18. For biochemical purposes, the viruses were plaque-
purified,   cultivated on HRT 18 and purified according to a
method described previously (Laporte et Bobulesco, 1981).

Primary foetal bovine kidney cells (PFBK) were cultivated in
Eagle's minimum essential medium (Eurobio, Paris) supplemented with
10 % foetal calf serum (FCS) (Flow Laboratories, France), 100 IU/ml
penicillin and 100 µg/ml streptomycin. These PFBK were used to
propagate BECV G110 (L'Haridon *et al*, 1982) and NCDCV (Mebus *et al*,
1973).

RP^d cells, a pig kidney cell-line, were cultivated as previously described (Laude, 1978) and used to grow HEV and TGEV.

Sac⁻ cells, a permanent rhabdosarcoma cell-line from mice,
was grown as previously described (Wege *et al*, 1979) and used to
cultivate MHV_4 - JHM and MHV_3.

Purification of the coronaviruses, immunization schedules, fusion procedures and partial characterization of monoclonal antibodies have been described previously (Roseto *et al*, 1982).

Radiolabelling and immuno-precipitation

Polypeptide specificities of monoclonal antibodies were determined by immunoprecipitation of ^{14}C-labelled viral polypeptides from HRT 18 cells infected with BECV G110 (Laporte *et al*, 1980). Confluent monolayers were infected by G110 at a m.o.i. of 10 PFU/cell At 16 h post-infection, the supernatant was discarded and replaced by fresh RPMI 1640 (Eurobio, France) containing 2 % FCS and 5μCi/ml of a ^{14}C-labelled amino-acid mixture (45 mCi/at. C - CEA, France). After a further 6 hours incubation, the medium was discarded, monolayers were washed twice with cold phosphate buffer saline pH = 7.2 (PBS) and the cells were solubilized in lysis buffer (Collins *et al*, 1982). The cytosol extract was centrifuged at 10,000 x g during 30 minutes to remove nuclear debris and aliquots were stored at - 80°C. Before immunoprecipitation, cytosol extracts were preabsorbed with *Staphylococcus aureus* to avoid non-specific binding. Briefly, cytosol extracts were mixed with a suspension of heat-killed formalin-fixed *Staphylococcus aureus* (Pansorbin, Calbiochem) to give a final concentration of 6 % in *Staphylococcus aureus*. After one hour at room temperature, bacteria were pelleted by centrifugation at 11,000 x g for 2 min. and the supernatant was used for immune precipitation. Fifty μl of cytosol extract, containing 150,000 TCA precipitable CPM, were mixed either with 10 μl of polyclonal antiserum or mouse ascitic fluid (MAF), or with 50 μl of undiluted hybridoma supernatant. The mixture was incubated for 1 hour at 37°C and 50 μl of sheep anti-mouse IgG (SAMIg) (Institut Pasteur, Paris) diluted 1/200 in TEN-OVA buffer (Tris 50 mM, pH = 7.2, 150 mM NaCl, 5 mM EDTA containing 2 % Aprotinin and 1 mg/ml ovalbumine), were added. After a further 1 hour incubation at 37°C, 100 μl of a 10 % suspension of heat-killed formalin-fixed *Staphylococcus aureus* were added to the mixture. Incubation was continued for an additional 45 min. at room temperature. Bacteria were pelleted by a 2 min. centrifugation at 11,000 x g, and washed 4 times in TEN-OVA. The final pellet was resuspended in sample preparation buffer containing 3 % sodium dodecyl sulfate (SDS) and heated at 56°C for 5 min. Reduction of viral polypeptides was achieved by incorporating 5 % 2-M.E. in sample buffer before heating. Bacteria were removed by centrifugation and samples were analyzed by electrophoresis on 10 % polyacrylamide slab-gels (Laemmli, 1970). Gels were stained by coomassie brilliant blue and processed for fluorography (Bonner and Laskey, 1974). Radioactivity was revealed by autoradiography of the slab gels on KODAK XAR-5 films. Controls included the precipitation of cytosol extracts from non-infected HRT 18 cells and precipitation of BECV polypeptides by monoclonal antibodies to an unrelated virus (Rotavirus).

Virus neutralization

Virus neutralizing activity of monoclonal antibodies was quantitated by a plaque reduction assay. Monoclonal antibodies in MAF
or TCF were first precipitated by ammonium sulfate at a final concentration of 50 %, resuspended in PBS and dialyzed during 24 h
against a 100 volume of the same buffer. The virus was diluted to
contain 100 PFU/0.1 ml and 0.2 ml were mixed with an equal volume
of diluted antibody. Virus-antibody mixtures were incubated during
1 hour at 37°C and plated onto HRT 18 cell monolayers in 6 wells
costar plates (COSTAR, Cambridge, Mass.). After an adsorption
of one hour at 37°C, the supernatant was discarded, monolayers were
washed once in RPMI 1640 medium and an agarose overlay was applied
as previously described (Vautherot, 1981). Forty to 48 h after
infection, plaques were revealed by adsorption of rat red-blood
cells (RRBC) (Vautherot, 1981). Neutralization titres were expressed as the reciprocal of the highest dilution giving a 50 % reduction in plaque number (PRD50). Studies on the kinetics of neutralization were performed according to a technique described previously
(Volk et al, 1982). All MAF were adjusted at an IgG concentration
of 0.1 mg/ml assuming an absortivity (1 % 1cm) for mouse Ig of 14
at 280 nm. In some experiments sheep anti mouse IgG, diluted 1/250,
was added to the virus antibody mixture after 30 min. at 37°C. This
mixture was further incubated during 30 min. at 37°C and then plated
on cells as described above.

Haemagglutination inhibition (HAI)

At first, purified BECV was titrated by an haemagglutination
assay (HA) using RRBC (Laporte et al, 1980). The HA titre of the
virus was expressed as the reciprocal of the last dilution which
gave a fully agglutination of RRBC. HAI was performed using TCF of
MAF preadsorbed with packed RRBC. Monoclonal antibody preparations
were diluted in PBS containing 2 mg/ml bovine serum albumin (BSA)
and 25 µl of each dilution were mixed with an equal volume of virus
suspension containing 4 HA units, in round-bottom microtitration
plates. Plates were incubated for 1 hour at 37°C and 50 µl of a
0.8 % RRBC suspension were added in each well. Plates were kept
at room temperature for an additional hour. HAI titres were expressed as the reciprocal of the last dilution inhibiting the haemagglutination.

ELISA

Enzyme-linked immunosorbent assays (ELISA) were performed using
a modification of a method previously described (Vautherot et al,
1981). Wells of microtitration plates (Microelisa, Dynatech) were
coated with 0.5 µg of purified BECV in 100 µl of 50 mM Pipes buffer
pH = 6.4, 150 mM NaCl. Plates were incubated overnight at 37°C.

Excess viral antigen was removed by 4 washes with PBS containing
0.05 % Tween 20 (PBS-Tween). Unbound sites of the solid phase were
saturated with 100 µl/well of a 1 % solution of Gelatin (Biomerieux,
France) in 10 mM Tris buffer pH = 7.4 containing 150 mM NaCl. After
1 hour at 37°C, plates were washed 4 times with PBS-Tween and 100 µl
of duplicate dilutions of monoclonal antibodies in PBS Tween were
added to the wells. Plates were then incubated at 37°C for 2 hours
and unbound antibodies were removed by 4 washes in PBS Tween. One
hundred microliters of anti-mouse IgG serum conjugated to Horse-
radish peroxidase were added to each well. Plates were incubated
for 2 hours at 37°C and washed 4 times in PBS Tween. Bound conjugated antibodies were detected by the addition of 100 µl of substrate solution,(10 mg of orthophenylene-diamin in 25 ml of 0.035M
citrate, 0.066M phosphate buffer pH = 5.0 containing 0.012 %
hydrogen peroxide). The colouring reaction was stopped after 12 min.
at room temperature by adding 50 µl/well of 5 N H_2SO_4. Optical
densities were read in a multichannel photometer (Flow laboratories
SA, France).

RESULTS

Characterization of monoclonal antibodies

        Twelve hybridomas secreting monoclonal antibodies to BECV strain
G110 were established from 271 hybrid colonies (Roseto et al, 1982).
Polypeptide specificity of the monoclonal antibodies was assayed by
two methods a) immunoprecipitation of ^{14}C-labelled viral polypeptides
and b) immunoperoxidase staining (IPS) of viral structural polypeptides separated by PAGE (Laporte et Bobulesco, 1981) and transferred
on nitrocellulose sheets by transverse electrophoresis (Towbin et al,
1979). Five monoclonal antibodies (A_9, A_{20}, B_5, I_7 and J_{18} - table
1) precipitated GP 105 together with a polypeptide of 150.000 daltons
in mol. wt. (Fig. 1). B_5, I_7 and J_{18} also stained GP 105 by IPS
whereas A_9 and A_{20} failed to react with SDS denatured structural
polypeptides. The three remaining anti GP 105 (C_{13}, F_7 and I_{16} -
table) only reacted in IPS and failed to precipitate GP 105
although they precipitated faintly the 150.000 daltons polypeptide
(Fig. 1). GP 105, both in the cytosol extract and in the whole
virus was found to differ from the major outer glycoprotein GP 125,
in that the latter was reduced to GP 65 when 2-M.E. was incorporated
in the sample preparation buffer.
        Monoclonal antibodies E_5, H_7, H_{19} and I_{12} neither precipitated
any of the radiolabelled polypeptides, nor reacted with transferred
viral proteins in IPS. Work is in progress to further characterize thes monoclonal antibodies.
        In order to correlate biological functions with polypeptides,
monoclonal antibodies were studied for their ability to neutralize
the virus and to inhibit haemagglutination with BECV G110 (Table 1).

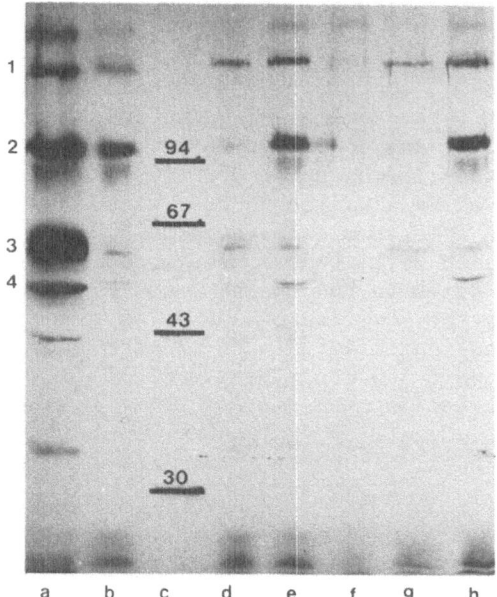

Fig. 1 :
Immunoprecipitation of viral
polypeptides with:
a) polyclonal hyperimmune
   serum precipitating 150 K
   (1), GP 105 (2), GP 65 (3)
   and VP 50 (4).
b and h) A_9, d) F_7, e) J_{18},
f) I_{12}, g) I_{16}.

Table 1 : Characterization of monoclonal antibodies to
          BECV G 110.

Monoclonal antibodies	Isotype	Specificity		Reciprocal titre		
		Immunoprecip. (a)	Immunostaining (b)	IIF	Neutralization	HAI
A_9	IgG_2b	GP105 & 150K	N.R. [(c)]	32	90	256
A_{20}	IgG_2a	GP105 & 150K	N.R.	128	4×10^3	0
B_5	IgG_2a	GP105 & 150K	GP 105	128	3.2×10^3	0
I_7	IgG_2a	GP105 & 150K	GP 105	32	1×10^3	0
J_{18}	IgG_2a	GP105 & 150K	GP 105	256	5.5×10^3	0
C_{13}	IgG_1	150K	GP 105	64	1×10^2	32
F_7	IgG_1	150K	GP 105	64	< 10	0
I_{16}	IgG_1	150K	GP 105	256	< 10	0
E_5	IgG_{2a}	N.R.	N.R.	128	< 10	0
H_7	IgG_{2a}	N.R.	N.R.	256	< 10	0
H_{19}	IgG_{2a}	N.R.	N.R.	64	< 10	0
I_{12}	IgG_{2a}	N.R.	N.R.	128	< 10	0

(a) *Immunoprecipitation of radiolabelled polypeptides from BECV infected cells.*

(b) *Immunoperoxidase staining of viral structural polypeptides, separated by electrophoresis
    on polyacrylamide gel and transferred on nitrocellulose sheets by transverse electrophoresis.*

(c) *N.R. = not reacting.*

Five monoclonal antibodies which precipitated GP 105 and 150K (A$_9$, A$_{20}$, B$_5$, I$_7$ and J$_{18}$) together with C$_{13}$ (anti GP 105 as revealed by IPS) neutralized the virus. However differences could be observed within this group regarding the persistence of a non-neutralized fraction. Monoclonal I$_7$ neutralized G110 without leaving any non-neutralized fraction, whereas a 3 % to 10 % non-neutralized fraction was always observed with the other neutralizing monoclonal antibodies. These data were confirmed by studies on the kinetics of neutrali- · zation (Fig. 2) and were independent of the protein concentration. The remaining two anti GP 105 monoclonal antibodies (I$_{16}$ and F$_7$) never displayed any neutralizing activity even when MAF were used instead of TCF. In order to detect a complement dependent neutralization (Collins *et al*, 1982) and to ascertain that the absence of neutralization was not due to low affinity binding of monoclonal antibodies, neutralization assays were performed in the presence of complement and/or sheep anti-mouse IgG (Table 2). The addition of complement had no visible effect on the neutralization by monoclonal antibodies except for A9 for which a two-fold increase in the neutralization titre was observed. The addition of sheep anti mouse IgG induced a 15-fold increase in the neutralizing titre of monoclonal antibody A$_9$, together with a reduction from 20 to 5 % of the non-neutralized fraction (Fig. 3).

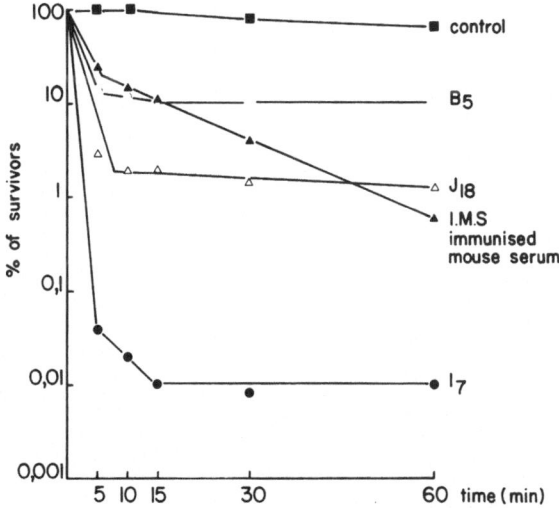

Fig. 2 : Kinetics of neutralization of BECV G 110
         by immunized mouse serum (IMS), and mono-
         clonal antibodies B$_5$, J$_{18}$ and I$_7$.

Table 2 : Neutralization of BECV G110 by monoclonal
antibodies in the presence of anti-mouse
IgG and/or complement.

| Monoclonal antibodies | Neutralization titre (PRD$_{50}$) | | | |
	Control	Complement[a]	AMIσ [b]	AMIσ + complement
A_9	8×10^2	1.8×10^3	1.25×10^4	1.25×10^4
A_{20}	1.5×10^5	1.5×10^5	1.5×10^5	1.5×10^5
B_5	1.3×10^6	1.3×10^6	1.3×10^6	1.3×10^6
I_7	5.5×10^3	N.T.	2.3×10^3	N.T.
J_{18}	2.2×10^5	N.T.	2.2×10^5	N.T.
C_{13}	1.1×10^4	1.1×10^4	1.1×10^4	1.1×10^4
F_7	< 100	N.T.	< 100	N.T.
I_{16}	< 100	< 100	< 100	< 100
E_5	< 100	N.T.	< 100	N.T.
H_7	< 100	N.T.	< 100	N.T.
H_{19}	< 100	N.T.	< 100	N.T.
I_{12}	< 100	< 100	< 100	< 100

(a) Guinea-pig complement

(b) Sheep anti-Mouse IgG (H + L)

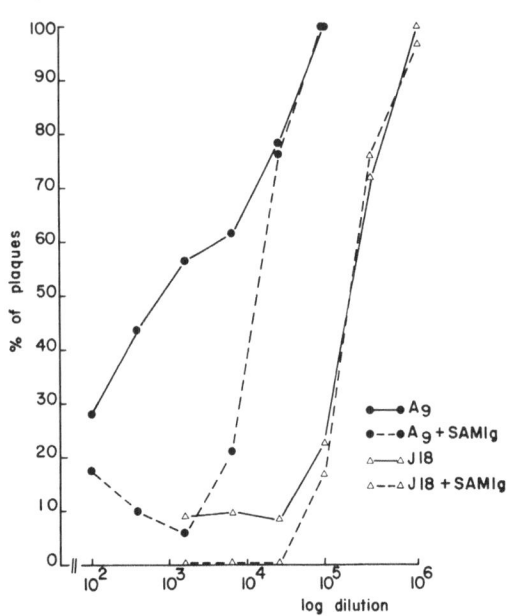

Fig. 3 : Comparative neutralization of BECV G110
by monoclonal anti-
bodies A9 and J$_{18}$ in
the presence or ab-
sence of sheep anti-
mouse IgG serum
(SAMIg).

This reduction of non-neutralized fraction from 10 % to 0 % was a common feature of monoclonal antibodies A_9, A_{20}, B_5, C_{13} and J_{18} when SAMIg was added. However monoclonal I_7, the one which neutralized without leaving any non-neutralized fraction, was never affected in its neutralizing activity by the addition of SAMIg. The addition of anti-immunoglobulins had no effect on non-neutralizing monoclonal antibodies. Together with the results on the kinetics of neutralization, these data suggest that the unneutralized fraction results from an equilibrium between bound and free antibody. Two monoclonal antibodies inhibited the agglutination of RRBC by BECV G110, A_9 and C_{13}, both of which neutralized the virus and were anti-GP 105. Absence of HAI by the other monoclonal antibodies was not due to an inability of the antibodies to bind to intact virions as binding was observed in ELISA assays (data not shown).

Monoclonal antibodies directed against GP 105 have been shown to inhibit both viral multiplication *in vitro,* and haemagglutination. The existence of monoclonal antibodies that outlined different functional domains on outer glycoproteins has been described for naked virus (Burstin *et al,* 1982) as well as enveloped virus (Kida *et al,* 1982). Whether these differences between monoclonal antibodies can be related to differences in affinity remains to be studied.

Cross-reactivity of monoclonal antibodies with coronaviruses of the OC$_{43}$ group and with TGE

BEC, HECV (two isolates of human enteric coronavirus) and a bovine respiratory coronavirus (Thomas *et al,* 1982) could not be distinguished by an indirect immunofluorescence assay (IIF) performed on monolayers of HRT 18 infected with these viruses and stained with monoclonal antibodies (Roseto *et al,* 1982) (table 3). However OC$_{43}$ and HEV, also grown on HRT18, differed from BECV as OC$_{43}$ was recognized by six non-neutralizing monoclonal antibodies (F_7, I_{16}, E_5, H_7, H_{19} and I_{12}) and HEV only by 5 monoclonal antibodies (I_{16}, E_5, H_7, H_{19} and I_{12}) (Table 3). The reactivity of monoclonal antibodies with HEV was not affected when this virus was grown on RPd cells (Laude, 1978). MHV4-JHM as well as MHV3 were recognized by 4 monoclonal antibodies (E_5, H_7, H_{19} and I_{12}) in an IIF test performed on acetone fixed Sac$^-$ monolayers (Table 3). Monoclonal antibodies to BECV failed to detect any viral antigen in RPd cells infected with TGE (Purdue strain) (data not shown).

Antigenic comparison of BECV isolates

The reactivity of monoclonal antibodies to G110 was assayed at first by IIF staining of HRT 18 monolayers infected by BECV isolates F_{15} (Laporte *et al,* 1979), NCDCV (Mebus *et al,* 1973), british and danish (Bridger *et al,* 1978). No differences could be detected between G110 and F15 (Table 4). However monoclonal anti-

Table 3 : Cross-reactivity of monoclonal antibodies to BECV
with coronaviruses of the OC 43 group.

Monoclonal antibodies	BECV G110	B. RCV (a)	HECV (b)	OC43 (c)	HEV (d)	MHV4 (e)
A_9	+	+	+	-	-	-
A_{20}	+	+	+	-	-	-
B_5	+	+	+	-	-	-
I_7	+	+	+	-	-	-
J_{18}	+	+	+	-	-	-
C_{13}	+	+	+	-	-	-
F_7	+	+			-	-
I_{16}	+	+			+	-
E_5	+	+	+		+	+
H_7	+	+	+	+	+	+
H_{19}	+	+	+	+	+	+
I_{12}	+	+	+	+	+	+

(a) Bovine Respiratory Coronavirus (tested on HRT cells)
(b) Human Enteric Coronavirus   (tested on HRT cells)
(c) Human Respiratory Coronavirus (tested on HRT cells)
(d) Hemagglutinating Encephalitis Coronavirus (tested on HRT and RPd cells)
(e) Mouse Hepatitis Virus strain JHM   (tested on SAC⁻ cells)

body A_9 never stained NCDCV infected cells (HRT_{18} or PFBK) ;
similarly F_7 failed to react with the third passage on HRT 18 of
the british and danish BECV isolates (Table 4).

Neutralization and HAI were used to further investigate the
cross-reactivity of monoclonal antibodies with G110, F_{15} and NCDCV.
Both assays confirmed the similarities between G110 and F15 (data
not shown) and that A_9 never reacted with NCDCV (Table 5). No
other difference could be observed between NCDCV and G 110
(Table 5).

The absence of binding of F_7 to the 4th passage of british
BECV isolate was also confirmed by an ELISA test (data not shown)
using purified virus as antigen. Comparison of the two viruses
(british and danish isolates) by neutralization did not reveal
any noticeable difference (Table 6). As during the first two
passages of the british isolate on HRT 18, monoclonal antibody F_7
stained a few infected cells, the virus was cloned in order to
investigate if different viral populations could be isolated from
the original inoculum. Plaque purification yielded 7 clones, 2 of
which reacted with F_7 whereas the remaining 5 were negative. Work
is in   progress to investigate the stability of these viral clones.

The absence of reactivity of monoclonal antibody A_9 with NCDCV and F_7 with the british and danish BECV isolates were the most obvious differences detectable among the BECV isolates tested.

Table 4 : Cross-reactivity of monoclonal antibodies
with BECV isolates (IIF staining).

Monoclonal antibodies	G110 and F_{15}	NCDCV	B.BECV and D.BECV
A_9	+	-	+
A_{20}	+	+	+
B_5	+	+	+
I_7	+	+	+
J_{18}	+	+	+
C_{13}	+	+	+
F_7	+	+	-
I_{16}	+	+	+
E_5	+	+	+
H_7	+	+	+
H_{19}	+	+	+
I_{12}	+	+	+

Table 5 : Reactivity of monoclonal antibodies with NCDCV.

Monoclonal antibodies	Neutralisation titre (PRD_{50})		HAI		ELISA	
	G110	NCDCV	G110	NCDCV	G110	NCDCV
A_9	90	0	256	0	2100 4×10^6*	0 0*
A_{20}	4×10^3	4×10^3	< 2	< 2	1.4×10^3	1.2×10^3
B_5	3.2×10^3	1×10^4	< 2	< 2	2×10^3	1.5×10^3
I_7	1×10^3	1×10^3	< 2	< 2	3×10^3	3.5×10^3
J_{18}	5.5×10^3	4×10^3	< 2	< 2	1.3×10^4	2×10^4
C_{13}	1×10^2	1×10^2	32	32	1×10^3	2×10^3
F_7	< 10	< 10	< 2	< 2	8×10^2	2.5×10^3
I_{16}	< 10	< 10	< 2	< 2	2.8×10^3	3×10^3
E_5	< 10	< 10	< 2	< 2	8×10^3	9.5×10^3
H_7	< 10	< 10	< 2	< 2	5×10^3	5×10^3
H_{19}	< 10	< 10	< 2	< 2	1.8×10^3	2.5×10^3
I_{12}	< 10	< 10	< 2	< 2	3×10^3	2.5×10^3

* Mouse ascitic fluid.

Table 6 : Neutralization of british and danish BECV
isolates by monoclonal antibodies.

Monoclonal antibodies	G 110	B.BECV	D.BECV
A_9	1.4×10^4 [a]	7.5×10^3 [a]	5.8×10^3 [a]
A_{20}	8.5×10^2	1.4×10^3	1.8×10^3
B_5	4.8×10^3	2.1×10^3	3.8×10^3
I_7	$> 8 \times 10^5$	$> 8 \times 10^5$	5×10^5
J_{18}	1.7×10^5	1.5×10^5	1.6×10^5
C_{13}	7×10^3 [a]	2.1×10^4 [a]	1.8×10^4 [a]
F_7	< 20	< 20	< 20
I_{16}	< 10	< 10	< 10
E_5	< 10	< 10	< 10
H_7	< 10	< 10	< 10
H_{19}	< 10	< 10	< 10
I_{12}	< 20	$< 2n$	< 10

(a) *Neutralization tests were performed in the presence of sheep anti-mouse IgG (H + L)*

CONCLUSION

     Monoclonal antibodies directed against GP 105 also precipitated
a 150 Kdaltons polypeptide. Whether this 150 Kpolypeptide is a glycosylated precursor to GP 105, as described for MHV4 (Siddell, 1982)
remains to be shown.
     Anti GP 105 monoclonal antibodies displayed neutralizing and
haemagglutination inhibition activities. Neutralization by anti
GP 105 was comparable to that described for monoclonal antibodies
anti MHV4-GP1 (Collins *et al*, 1982). The presence of a non-neutralized fraction,presumably resulting from an equilibrium between free
and bound antibody, was reported for other monoclonal antibodies
(Volk *et al*, 1982). The addition of anti mouse IgG to neutralizing
monoclonal antibodies to BECV consistently decreased this non -
neutralized fraction from 10 % to 0 %.
     Detailed results on the biological activity of monoclonal
antibodies to the other outer glycoproteins of BECV are not yet
available. However this report shows that GP 105, a minor component
of the peplomers, is involved in virus to cell interactions as well
as in viral-induced haemagglutination. Previous publications described an HA activity of BECV (King and Brian, 1982) and HEV
(Pocock, 1978) associated with GP65/125 as shown by bromelain
treatment and sensitivity to reducing agents. Two anti-GP 105
displayed HAI activity showing that either GP 105 is closely asso-

ciated with the haemagglutinin, or that GP 105 itself carries a part, if not all, of the viral receptor for RRBC.

Antibodies against GP 105 defined at least two functional domains, one outlined by neutralizing monoclonal antibodies (A_{20}, B_5, I_7, J_{18}) and the other one being recognized by monoclonal antibodies with neutralizing and HAI activity (A_9 and C_{13}).

The reactivity of monoclonal antibodies to BECV with other coronaviruses showed that monoclonal antibodies E_5, H_7, H_{19} and I_{12} outlined antigenic determinant(s) common to MHV, OC_{43}, HEV and BECV. However OC_{43} and HEV were also recognized by monoclonal antibodies I_{16} and F_7 which both are directed against the structural GP 105.

A bovine respiratory coronavirus (Thomas *et al*, 1982) was found to be similar to BECV G110 in its reactivity with monoclonal antibodies. Experimental studies on the compared pathogenicity of this virus and BECV confirmed this similarity (Reynolds, 1982).

HECV, isolated from diarrhoeic babies (Bobulesco, 1983) and from young adults (J. Laporte, unpublished results), did not differ from BECV regarding their reactivity with monoclonal antibodies. Storz *et al* (1981) reported an accidental contamination of man by BECV and Patel *et al*, (1982) succeeded in infecting gnoto-biotic calves with an HECV isolate. Whether BECV and HECV are different is not yet resolved but cross contamination was clearly demonstrated. HECV can easily be differentiated from OC_{43} and is more closely related to BECV than to human respiratory coronavirus.

Antigenic analysis of BECV isolates revealed minor changes on GP 105. The US isolate (NCDCV) failed to react with A_9 and the british isolate was found to contain at least two viral populations which could be selected by plaque purification. These antigenic changes were the only ones which could be detected as all the other monoclonal antibodies reacted with the different isolates in a very similar manner.

ACKNOWLEDGMENTS

We would like to thank Dr Janice Bridger, Hubert Laude, Stuart Siddell for providing different viruses and cell-lines ; Françoise Rossi and Yann Fedon for excellent technical assistance and Nicolle Leblanc for typing the manuscript.

REFERENCES

Bobulesco, P.,1983, Etude des proteines structurales du coronavirus
    entéritique bovin. Comparaison structurale et antigénique
    avec une souche de coronavirus entéritique d'origine humaine
    Thèse de Doctorat de Troisième Cycle, Université Paris VII,
    Paris.
Bonner, W.M., and Laskey, R.A., 1974, A film detection method for
    tritium labelled proteins and nucleic acids in polyacryla-
    mide gels. Europ. J. of Biochemistry, 46:83.
Bridger, J.C., Woode, G.N., and Meyling, A., 1978, Isolation of
    coronaviruses from neonatal calf diarrhoea in Great Britain
    and Denmark. Vet. Microbiol., 3:101.
Burstin, S.J., Spriggs, D.R., and Fields, B.N., 1982, Evidence for
    functional domains on the reovirus type 3 hemagglutinin.
    Virology, 117:146.
Collins, A.R., Knobler, R.L., Powell, H., and Buchmeier, M.J., 1982,
    Monoclonal antibodies to Murine Hepatitis Virus-4 (Strain
    JHM) define the viral glycoprotein responsible for attach-
    ment and cell-cell fusion. Virology, 119:358.
Gerna, G., Battaglia, M., Cereda, P.M., and Passarani, N., 1982,
    Reactivity of Human Coronavirus OC43 and Neonatal Calf
    Diarrhoea Coronavirus Membrane-associated antigens. J. gen.
    Virol., 60:385.
Horzinek, M.C., Lutz, H., and Pedersen, N.C., 1982, Antigenic
    relationships among homologous structural polypeptides of
    porcine, feline and canine coronaviruses. Infect. Immun.,
    37 (3):1148.
Kida, H., Brown, L.E., and Webster, R.G., 1982, Biological acti-
    vity of monoclonal antibodies to operationally defined an-
    tigenic regions on the hemagglutinin molecule of A/Seal/
    Massachusetts/1/80 (H7N7) Influenza Virus. Virology, 122:38.
King, B., and Brian, D.A., 1982, Bovine coronavirus structural
    proteins. J. Virol. 42(2):700.
Laemmli, U.K., 1970, Cleavage of structural proteins during the
    assembly of the head of bacteriophage T_4. Nature, London,
    227:680.
Laporte, J., L'Haridon, R., and Bobulesco, P., 1979, *In vitro*
    culture of Bovine Enteric Coronavirus (BEC). Les Colloques
    de l'INSERM, Entérites virales, 90:99.
Laporte, J., Bobulesco, P., Rossi, F., 1980, Une Lignée cellu-
    laire particulièrement sensible à la réplication du Corona-
    virus entéritique bovin : les cellules HRT18. C.R. Acad.
    Sc. Paris, 290, série D:623.
Laporte, J., and Bobulesco, P., 1981, Polypeptide structure of
    bovine enteric coronavirus : comparison between a wild
    strain purified from feces and a HRT 18 cell adapted strain
    in : Biochemistry and Biology of Coronaviruses, V. ter
    Meulen, S. Siddell and H. Wege ed., Plenum Publishing corp.

Laude, H., 1978, Virus de la peste porcine classique : isolement
    d'une souche cytolytique à partir de cellules IB-Rs 2.
    Ann. Microbiol. (Inst. Pasteur). 129 A:553.
L'Haridon, R., Scherrer, R., Vautherot, J.F., La Bonnardière, C.,
    Laporte, J., Cohen, J., 1981, Adaptation d'un isolement de
    coronavirus entérique bovin à la culture cellulaire et carac-
    térisation de la souche obtenue. Ann. Rech. Vét. 12(3):243.
Mebus, C.A., Stair, E.L., Rhodes, M.B., and Twiehaus, M.J., 1973,
    Neonatal calf diarrhea : propagation, attenuation, and cha-
    racteristics of a coronavirus-like agent. Am. J. Vet. Res.
    34(2):145.
Patel, J.R., Davies, H.A., Edington, N., Laporte, J., and Macnaugton,
    M.R., 1982, Infection of a calf with the enteric coro-
    navirus strain Paris. Arch. Virol. 73:319.
Pedersen, N.C., Ward, J., and Mengeling, W.L., 1978, Antigenic
    relationship of the Feline Infectious Peritonitis Virus to
    coronaviruses of other species. Arch. Virol. 58:45.
Pocock, D.H., 1978, Effect of sulphydryl reagents on the biological
    activities, polypeptide composition and morphology of haemag-
    glutinating encephalomyelitis virus. J. gen. Virol. 40:93.
Reynolds, D.J., in press, Coronavirus replication in the intes-
    tinal and respiratory tracts during experimental and natural
    infections of calves, in : E.E.C. Seminar on gastro-intesti-
    nal diseases in the young pig and calf.
Roseto, A., Vautherot, J.F., Bobulesco, P., et Guillemin, M.C.,
    1982, Isolement d'hybrides cellulaires secrétant des anti-
    corps spécifiques du coronavirus entérique bovin. C.R. Acad.
    Sc. Paris. 294, série III:347.
Sharpee, R.L., Mebus, C.A., and Bass, E.P., 1976, Characterization
    of a calf diarrheal coronavirus. Am. J. Vet. Res. 37(9):1031.
Siddell, S.G., 1982, Coronavirus JHM : tryptic peptide finger-
    printing of virion proteins and intracellular polypeptides.
    J. gen. Virol. 62:259.
Stair, E.L., Rhodes, M.B., White, R.G., and Mebus, C.A., 1972,
    Neonatal calf diarrhea : purification and electron micros-
    copy of a coronavirus-like agent. Am. J. Vet. Res. 33(6):1147.
Storz, J., and Roth, R., 1981, Reactivity of antibodies in
    human serum with antigens of an enteropathogenic bovine
    coronavirus. Med. Microbiol. Immunol. 169:169.
Thomas, L.H., Gourlay, R.N., Stott, E.J., Howard, C.J., and Bridger,
    J.C., 1982, A search for new microorganisms in calf pneumonia
    by the inoculation of gnotobiotic calves. Res. Vet. Sci.
    33:170.
Tompkins, W.A.F., Watrach, A.M., Schmale, J.D., Schultz, R.M., and
    Harris, J.A., 1974, Cultural and antigenic properties of new-
    ly established cell strains derived from adenocarcinomas of
    the human colon and rectum. J. Natl. Cancer Inst. 52(4):1101.
Towbin, H., Staehelin, T., and Gordon, J., 1979, Electrophoretic
    transfer of proteins from polyacrylamide gels to nitro-

cellulose sheets : procedure and some applications. Proc. Natl. Acad. Sci. USA, 76 (9):4350.

Vautherot, J.F., 1981, Plaque assay for titration of Bovine Enteric Coronavirus. J. gen. Virol. 56:451.

Vautherot, J.F., L'Haridon, R., Scherrer, R., Laporte, J., 1981, Titrage des anticorps anti-coronavirus bovin par la méthode ELISA et l'immunofluorescence indirecte. in : Réunion de la Société Française de Microscopie. Méthodes de diagnostic rapide.

Volk, W.A., Snyder, R.M., Benjamin, D.C., and Wagner, R.R., 1982, Monoclonal antibodies to the glycoprotein of vesicular stomatitis virus : comparative neutralizing activity. J. Virol. 42:220.

Wege, H., Wege, H., Nagashima, L., and Ter Meulen, V., 1979, Structural polypeptides of the murine coronavirus JHM. J. gen. Virol., 42:37.

Weiss, S.R., 1983. Coronaviruses SD and SK share extensive nucleotide homology with murine coronavirus MHV-A59, more than that shared between human and murine coronaviruses. Virology. 126:669.

PLAQUE ASSAY, POLYPEPTIDE COMPOSITION AND IMMUNOCHEMISTRY OF FELINE INFECTIOUS PERITONITIS VIRUS AND FELINE ENTERIC CORONAVIRUS ISOLATES

John F. Boyle[1], Niels C. Pedersen[1], James F. Evermann[2], Alison J. McKeirnan[2], Richard L. Ott[2] and John W. Black[3]

[1]Department of Medicine, School of Veterinary Medicine
University of California, Davis, CA 95616

[2]Department of Veterinary Clinical Medicine and Surgery
School of Veterinary Medicine, Washington State Univ.
Pullman, WA 99164

[3]Specialized Assays, P.O. Box 25110
Nashville, TN 37202

INTRODUCTION

The coronaviral nature of feline infectious peritonitis virus (FIPV) and feline enteric coronavirus (FECV) has been well documented by morphological, physicochemical and antigenic studies[1-10]. However, biochemical and detailed immunochemical analyses of FIPV and FECV have been difficult due to the inability to prepare sufficient quantities of viral material. Recently, we have been able to propagate FIPV and FECV in continuous cell culture of feline origin[8,11-13].

The purpose of this report is to describe the purification of feline coronaviruses from infected cell culture and to compare five strains with respect to: 1) plaque characteristics, 2) viral structural polypeptide composition and 3) serologic reactivity of experimentally infected cats against the structural polypeptides of homologous and heterologous strains.

MATERIALS AND METHODS

Cells and virus

Fetal cat whole fetus (fcwf-4) cells were used to propagate all feline coronavirus strains. Cells were cultured with Eagle's

133

minimum essential medium supplemented with 20% Leibovitz's L-15
medium, L-glutamine, antibiotics and 10% fetal bovine serum
(FBS). The isolation and pathogenic characterization of FIPV-UCD1
(UCD1), FIPV Black High passage (BHP), FIPV-Black Low Passage
(BLP), FIPV-79-1146 and FECV-79-1683 have been previously
described[8,9,11-15].

Titration of virus infectivity

Feline coronaviruses were titered by either dilution to
endpoint of infectivity or by plaque assay. For dilution to
endpoint titrations, a standard tissue culture infectious dose
assay was used. Tissue culture infectious doses for 50% of the
cultures (TCID50) were calculated by the method of Reed and
Muench[16].

Plaque assays were performed in 6 or 12 well Costar cluster
plates (Costar, Cambridge, MA). Monolayers of fcwf-4 cells were
prepared in the plates. The culture medium was aspirated from the
wells, and serial five or ten-fold dilutions of virus in Hank's
balanced salt solution were inoculated onto the cultures. The
inocula were adsorbed for 45 minutes at 37 degrees C, with
occasional rocking. At the end of the adsorption period, the cultures were overlaid with medium containing 0.5% Noble agar and
incubated at 37 degrees C for 1 to 5 days. Overlay medium was
then removed, the monolayer rinsed with water, and stained with
crystal violet.

Strains UCD1, BLP, BHP, 79-1146 and 79-1683 of feline coronavirus were cultured and plaque picked three times under 0.5%
agar. After the third pick, the virus was inoculated onto monolayers of fcwf-4 cells, allowed to replicate until CPE became
apparent and then freeze-thawed at -70 degrees C twice. Clarified
culture supernatants were aliquoted and stored at -70 degrees C
for later use as stock virus.

Enzyme-linked immunosorbent assay (ELISA)

An indirect method of ELISA was used for the detection of
coronavirus antigen at various stages in the purification. This
assay was performed essentially as previously described by
Osterhaus et al[17] and Horzinek et al[10].

Protein determinations

The Coomassie Blue dye binding method of Bradford[18] was
adapted for use in 96 well round bottom microplates.

Metabolic radiolabeling of virus

Confluent monolayers of fcwf-4 cells were prepared in

plastic cell culture flasks (Costar, Cambridge, MA). The
medium was removed and the cultures were inoculated with a 1:5
dilution of the appropriate stock virus. The virus was
adsorbed at 37 degrees C for 45 minutes with occasional rocking. The inocula were then removed, and Eagle's MEM containing
25% normal concentration of amino acids and 2% dialyzed FBS was
added (10 ml/75 cm^2). The cultures were incubated for 4 hours
at 37 degrees C, after which time 2 uCi/ml of [3H] amino acids
was added to the medium. The cultures were harvested soon
after CPE was apparent.

Virus purification

Virus was purified by polyethylene glycol precipitation, a
discontinuous sucrose gradient centrifugation step and
isopycnic centrifugation in a 20-50 percent (wt/wt) linear
sucrose gradient essentially as described by Sturman et al[19].

SDS - polyacrylamide gel electrophoresis (SDS-PAGE)

Polyacrylamide gradient slab gels (8-16%), with 3%
stacking gels, were run using the discontinuous system of
Laemmli[20]. The acrylamide gradient was stablized during
pouring with glycerol. Samples were disrupted in treatment
buffer for 15 minutes at 25 degrees C. The final concentration
of the components of the sample treatment buffer were 62.5 mM
Tris, 2% SDS, 2% 2-mercaptoethanol, 10% glycerol, 0.01%
bromophenol blue, pH 6.8. The gels were electrophoresed at 15
mA per gel. Molecular weights were determined using a series
of eight molecular weight standards (200kd - 14.4kd, Bio Rad,
Richmond, CA).

Radioactivity profiles were generated by electrophoresing
the proteins of metabolically labeled purified virus in a 1.5
mm thick 25 cm long SDS-polyacrylamide gel. The appropriate
lane of the slab gel was cut from the gel and sliced
horizontally to generate 1.5 cm x .15 cm x .4 cm pieces. The
gel fractions were digested at 37 degrees C for 2 hours with
0.4 ml of NCS tissue solubilizer (9 parts NCS: 1 part water,
Amersham Corp., Arlington Heights, IL). Ten milliliters of 2
parts PCS: 1 part xylene was used as scintillation fluid.
Disintegrations per minute were calculated from counts per minute using the external standard channels ratio method.

Immunoblots

The electrophoretic transfer of proteins from polyacrylamide gels to nitrocellulose paper and the immunologic
detection of the blotted proteins (immunoblotting) was
performed similar to the method of Towbin et al[21]. Serum

samples were diluted 1:50 in dilution buffer consisting of 0.15
M NaCl, 0.05 M Tris, pH 7.4, 0.005 M EDTA, 0.1% bovine serum
albumin and 0.05% tween 20. 125_I labeled rabbit anti-feline
IgG was prepared by the chloramine T method[22] and used at a
final concentration of 1 - 5 x 10^5 cpm/ml in dilution buffer.

RESULTS AND DISCUSSION

Plaque assay of feline coronaviruses

Plaques produced by 79-1146 and 79-1683 could readily be
observed 2 days post infection, while UCD1, BLP and BHP usually
took up to 5 days to become large enough to be viewed without
the microscope.   Plaque size varied considerably between
strains but was consistent for each strain. UCD1 and BLP
produced small plaques, about 1-2 mm 5 days post-infection.
FIPV-BHP which originated from FIPV-BLP stocks, but was
passaged in cell culture more than 50 times, has the ability to
form slightly larger plaques (3mm in 5 days). FIPV-79-1146 and
FECV-79-1683 produced much larger plaques, > 3mm 2 days post
infection (Figure 1).   Early CPE produced by the five strains
consisted of syncytia formation, while later CPE was
characterized by rounding of polykaryons and detachment from
the plastic substrate (Figure 2).   Titers of the stock virus
also varied between strains: UCD1 and BLP having low titers
(<10^4 pfu/ml), BHP and 79-1146 having moderate titers (about
10^5 pfu/ml) and 79-1683 having the highest titer (>10^6 pfu/ml).

The results of the plaque assay of the five strains of
feline coronavirus we have investigated indicate a great
difference in their plaque forming characteristics.   Two
strains, FIPV-UCD1 and FIPV-BLP, form small plaques and do not
replicate to high titer in the culture system used. FIPV-BHP
forms a slightly larger plaque and produces moderate titers of
virus.   The continuous passage of BHP has also caused it to
attenuate to the extent that it is no longer pathogenic to
cats[14]. Strains 79-1146 and 79-1683, on the other hand, form
large plaques and replicate to high titers. In culture without
agar overlay, these strains show extensive CPE 24 hours after
infection.   This is unlike the other feline coronavirus
isolates grown in monolayers without agar overlay. These other
isolates do not show CPE until at least 48 hours post
infection.   The CPE is then limited to small foci of infection
which does not appear to spread to other areas of the
monolayer, unless the infected cell cultures are passed.   This
may be due to the low multiplicities of infection (MOI) used,
since it is difficult to obtain MOIs greater than 0.002 for
these low titer virus strains. Another possible explanation is
that FIPV-UCD1 and the Black isolates are highly cell
associated, and that transmission to adjacent normal cells

occurs primarily via fusion with infected cells. On the other
hand, FIPV-79-1146 and FECV-79-1683 progeny virions may be more
freely released into the medium, thereby infecting cells in
more distant areas of the monolayer.

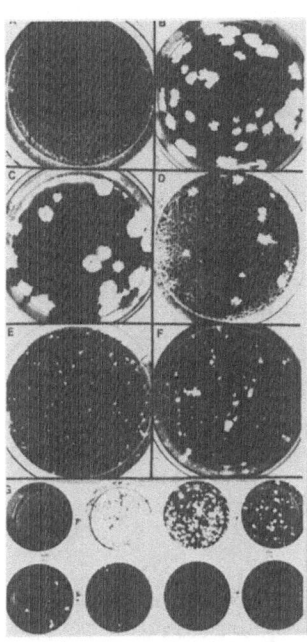

Figure 1.   Plaques pro-
duced by feline coronaviruses: uninfected monolayer of fcwf cells (A),
two   days   post-infection
FIPV-79-1146 (B) and FECV-
79-1683 (C),   five   days
post-infection   FIPV-BHP
(D),   FIPV-BLP   (E)   and
FIPV-UCD1 (F).   Plaque
assay of FIPV-UCD2, first
well   was   sham   inoculated
control, subsequent wells
inoculated   with   serial
five-fold dilutions (G).

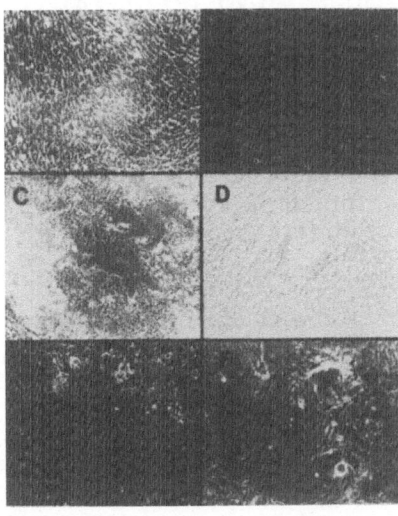

Figure 2.   Cytopathic
effect of feline coronaviruses: uninfected monolayer of fcwf cells (A),
FECV-79-1683;   18   hours
post infection (B) and 48
hours post-infection (C),
FIPV-UCD1; 48 hours post-
infection (D) and 5 days
post-inoculation   (E),
FIPV-BHP; five days post-
inoculation (F).

Purification of feline coronavirus from infected cell cultures

The procedure of Sturman et al 19 was used to purify feline coronavirus from infected cell cultures of feline origin. The virus routinely banded at 1.18 g/ml in isopycnic sucrose density gradients (Figure 3), which has been observed for other members of the Coronaviridae 23,24.

The recovery of infectious virus from a representative purification is summarized in Table 1. Despite the low percentage of infectious virus recovered from the band in the final centrifugation step (usually about 2%), the amount of infectious virus per milligram of protein was increased 30 fold. Using methods similar to those applied here, other investigators have reported a much higher percentage recovery of infectious particles after purification than the 2% observed for FIPV-BHP, i.e., 25% for TGEV[25]; 32% for hemagglutinating encephalomyelitis virus (HEV) of swine[26], and 66% for mouse hepatitis virus A59 (MHV-A59)[19]. This may be due the innate lability of the virion. Indeed, negative stain electron microscopy of FIPV-BHP and TGEV purified identically shows that many of the virions in the FIPV preparations are broken open, whereas virions in the TGEV preparations are uniformly intact[27].

Feline coronavirus polypeptides

The structural proteins that compose the virion of various coronaviruses have been analyzed by several laboratories[28]. In general, the coronavirus particle appears to have 4 to 7 proteins. A simple model for the structure of the coronavirion has been proposed by Sturman et al[19], who suggest that the major viral protein (N; apparent molecular weight (Mr)=50kd) is associated with the RNA. The nucleocapsid is surrounded by a lipid envelope containing a transmembrane integral glycoprotein (E1; Mr=23kd) which associates with the nucleocapsid in the interior of the virion while simultaneously exposing a portion of its structure to the external environment. The third and fourth major polypeptides are glycoproteins (E2; Mr=90kd and 180kd). The 180kd molecule is a dimer of the 90kd polypeptide, and together they comprise the characteristic peplomers of the coronavirion[29].

Radiolabeled polypeptides of UCD1 and BHP were analyzed by SDS-PAGE. Figures 4 and 5 showed that these two strains of feline coronavirus shared the 3 major polypeptides found in many members of the coronaviridae. The major polypeptide, with an apparent molecular weight of 45,000 daltons (45kd) is likely to be the nucleocapsid protein (N). The small polypeptide, which migrated as a broad band in the range of 33,000 to 27,000

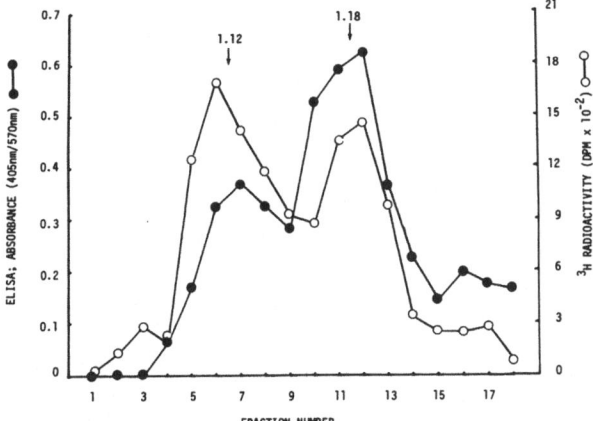

Figure 3. Enzyme-linked immunosorbent assay reactivities and ^{3}H radioactivities of fractions from a representative 20-50% (w/w) linear sucrose gradient used to purify metabolically radiolabeled FIPV-BHP.

daltons is probably the envelope protein (E1), while the large polypeptide, Mr of 210,000 daltons, is most likely the peplomer protein. At the top of the gel, a very large protein was sometimes observed. The molecular weight of this component was difficult to determine precisely, as the highest molecular weight standard used was 200kd, but it is estimated to be at least 400kd. A minor protein, Mr 42kd, was also reproducibly seen.

TABLE 1 - FIP virus purification and recovery of infectious virus.

Virus sample	Infectivity $(TCID_{50} \times 10^5/ml)$	Volume (ml)	% Recovery of infectivity	Total protein (mg)	$TCID_{50} \times 10^5$ mg of protein
Clarified infected cell culture super-natant	2.3	160	100	325	1.1
Polyethylene glycol precipitate	26	8	57	19.6	11
Interphase from 20/50% discontinuous sucrose gradient	18	3	15	1.87	29
Band from 20-50% continuous sucrose gradient $(1.175 - 1.19 \text{ g/cm}^3)$	3.5	2	2	0.23	30

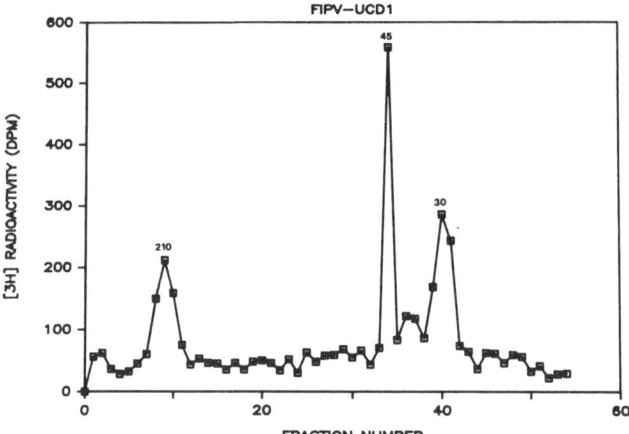

Figure 4. SDS-Polyacrylamide gel electrophoresis profile of ^{3}H amino acid labeled FIPV-UCD1. Numbers above the individual peaks represent molecular weight in kilodaltons.

The polypeptide structure of the feline coronaviruses was confirmed by coupling SDS-PAGE with the ability to detect resolved viral proteins immunologically once they were trans-ferred to nitrocellulose paper (immunoblots). Cell culture material which had been sham inoculated (no virus) and prepared

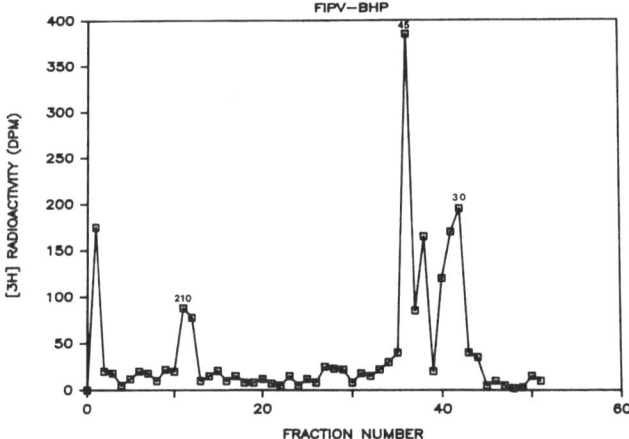

Figure 5. SDS-Polyacrylamide gel electrophoresis profile of ^{3}H amino acid labeled FIPV-BHP. Numbers above the individual peaks represent molecular weight in kilodaltons.

identically to feline coronavirus preparations was used as a virus negative control. Figure 6 shows the results of an immunoblot in which isopycnically banded FIPV-BHP was detected with various feline anti-coronavirus serum samples. Figures 7 through 9 represent the results of experiments in which five strains of feline coronavirus and sham inoculated cell preparations were electrophoresced in preparative gels, the separated proteins transferred to nitrocellulose and the polypeptides detected with serum samples from various cats. The viral antigen used to generate the blots in figures 7 through 9 was from the 20/50% interface of a discontinuous sucrose gradient. Table 2 summarizes the apparent molecular weights of the proteins for each strain. The nomenclature of Sturman et al[11] has been used to classify the polypeptides. The most prominent protein (N; Mr 45kd) was recognized by all serum samples used. The broad 30kd band (E1) seen in radioactivity profiles was resolved as a broad triplet. The precise nature of the relationship between the individual components of the E1 complex has not been investigated, but it is likely that differences in the glycosylation in the amino-terminal domain contributes to the polymorphism, as has been demonstrated by Stern et al[30] for the infectious bronchitis virus (IBV) E1 family.

The large 210kd peplomer protein was detected only when certain serum samples were used. Although the E2 polypeptide was easily seen in [^{3}H] SDS-PAGE profiles of metabolically labeled virus, it was barely detectable in the immunoblots. Three possibilities could contribute to this: (1) inefficient transfer to nitrocellulose paper during blotting, (2) lack of humoral response to this polypeptide by cats infected with feline coronaviruses or (3) loss of critical antigenic determinants during SDS-PAGE or electrophorectic transfer. The first possibility seems least likely, however, since Coomassie Blue staining of gels and amido black staining of nitrocellulose paper after blotting shows that the majority of even the larger molecular weight proteins have left the gel and bound to the nitrocellulose. Also of interest is the fact that no protein was seen which would serve as a likely candidate for a monomer E2 polypeptide as has been demonstrated in the murine coronavirus system[29].

Other proteins were also readily detected by this technique; Mr: 400kd, 190kd, 162kd, 76kd, 66kd, 57kd, 15kd, 11kd and 8kd. However, these are not likely to be viral polypeptides, because: 1) blots using sham inoculated culture material as antigen also contain bands of 190, 162, 76, 66 and 75kd (Figure 7), 2) infected animals' antibody responses to the 15, 11 and 8kd proteins do not increase through the course of infection (Figure 9) and (3) these proteins are not seen in metabolically labeled virus preparations (Figures 4 and 5).

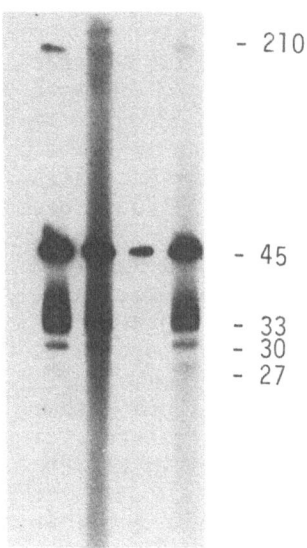

- 210

- 45

- 33
- 30
- 27

Figure 6. Immunoblot of highly purified FIPV-BHP from the 1.18 g/ml fraction of an isopyknic sucrose gradient, reacted with various feline serum samples. Values are apparent molecular weights in kilodaltons.

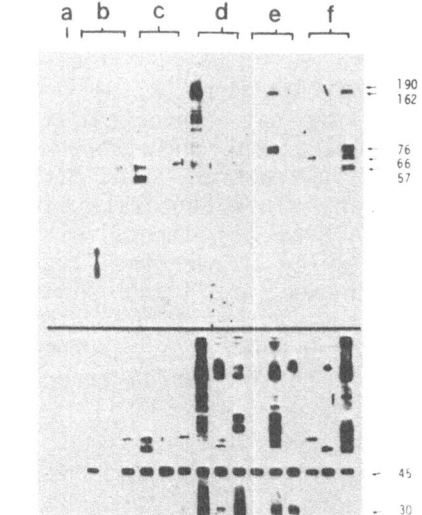

a b c d e f

A

190
162

76
66
57

B

- 45

- 30

Figure 7. Immunoblots of sham inoculated fcwf cell culture material (panel A) and FIPV-UCD1 inoculated culture material (panel B), reacted with serum samples from cats with the following natural histories: pre-infec- tion (a lane), died FIP; 79-1146 (b lanes), convalescent FECV; 79- 1683 (c lanes), con- valescent FIP; UCD1 (d lanes), died FIP; UCD1 (e lanes) and conva- lescent FECV; UCD1 (f lanes). Values are ap- parent molecular weights in kilodaltons.

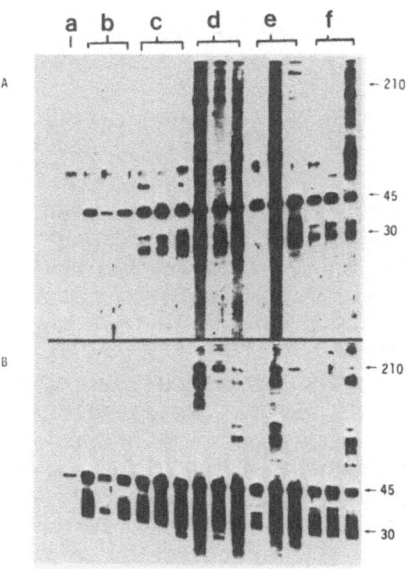

Figure 8. Immunoblots of FIPV-BLP (panel A) and FIPV-BHP (panel B) inoculated cell culture material, reacted with serum samples from cats with the following natural histories: pre-infection (a lane), died FIP: 79-1146 (b lanes), convalescent FECV; 79-1683 (c lanes), convalescent FIP; UCD1 (d lanes), died FIP; UCD1 (e lanes) and convalescent FECV; UCD1 (f lanes). Values are apparent molecular weights in kilodaltons.

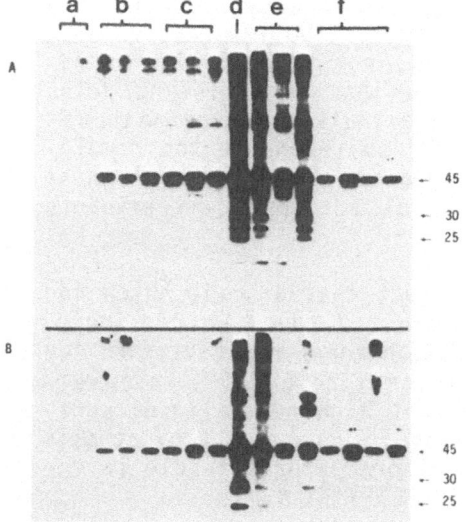

Figure 9. Immunoblots of FIPV-79-1146 (panel A) and FECV-79-1683 (panel B) inoculated cell culture material, reacted with serum samples from cats with the following natural histories: pre-infection (a lanes), died FIP; 79-1146 (b lanes), convalescent FECV; 79-1683 (c lanes), convalescent FIP; UCD1 (d lane), died FIP; UCD1 (e lanes) and convalescent FECV; UCD1 (f lanes). Values are apparent molecular weights in kilodaltons.

It therefore appears that the protein structure of the feline coronaviruses is similar to other members of the Coronaviridae[28].

Comparison of feline serological response to various feline coronaviruses

Serum samples were collected from cats which had been inoculated pronasally with various strains of feline coronavirus[9,13,14]. Figures 7 through 9 show the results of immunoblots using convalescent or pre-mortem serum samples from cats infected with the FIPV UCD1, FECV UCD, 79-1146 and 79-1683 to detect homologous and heterologous antigen. Table 3 summarizes the cross-reactivity between heterologous and homologous feline sera and viral antigen preparations. The humoral response of cats to the individual polypeptides of homologous and heterologous virus preparations, as determined by immunoblotting, appeared to be fairly consistent. Animals infected with FIPV-UCD1, FECV-UCD, FIPV-79-1146 and FECV-79-1683 all had serum antibodies which recognized the N and E1 proteins of all coronavirus strains used, i.e., FIPV-UCD1, FIPV-BLP, FIPV-BHP, 79-1146 and 79-1683. However, the anti-FIPV-UCD1 and anti-FECV-UCD1 samples tended to react more strongly with all of the virus strains. This is most likely due to the fact that these samples had higher titers to coronaviral antigen, as determined by indirect fluorescent and ELISA antibody tests (data not shown).

On the other hand, most animals had very low or undetectable levels of antibodies to the E2 peplomer protein. The only animals that responded to this polypeptide were those infected with FIPV-UCD1 and FECV-UCD1, and these antibodies reacted only with FIPV-UCD1, FIPV-BLP and FIPV-BHP, not with 79-1146 or 79-1683. This does not necessarily indicate more distant relationship of these strains, because animals infected with 79-1146 and 79-1683 also did not appear to recognize the homologous E2 antigen. This may be due to the low titers of these serum samples or to loss of critical antigenic determinants during SDS disruption of antigen.

Of particular interest is the fact that animals which had died of feline infectious peritonitis and those we considered to be immune to FIP showed comparable humoral reactivity to the individual polypeptides of the virion (Table 3). This evidence, along with the observation that high neutralizing antibody titers to FIPV are not protective, supports the hypothesis that cell mediated immunity plays a more important role in the recovery of a cat from infection with FIPV[14,15].

Table 2.   Apparent molecular weights of FIPV, FECV and TGEV polypeptides. Values represent kilodaltons, NS = not seen.

| | POLYPEPTIDE | | |
STRAIN	N	E1	E2
FIPV-UCD1	45	32	210
		30	
FIPV-BLP	45	33	210
		30	
		27	
FIPV-BHP	45	33	210
		30	
		27	
79-1146	45	30	NS
		27	
		25	
79-1683	45	30	NS
		27	
		25	
TGEV (Miller)	48	31	200
		27	

Table 3.   Summary of cross-reactivity of serum samples from cats infected with various strains of feline coronavirus to heterologous and homologous viral antigen preparations. Convalescent samples were from cats having recovered from experimental infection. Pre-mortem samples were taken from cats in the terminal stages of FIP (experimentally induced) just prior to euthanasia. Cross-reactivity was broken down into 6 categories, by density of the individual bands on the autoradiographs: ++++ = greatest reactivity, 0 = no reactivity.

| | | | Natural history of serum sample | | |
Viral Antigen	Died 79-1146	Conval. 79-1683	Conval. FIPV-UCD1	Died FIPV-UCD1	Conval. FECV-UCD1
79-1146					
N	++	++	++++	+++	++
E1	+	++	+++	+++	+
E2	0	0	0	0	0
79-1683					
N	+	++	+++	+++	+
E1	0	+	++	++	+
E2	0	0	0	0	0
FIPV-UCD1					
N	+++	+++	+++	+++	+++
E1	+	++	++	++	+
E2	0	0	+	+/-	0
FIPV-BHP					
N	+++	+++	+++	+++	+++
E1	++	++	+++	++	++
E2	0	0	++	++	+
FIPV-BLP					
N	++	+++	+++	+++	+++
E1	+	++	+++	+++	++
E2	0	0	+	+	+

REFERENCES

1. Ward, J.M. 1970. Morphogenesis of a virus in cats with ex-
    perimental feline infectious peritonitis. Virol. 41:191-194.
2. Zook, B.C., King, N. W., Robison, R.L. and McCombs, H.L.
    1968. Ultrastructural evidence for the viral etiology of
    feline infectious peritonitis. Path. Vet. 5:91-95.
3. Ward, J.M., Munn, R.J., Gribble, D.H. and Dungworth, D.L.
    1968. An observation of feline infectious peritonitis. Vet.
    Record. 83:416-417.
4. Pedersen, N.C. 1976. Morphologic and physical character-
    istics of feline infectious peritonitis virus and its growth
    in autochthonous peritoneal cell cultures. Amer. J. Vet.
    Res. 37:567-572.
5. Horzinek, M.C., Osterhaus, A.D.M.E. and Ellens, D.J. 1977.
    Feline infectious peritonitis. Zbl. Vet. Med. B. 24:398-405.
6. Reynolds, D.J., Garwes, D.J. and Gaskell, C.J. 1977. Detec-
    tion of transmissible gastroenteritis neutralizing antibody
    in cats. Arch. Virol. 55:77.
7. Pedersen, N.C., Ward, J. and Mengeling, W.L. 1978. Antigenic
    relationship of the feline infectious peritonitis virus to
    coronaviruses of other species. Arch. Virol. 58:45-53.
8. McKeirnan, A.J., Evermann, J.F., Hargis, A., Miller LM, Ott
    RL: 1981. Isolation of feline coronaviruses from two cats
    with diverse disease manifestations. Fel. Prac. 11(3):16-20.
9. Pedersen, N.C., Boyle, J.F. and Floyd, K., Fudge, A. and
    Barker, J. 1981b. An enteric coronavirus infection of cats
    and its relationship to feline infectious peritonitis. Amer.
    J. Vet. Res. 42(3):368-377.
10. Horzinek, M.C., Lutz, H. and Pedersen, N.C. 1982. Antigenic
    relationship among homologous structural polypeptides of
    porcine, feline and canine coronavirus. Infec. Immun.
    37:1148-1155.
11. Black, J.W. 1980. Recovery and in vitro cultivation of a
    coronavirus from lab-induced cases of feline infectious peri-
    tonitis. Vet. Med./Sm. Anim. Clin. 75(5):811-814.
12. Evermann, J.F., Baumgartener, L., Ott, R.L., Davis, E.V. and
    McKeirnan, A.J. 1981. Characterization of a feline infecti-
    ous peritonitis virus isolate. Vet. Pathol. 18:256-265.
13. Pedersen, N.C., Boyle, J.F. and Floyd, K. 1981a. Infection
    studies in kittens, using feline infectious peritonitis virus
    propagated in cell culture. Amer. J. Vet. Res. 42(3):363-367.
14. Pedersen, N.C. and Black, J.W. 1983. Attempted immunization
    of cats against feline infectious peritonitis using either
    avirulent live virus of sublethal amounts or virulent
    virus. Am. J. Vet. Res. 44:229-234.
15. Pedersen, N.L., Black, J.W., Boyle, J.F., Everman, J.F.,
    McKeirnan, A.J. and Ott, R.L.: 1983. Pathogenic differences
    between various coronavirus isolates. This volume.

16. Reed, L.J. and Muench, H. 1983. A simple method of estimating fifty percent endpoints. Amer. J. Hygiene. 27:493-497.

17. Osterhaus, A., Kroon, A. and Wirahadiredja, R. 1979. ELISA for the serology of FIP virus. Vet. Quarterly. 1:59-62.

18. Bradford, M.M. 1976. A rapid and sensitive method for the quantitation of protein utilizing the principle of protein-dye binding. Anal. Biochem. 72:248.

19. Sturman, L.S., Holmes, K.V. and Behnke, J. 1980. Isolation of coronavirus envelope glycoproteins and interaction with the viral nucleocapsid. J. Virol. 33(1):449-462.

20. Laemmli, U.K. 1970. Cleavage of structural proteins during the assembly of the head of bacteriophage T4. Nature. 227:680-685.

21. Towbin, H., Staehelin, T. and Gordon, J. 1979. Electrophoretic transfer of proteins from polyacrylamide gels to nitrocellulose sheets: Procedure and some applications. Proc. Nat. Acad. Sci. 76(9):4350-4354.

22. Garvey, J.S., Cremer, N.E. and Sussdorf, D.H., Eds. 1977. 1251 or 1311 labeled proteins. In: Methods in Immunology. W.A. Benjamin, Inc., Massachusetts.

23. Robb, J.A. and Bond, C.W. 1979. Coronaviridae. In Comprehensive Virology. Vol. 14, pp 193-247. Edited by H. Fraenkel-Conrat and R. R. Wagner. New York: Plenum Press.

24. Tyrrell, D.A.J., Tyrrell D.A.J., Alexander D.J., Almeida J.D., Cunningham C.H., Easterday B.C., Garwes D.J., Hierholzer J.C., Kapikian A., MacNaughton M.R. and McIntosh K.: 1978. Coronaviridae: Second report. Intervirology. 10:321-328.

25. Garwes, D.J. and Pocock, D.H. 1975. The polypeptide structure of transmissible gastroenteritis virus. J. Gen. Virol. 29:25-34.

26. Pocock, D.H. and Garwes, D.J. 1977. The polypeptides of hemagglutinating encephalomyelitis virus and isolated subviral particles. J. Gen. Virol. 37:487-499.

27. Boyle, J.F. 1982. Ph.D. dissertation: Aspects of the pathogenesis and biology of feline infectious peritonitis virus and feline enteric coronavirus. University of California, Davis.

28. Mahy, B.W.J. 1981. Biochemistry of coronaviruses 1980. In: Biochemistry and Biology of Coronaviruses. V. ter Meulen, S. Siddell and H. Wedge, Eds. Plenum Press. New York.

29. Sturman, L.S. and Holmes, K.V. 1977. Characterization of a coronavirus. II. Glycoproteins of the viral envelope: Tryptic peptide analysis. Virol. 77:650-660.

30. Stern, D.F., Burgess, L. and Stefton, B. 1982. Structural analysis of virion proteins of the avian coronavirus infectious bronchitis virus. J. Virol. 42(1): 208-219.

ASSEMBLY OF 229E VIRIONS IN HUMAN EMBRYONIC LUNG FIBROBLASTS AND
EFFECTS OF INHIBITION OF GLYCOSYLATION AND GLYCOPROTEIN TRANSPORT
ON THIS PROCESS

M.C. Kemp[1,2,3], A. Harrison[4], J.C. Hierholzer[4] and
J.S. Burks[1,2,3]

[1]Center for Neurological Diseases/Rocky Mountian Multiple
Sclerosis Center, [2]Veterans Administration Medical Center
[3]University of Colorado School of Medicine, Denver,
Colorado. Division of Viral Diseases, [4]Centers for
Disease Control, Atlanta, Georgia, U.S.A.

Assembly of virions in 229E infected cells were studied along
with the effect(s) of an inhibitor of glycosylation (tunicamycin)
and an inhibitor of glycoprotein transport (monensin) on this process. The results of these studies are summarized herein.

There were no significant differences observed between untreated and monensin- or tunicamycin-treated cells early in the
infectious cycle. One hour post infection (PI) virus particles were
seen in close proximity to the plasma membrane and projections from
the viral envelope, presumably viral glycoproteins, appeared to be
making membrane contact. A few particles were seen to be in various
stages of being engulfed by a process of viropexis. By two hours
PI a small number of intact spherical enveloped particles
(80-150nm) were seen within intracytoplasmic vacuoles, some,
however, were oval or dumb-bell shaped. All particles, consisted of
a double membrane surrounding a core of varying electron density.
Densely stained viral particles were observed in lysosomes in
untreated and treated cells, but lysosomal activity was more
pronounced in treated cells.

At 6 hours PI when viral protein synthesis was first detected
(1) and before viral assembly was observed, roughly circular,
electron lucent structures with dense limiting membranes (2) were
seen in untreated and treated cells.

Budding of virus particles from the intracytoplasmic membranes
was first observed in all cells at 8hr PI. In tunicamycin treated

149

cells, aggregation of ribosomes and increased numbers of virions within the golgi complex were observed. Virions assembled in tunicamycin treated-cells were enveloped but the particles appeared smooth, whereas, in untreated or monensin-treated cells delicate projections radiated from the viral membrane.

Viral particles assembled in monensin-treated cells contained translucent cores. Similar particles were observed in untreated and tunicamycin-treated cells but they were far less numerous. Particles having a translucent core are not devoid of nucleic acid since the ribonucleoprotein complex was seen underlying the capsid structure. It is probable that the translucent particles are immature virions.

Vacuolization of all cells increased with time. But, monensin caused the formation of large dilated vesicles, which did not contain any viral particles.

At 12hr. PI cytoplasmic inclusions similar to those described by Oshiro et al (3), composed of densely staining particles within a granular matrix and enclosed by a double membrane were seen in cells.

As early as 12hr PI in untreated cells, large virus containing vacuoles could be seen to be fusing with the plasma membrane and in the process of rupturing, thereby, releasing virions. Numerous virions were observed in extracellular spaces surrounding untreated cells. But, in treated cells membrane bound aggregates of virions were observed in the extracellular spaces. By 24hr PI many untreated cells were lysed thus releasing virus. Of particular interest was the large accumulation of spherical and dumb-bell shaped particles in the perinuclear space late in the infection.

From these studies it may be concluded that glycosylation and glycoprotein transport effect the agress of 229E virions but not the assembly.

REFERENCES

1.   M.C. Kemp, A. Harrison, J.C. Hierholzer, and J.S. Burks,
     Characterization of Viral Proteins Synthesized in 229E In-
     fected Cells and Effect(s) of Inhibition of Glycosylation and
     Glycoprotein Transport (See these proceedings).
2.   M.C. Kemp, A. Harrison, J.C. Hierholzer, and J.S. Burks,
     Electron Lucent Structures Induced by Coronaviruses (See these
     proceedings).
3.   L.S. Ohiro, J.H. Schieble, and E.H. Lennette, Electron Micro-
     scopic Studies of Coronavirus, J. gen. Virol 12:161(1971).

AMPHOTERICIN INHIBITS CORONAVIRUS SD, SK AND A59 GROWTH

B.L. DeVald, J.C. Gerdes, J.S. Burks, and M.C. Kemp

Center for Neurological Diseases/Rocky Mountain Multiple
Sclerosis Center, Veterans Administration Medical Center
University of Colorado School of Medicine
Denver, Colarado, U.S.A.

Fungizone (AMB) a clinical formulation of Amphotericin B
has been widely used as an antifungal agent. The synthetically
derived analogue Amphotericin B Methyl Ester (AME) has a similar
antifungal activity.

The biological effects of polene macrolide antimicrobial
agents (AMB, AME) depend on their high affinity for sterols in
the cell membrane. Therefore, they have been shown to inhibit
growth of certain enveloped viruses. Antiviral activity was not
demonstrated against non-enveloped viruses (2).

In our viral isolation studies, we routinely collected human
brain tissue at autopsy in cold sterile Hanks balance salt solution (HBSS) with double strength penicillin and streptomycin. To
decrease the potential of fungal contamination, we began adding AMB
at 25 mcg/ml (the manufacturers recommended concentration) to HBSS
at the time of collection of brain at autopsy. We have never added
AMB or AME to our tissue culture. Before we began adding AMB to
HBSS, coronaviruses were isolated while working with human tissue
in 2 of 4 autopsies. After adding AMB to the isolation protocol,
20 consecutive autopsies on MS patients were negative for viral
isolation. The possibility of inhibition of coronavirus growth by
AMB or AME was explored in this study.

Coronaviruses SD, SK and A59 (200 pfu/ml) were mixed with AMB
or AME in equal volumes of media with or without fetal calf serum.
The antifungal agents were diluted to a final concentrations of 1,
10, 25, 50 or 100 mcg/ml. All mixtures of virus and antifungal
agents were assayed in triplicate. A 50% reduction in the number of

virus plaques by the antifungal agents was considered to be the minimal inhibitory concentration (MIC).

Using AMB and AME in the tissue culture system, inhibition of all three coronaviruses was noted when the cultures were incubated with serum free medium (Table 1). The addition of 2% fetal calf serum, eliminated inhibition of SK and A59. However, SD growth was still inhibited at MIC of 10 mcg/ml.

Since fungal contamination is an inherent problem associated with primary viral isolation studies using autopsy material, the choice and concentration of AMB or AME must be considered. As we have demonstrated, AME and AMB inhibit coronavirus SD, SK and A59 multiplication. Therefore, we have eliminated these agents from our autopsy tissue procurement procedure.

TABLE I

MINIMAL INHIBITORY CONCENTRATION

VIRUS	% SERUM	AMPHOTERICIN B	AMPHOTERICIN B METHYLESTER
A59	0	100mcg/ml	25mcg/ml
SD	0	1mcg/ml	1mcg/ml
SK	0	1mcg/ml	1mcg/ml
A59	2	No Inhibition	No Inhibition
SD	2	No Inhibition	10mcg/ml
SK	2	No Inhibition	No Inhibition
SD	10		No Inhibition

REFERENCES

1. Bonner, D.P., W. Mechlinski and C.P. Schaffner. 1972 Polyene Macrolide Derivatives I-III. J. Antiobio. XXV: 256-262.
2. Stevens, N.M., C.G. Engle, P.B. Fisher, W. Mechlinski, and C.P. Schaffner. 1975. In Vitro Antiherpetic Activity of Water Soluble Amphotericin B Methyl Ester. Arch. Virol. 48:391-394.

This work was supported by the Kroc Foundation and the Veterans Administration.

ELECTRON LUCENT STRUCTURES INDUCED BY CORONAVIRUSES

M.C. Kemp[1,2,3], A. Harrison[4], J.C. Hierholzer[4], and
J.S. Burks[1,2,3]

[1]Center for Neurological Diseases/Rocky Mountain Multiple Sclerosis Center, [2]Veterans Administration Medical
Center, [3]University of Colorado School of Medicine,
Denver, Colorado. [4]Division of Viral Diseases, Centers
for Disease Control, Atlanta, Georgia, U.S.A.

Viral inclusion bodies have long been considered pathognomo-
ic. Coronaviruses cause the formation of cytoplasmic inclusions
consisting of densely staining particles contained within a
granular matrix enclosed by a double membrane (1). During studies
on the assembly of 229E in human embryomic lung fibroblasts
roughly circular electron lucent structures with dense limiting
membranes, sometimes empty but frequently containing net-like
beaded strands, were seen in the cytoplasm of infected cells that
differed from the previously described inclusions. These
structures vary in size from 300-900nm in diameter (Fig. 1) and
appear at approximately 6hr post-infection (PI), i.e. at a time
when viral protein synthesis is initiated (2) and before the
assembly of virions (3).

Similar structures were seen in suckling mouse brain infected
with coronaviruses OC-43 (Fig. 2), OC-38, calf diarrhia (Fig. 3)
and mouse hepatitis. These structures were also seen in 3T3 cells
infected with SK virus, a coronavirus isolated while working with
multiple sclerosis autopsy brain tissue (4).

Formation of the electron lucent structures was not inhibited
by incubation of the cells with an inhibitor of glycosylation
(tunicamycin) or glycoprotein transport (monensin). The structures
may correspond to the CPV-1 structures described by Grimley et al
(5) for Semliki Forest virus infected cells.

Demonstration of such structures in infected tissues may

prove useful for the diagnosis of coronavirus infection.

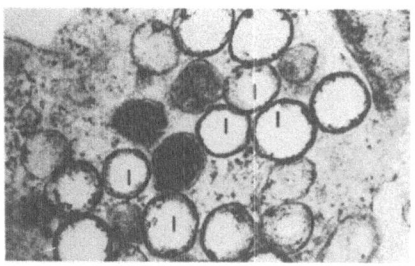

Figure 1: Electron micrograph of 229E
infected cells. Virions located in
lysosomes (L) are surrounded by
numerous electron lucent structures
(1) with dense limiting membranes.

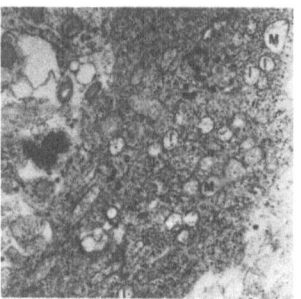

Figure 2: Suckling mouse
brain infected with OC-43.
Numerous electron lucent
structures (1) are distri-
tributed throughout the
cytoplasm and are easily
differentiated from
mitochondria (M).

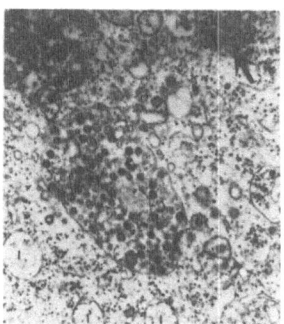

Figure 3: An electron micrograph of
calf diarrhia virus infected
suckling mouse brain. Electron
lucent structures (1) containing
net-like beads can be seen. Arrow
indicates the inclusion structures
described by Oshiro et al (1).

REFERENCES

1. L.S. Oshiro, J.H. Schieble, and E.H. Lennette, Electron Micro-
    scopic Studies of Coronavirus, J. Gen Virol. 12:161(1971).
2. M.C. Kemp, J.C. Hierholzer, A. Harrison, and J.S. Burks,
    Characterization of Viral Proteins Synthesized in 229E
    Infected Cells and Effect(s) of Inhibition of Glycosylcation
    and Glycoprotein Transport on This Process (See these
    proceedings).
3. M.C. Kemp, A. Harrison, J.C. Hierholzer, and J.S. Burks, As-
    sembly of 229E Virions in Human Embryonic Lung Fibroblasts
    and Effects of Inhibition of Glycosylation and Glycoprotein
    Transport on This Process (See these proceedings).
4. J.S. Burks, B. L. DeVald, L.D. Jankovsky, and J.C. Gerdes,
    Two Coronaviruses Isolated from Central Nervous System of Two
    Multiple Sclerosis Patients, Science 209:933(1980).
5. P.M. Grimley, I. K. Berezesky, and R.M. Friedman, Cytoplasmic
    Structures Associated with an Arbovirus Infection: Loci of
    Viral Ribonucleic Acid Synthesis, J. Virol. 2:1326(1968).

CLONING AND SEQUENCING THE NUCLEOCAPSID AND E1 GENES
OF CORONAVIRUS

John Armstrong, Sjef Smeekens[+1], Willy Spaan[+],
Peter Rottier[+] and Ben van der Zeijst[+]

European Molecular Biology Laboratory
Postfach 10.2209, 69 Heidelberg, FRG
[+]Institute of Virology, Veterinary Faculty, State University
of Utrecht, 3508 TD Utrecht, The Netherlands
[1]Present address: Molecular Cell Biology Group
State University of Utrecht, Padualaan 8, 3808 CH Utrecht

INTRODUCTION

The widespread medical and veterinary importance of Coronaviruses provided the initial reason for studying these viruses at the molecular level. However, two unusual features of the viral life cycle are of particular interest for "pure" molecular biology. First, the intracellular budding site of Coronaviruses, apparently associated with the restricted intracellular distribution of the E1 glycoprotein[1] suggests that this protein may provide a model to study the transport and sorting of membrane proteins of the endoplasmic reticulum and Golgi apparatus. Secondly, the unusual "nested set" structure of the viral RNA's[2,3,4,5](Spaan et al., this volume) implies a replication mechanism unlike that of other RNA viruses.

With the aim of learning more about both these aspects of Coronavirus molecular biology, we have prepared cDNA clones whose sequences span the nucleocapsid and E1 genes of MHV-A59.

MATERIALS AND METHODS

Preparation of cDNA from mRNA of MHV-A59-infected cells, cloning and sequence determination were as described previously[6]. Further clones were isolated from the same cDNA preparation by digestion with the restriction enzymes BalI (BRL) or RsaI (New England Biolabs) and ligation to the plasmid vector pEMBL8[7]. Single-stranded DNA from recombinant clones was prepared according to Dente et al.[7] but using wild-type phage fd for superinfection.

RESULTS

Corrected sequence of the nucleocapsid gene

Comparison of the original sequence of the nucleocapsid gene[6] with that of the corresponding gene from MHV JHM strain (Skinner and Siddell, this volume) revealed, among other differences, an apparent change of reading frame between nucleotides 478 and 795 (numbering as 6); two of the three possible reading frames lack terminator codons throughout this region. Re-examination of the sequencing autoradiograms, however, clearly shows that the apparent difference is due to two errors in the sequence reported for A59; the corrected sequence includes an additional C between bases 477 and 478, and lacks the G at position 795. The resulting amino acid sequence of the nucleocapsid is shown in Fig.1.

MSFVPGQENAGGRSSSVNRAGNGILKKTTWADQTERGPNNQNRGRRNQPKQTATTQPNSGSVVPHY

SWFSGIFTQFQKGKEFQFAEGQGVPIANGIPASEQKGYWYRHNRRSFKTPDGQQKQLLPRWYFYYL

GTGPHAGASYGDSIEGVFWVANSQADINTRSDIVERDPSSHEAIPIRFAPGTVLPQGFYVEGSGRS

APASRSGSRSQSRGPNNRARSSSNQRQPASTVKPDMAEEIAALVLAKLGKDAGQPKQVIKQSAKKV

RQKILNKPRQKRIPNKQCPVQQCFGKRGPNQNFGGSEMLKLGTSDPQFPILAELAPTVGAFFFGSK

LELVKKNSGGADEPTKDVYELQYSGAVRFDSTLPGFETIMKVLNENLNAYQKDGGADVVSPKPQRK

GRRQAQEKKDEVDNVSVAKPKSSVQRNVSERLTPEDRSLLAQILDDGVVPDGLEDDSNV

Figure 1.   Amino-acid sequence of MHV-A59 nucleocapsid protein.

Sequence of the E1 gene

Digestion of cDNA with the restriction enzymes BalI and RsaI gave clones whose sequences encompassed the E1 gene (Fig.2). Clone R55 contains part of the leader region common to the 5' end of all the viral RNA's (Spaan et al., this volume). Clones R55 and PR9 have subsequently been shown to be adjacent, by subcloning and sequencing of a full-length E1 clone (Niemann, this volume). A previously unidentified clone, F11, also comes from within the E1 gene (Fig.2).

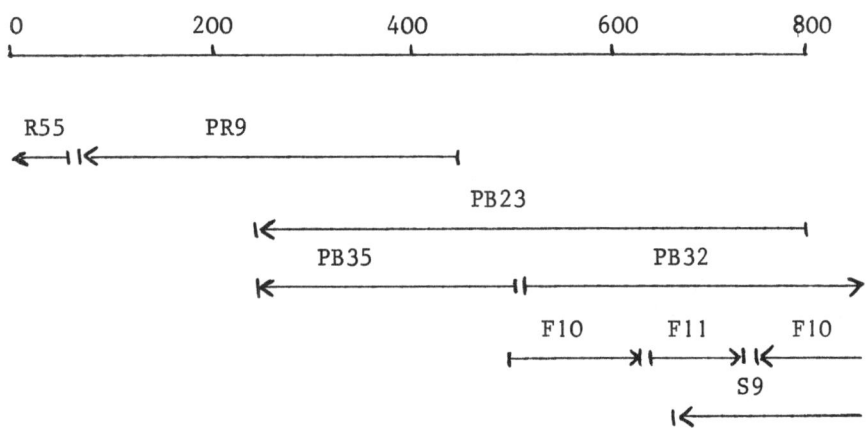

Figure 2.   Arrangement of clones spanning the E1 gene of MHV-A59.
            Arrows show the direction in which the sequence was
            determined. Numbering is as Fig. 3. cDNA was digested
            with RsaI (R), BalI (B), Fnu DII (F) or S1 nuclease (S),
            and cloned in M13 mp8 or pEMBL8 (P).

    Analysis of clones from the nucleocapsid region had revealed
two, S9 and F10, whose sequences diverged at their 5' ends at almost
exactly the inferred site of fusion between the leader sequence and
the nucleocapsid-coding region of RNA7[6], suggesting that one of these
clones originated from RNA7 and the other from a larger RNA. Comparison of the two sequences with those from the E1 gene, and with
sequences determined directly from RNA7 and the viral genome (Spaan
et al., this volume) shows that clone S9 originates from one of the
six larger RNA's and covers the region from the 3' end of the E1
gene to the 5' end of the nucleocapsid gene. Clone F10, however,
represents a fusion of an internal portion of the E1 gene to the 5'
end of the nucleocapsid, in opposite orientations (Fig.2); presumably it arose from artefactual synthesis of a "third" DNA strand
during synthesis of the second strand of the cDNA.

    The sequence of the E1 gene, and the translated amino acid
sequence of the protein are shown in Fig.3.

```
                                              M  S  S  T  T  Q
ACCTCTCAACTCTAAAACTCTTGTAGTTTAAATCTAATCCAAACATTATGAGTAGTACTACTCA

  A  P  E  P  V  Y  Q  W  T  A  D  E  A  V  Q  F  L  K  E  W  N
GGCCCCAGAGCCCGTCTATCAATGGACGGCCGACGAGGCAGTTCAATTCCTTAAGGAATGGAAC
                                    40
  F  S  L  G  I  I  L  L  F  I  T  I  I  L  Q  F  G  Y  T  S  R
TTCTCGTTGGGCATTATACTACTCTTTATTACTATCATACTACAGTTCGGTTACACGAGCCGTA
                                          60
  S  M  F  I  Y  V  V  K  M  I  I  L  W  L  M  W  P  L  T  I  V  L
GCATGTTTATTTATGTTGTGAAAATGATAATCTTGTGGTTAATGTGGCCACTGACTATTGTTTT
                                    80
  C  I  F  N  C  V  Y  A  L  N  N  V  Y  L  G  F  S  I  V  F  I
GTGTATTTTCAATTGCGTGTATGCGCTAAATAATGTGTATCTTGGATTTTCTATAGTGTTTACT
                              100
  I  V  S  I  V  I  W  I  M  Y  F  V  N  S  I  R  L  F  I  R  T
ATAGTGTCCATTGTAATCTGGATTATGTATTTTGTTAATAGCATAAGGTTGTTTATCAGGACTG
                        120
  G  S  W  W  S  F  N  P  E  T  N  N  L  M  C  I  D  M  K  G  T  V
GTAGCTGGTGGAGCTTCAACCCCGAAACAAACAACCTTATGTGTATAGATATGAAAGGTACCGT
                  140
  Y  V  R  P  I  I  E  D  Y  H  T  L  T  A  T  I  I  R  G  H  L
GTATGTTAGACCCATTATTGAGGATTACCATACACTAACAGCCACTATTATTCGTGGCCACCTC
            160
  Y  M  Q  G  V  K  L  G  T  G  F  S  L  S  D  L  P  A  Y  V  T
TACATGCAAGGTGTTAAGCTAGGCACCGGTTTCTCTTTGTCTGACTTGCCCGCTTATGTTACAG
            180
  V  A  K  V  S  H  L  C  T  Y  K  R  A  F  L  D  K  V  D  G  V  S
TTGCTAAGGTGTCACACCTTTGCACTTATAAGCGCGCATTCTTAGACAAGGTAGACGGTGTTAG
      200
  G  F  A  V  Y  V  K  S  K  V  G  N  Y  R  L  P  S  N  K  P  S
CGGTTTTGCTGTTTATGTGAAGTCCAAGGTCGGAAATTACCGACTGCCCTCAAACAAACCGAGT
  220
  G  A  D  T  A  L  L  R  I
GGCGCGGACACCGCATTGTTGAGAATCTAATCTAAACTTTAAGGATG
```

Figure 3.   Sequence of the MHV-A59 E1 gene and protein, including
            part of the leader region. Clone R55 contains an addi-
            tional 5 nucleotides in the leader, as shown in Fig. 4.
            The last three bases shown correspond to the initiation
            codon of the nucleocapsid gene. E1 protein has a pre-
            dicted molecular weight of 26000.

DISCUSSION

Topography of the E1 protein

The assembly of the E1 protein into microsomal membranes, and its disposition across the lipid bilayer, have been investigated by Rottier et al. (this volume). Several of its features can be compared with the sequence shown in Fig.3.

1. In contrast to the majority of membrane proteins, E1 lacks a cleaved "leader" peptide: inspection of the N-terminal region of the sequence shows no good candidates for a cleavage site[8].

2. The N-terminal portion carries the unusual O-linked sugars found in the mature protein[9]; assuming the terminal Met is removed (usually the case in eukaryotes), the N-terminal sequence is Ser-Ser-Thr-Thr, an obvious site for potential O-glycosylation.

3. Only approximately 2.5kD of polypeptide are susceptible to proteolysis from the N-terminus, on the inside of the microsomal vesicle, and 1.5kD from the C-terminus on the outside, implying that the rest of the protein is buried in the membrane. A sequence of 22 uncharged residues, from positions 26 to 47, represents a potential membrane-spanning region; the first 25 residues would then correspond to the portion removed by protease. A further sequence of uncharged residues, from positions 57 to 106, is sufficiently long to represent second and third membrane-spanning segments. There are no further hydrophobic sequences, implying that the region from residues 107 to approximately 190 is either folded in the membrane to neutralise charges, or, more plausibly, is adjacent to the membrane, but resistant to proteolysis. The remaining C-terminal portion would then correspond to the proteolysed terminus.

Thus, the sequence in general confirms the various unusual characteristics of the E1 glycoprotein, any of which may be related to its restricted intracellular distribution. The availability of cDNA to the E1 gene, in a single clone (Niemann, this volume) presents the opportunity to dissect the functions of the molecule, by mutagenesis and expression of the gene.

Synthesis of Coronavirus mRNA's

It is now clear that the subgenomic RNA's of MHV-A59 share a short 5' "leader" region, probably corresponding to the 5' end of the genome RNA[5,10] (and Spaan et al., this volume). Assuming that all the RNA's are synthesized from a full-length negative-strand template[11], and that they are not produced from genome-length precursors[12], a possible mechanism for RNA synthesis would be completion of the leader region, followed by "jumping" of the viral polymerase to one of several sites within the template, upstream of each gene: synthesis would then continue until the end of the template was reached. How could such sites be recognized, and how would their efficiencies be regulated to ensure synthesis of the RNA's in the correct proportions?

```
                                            Met(Nucleocapsid)
  RNA7          uuuaAAUCUAAUCUAAACuuuaaggaug
  Clone S9      ugagAAUCUAAUCUAAACuuuaaggaug
                     (E1)Stop
                                       Met(E1)
  RNA6          uuuaAAUCUAAUCcAAACauuaug
  RNA6,
  clone R55  uuuaAAUCUAAUCUAAUCcAAACauuaug
```

Figure 4.   Conserved sequences upstream of coding regions in MHV-A59. The sequence adjacent to the nucleocapsid gene in RNA7 (Spaan et al., this volume) is aligned with the corresponding region in the larger RNA's (clone S9), and with the two sequences upstream of the E1 gene; from a full-size E1 clone (Niemann, this volume) and from clone R55.

Comparison of the various sequences upstream of the nucleocapsid and E1 genes shows some features of interest (Fig.4). A sequence of 14 bases, with one mismatch, is present on the 5' side of the E1 gene in RNA6, and in the intergenic region between the E1 and nucleocapsid genes, suggesting that this represents a site for re-initiating RNA synthesis, and will be found on the 5' side of all the viral genes. However, one clone from the 5' end of the E1 gene, clone R55, contains an additional 5 nucleotides next to the sequence of 14 (Fig.4), reminiscent of the sequence of RNA7 from the JHM strain (Skinner and Siddell, this volume). Thus, there is apparent heterogeneity in the site of fusion between the leader and the E1-coding region in RNA6, consistent with the low molar yield of an oligonucleotide from this region isolated by Lai et al.[10].

A possible mechanism which accommodates these data is that the sites for re-initiation of RNA synthesis are recognized by base-pairing of the leader sequence to internal sites within the negative-strand template. This would be possible if part of the 14-base sequence of Fig.4 was also present in the leader itself. This is illustrated, for RNA6, in Fig.5. A consequence of the sequence of this region, however, is that the leader could base-pair in an alternative position, generating the lengthened sequence found in clone R55 (Fig.5).

```
          3'-UUAGAUUAGGUUUGUAAUAC-5'    Template
       5'-uuuaaaucuaaucCAAACAUUAUG-3'   RNA6
   5'-uuuaaaucuaaucUAAUCCAAACAUUAUG-3'  RNA6,CLONE R55
```

Figure 5. Hypothetical base-pairing between the leader RNA (small letters) and the negative-strand template. Alternative positions of base-pairing could generate the alternative sequences observed in two RNA6 clones.

Clearly this model is at present very speculative, but it implies a possible mechanism for regulating the relative levels of synthesis of the RNA's: variations in the length, precision and number of positions of base-pairing between the leader and the template could determine the probability of re-initiation at a particular site. Further sequence analysis of the MHV-A59 RNA's, in particular of the 5' end of the genome, are now required to test this, and other possible models for the generation of Coronavirus mRNA's.

REFERENCES

1. K. Holmes and J.N. Behnke, Biochemistry and Biology of Corona-viruses, in "Advances in Experimental Medicine", V. Ter Meulen, S. Siddell and H. Wege, eds., vol. 142, Plenum Press, New York (1981).

2. D.F. Stern and S.I.T. Kennedy, Coronavirus multiplication strategy II. Mapping the avian infectious bronchitis virus intracellular RNA species to the genome, J. Virol. 36, 440-449 (1980)

3. M.M. Lai, P.R. Brayton, R.C. Armen, D.D. Patton, C. Pugh and S.A. Stohlman, Mouse hepatitis virus A59: mRNA structure and genetic localization of the sequence divergence from hepatotropic strain MHV-3, J. Virol. 39, 823-834 (1981)

4. S. Cheley, R. Anderson, M.J. Cupples, E.C.M. Lee Chan and V.L. Morris, Intracellular murine hepatitis-virus-specific RNA's contain common sequences, Virology 112, 596-604 (1981)

5. W.J.M. Spaan, P.J.M. Rottier, M.C. Horzinek and B.A.M. van der Zeijst, Sequence relationships between the genome and the intracellular RNA species 1,3,6 and 7 of mouse hepatitis virus strain A59, J. Virol. 42, 432-439 (1982)

6. J. Armstrong, S. Smeekens and P. Rottier, Sequence of the nucleocapsid gene from murine coronavirus MHV-A59, Nucl. Acids Res. 11, 883-891 (1983)

7. L. Dente, G. Cesareni and R. Cortese, pEMBL: a new family of
    single stranded plasmids, Nucl. Acids Res. 11, 1645-1655 (1983)
8. G. von Heijne, Patterns of amino acids near signal-sequence
    cleavage sites, Eur. J. Biochem. 133, 17-21 (1983)
9. H. Niemann and H.-D. Klenk, Coronavirus glycoprotein E1, a new
    type of viral glycoprotein, J. Mol. Biol. 153, 993-1010 (1981)
10. M.M. Lai, C.D. Patton and S.A. Stohlman, Further characterisa-
    tion of mRNA's of mouse hepatitis virus: presence of common 5'-
    end nucleotides, J. Virol. 41, 557-565 (1982)
11. M.M. Lai, C.D. Patton and S.A. Stohlman, Replication of mouse
    hepatitis virus: negative-stranded RNA and replicate form RNA
    are of genome length, J. Virol. 44 , 487-492 (1982)
12. L. Jacobs, W.J.M. Spaan, M.C. Horzinek and B.A.M. van der Zeijst
    Synthesis of subgenomic mRNA's of mouse hepatitis virus ls
    initiated independently: evidence from UV transcription mapping,
    J. Virol. 39, 401-406 (1981)

ACKNOWLEDGEMENTS

We thank Michael Skinner and Heiner Niemann for sharing data and
Annie Steiner for preparation of the manuscript. J.A. was the recipient of a European Fellowship from the Royal Society. P.R. was
supported at the EMBL by a short-term EMBO fellowship.

NUCLEOTIDE SEQUENCING OF MOUSE HEPATITIS VIRUS

STRAIN JHM MESSENGER RNA 7

Michael Skinner and Stuart Siddell

Institute of Virology
University of Würzburg, F.R.G.

INTRODUCTION

Determination of the nucleic acid sequence of MHV genomic and subgenomic RNAs is clearly a way of predicting the primary structure of encoded polypeptides and at the same time identifying non-coding regions, which may be relevant to the regulation of the viral genes and to the replication of the viral RNA. A comparative analysis of the sequences of different MHV strains, or mutants with altered phenotypes, and of other coronaviruses will also be a method of identifying functionally important regions by their conserved sequences. Such analysis will also be required to relate changes in nucleotide sequence to changes, for example, in host range and pathogenicity.

As the first stage of a project to clone and sequence DNA copies of MHV-JHM RNA, we decided to clone the smallest and most abundant viral mRNA found in JHM-infected cells (mRNA7), the messenger which represents the 1800 bases of 3' terminal viral sequence encoding the nucleocapsid (N) protein. The N protein of JHM has an apparent molecular weight, on SDS-polyacrylamide gels, of approximately 60,000[1] and has been shown to be a basic protein[2]. It is the only phosphoprotein found in the virion, being phosphorylated at serine residues[3]. It can also serve as a substrate for a kinase associated with the purified virion[4]. Little is known about the role of N protein in the assembly of the MHV capsid but it has been suggested[3] that the degree of phosphorylation of the protein might regulate its interaction with the viral RNA and hence the maturation of virus particles.

METHODS

Synthesis and Cloning of cDNA

Polyadenylated RNA was isolated from Sac(-) cells that had
been infected with MHV-JHM, as previously described[1]. Double-
stranded cDNA was prepared from 10 ug of polyadenylated RNA,
using oligo dT and oligo dG to prime first and second strand
synthesis, respectively, then oligo dC-tailed, double-stranded
cDNA was annealed to PstI-cleaved, oligo dG-tailed pAT153,
according to protocols described by Land et al[5]. Escherichia
coli HB101 was transformed with the annealed plasmid/cDNA using
the method of Dagert and Ehrlich[6]. Tetracycline-resistant,
ampicillin-sensitive bacterial clones, from two independent cDNA
cloning experiments, were screened for JHM-specific sequences
by hybridization with a single-stranded cDNA probe, containing ^{32}P,
that had been copied from genome RNA isolated from purified virions.

Characterization of cloned cDNA

The size of inserts in plasmids from strongly-hybridizing
clones was determined by gel electrophoresis of DNA extracted
by the method of Holmes and Quigley[7]. Plasmids containing the
largest inserts were prepared from 1 litre cultures and were purified by equilibrium centrifugation in ethidium bromide/caesium
chloride. Inserts were excised from the plasmids using PstI and
were recovered from agarose gels by electroelution. The inserts
were mapped by partial digestion with restriction enzymes of DNA
that had been labelled using ^{32}P cordycepin triphosphate and
terminal deoxynucleotidyl transferase.

Nucleotide sequencing

Fragments of two cDNA inserts were generated by a variety
of restriction enzymes and cloned into the M13 vectors mp 8 and
mp 9[8]. The fragments were sequenced using the chain terminator
method of Sanger et al.[9]. 77 % of the cDNA was sequenced on both
strands, a further 14 % on different but overlapping fragments
of the same strand and the remainder was sequenced at least twice.
Towards the end of the sequencing project specific clones were
identified by their hybridization to a panel of characterized M13
clones. M13 hybridization probes were prepared by the method of
Hu and Messing[10].

Translation in vitro, hybrid-arrested translation and polyacrylamide gel electrophoresis

Polyadenylated RNA from cells infected with MHV-JHM was translated in a rabbit reticulocyte lysate as previously described[1]. Hybrid-arrested translation experiments, using purified cDNA insert and polyadenylated RNA from cells infected with MHV-JHM, were performed according to the method of Paterson and Kuff[11], using a rabbit reticulocyte lysate. Translation products were analysed on 15 % polyacrylamide gels[12].

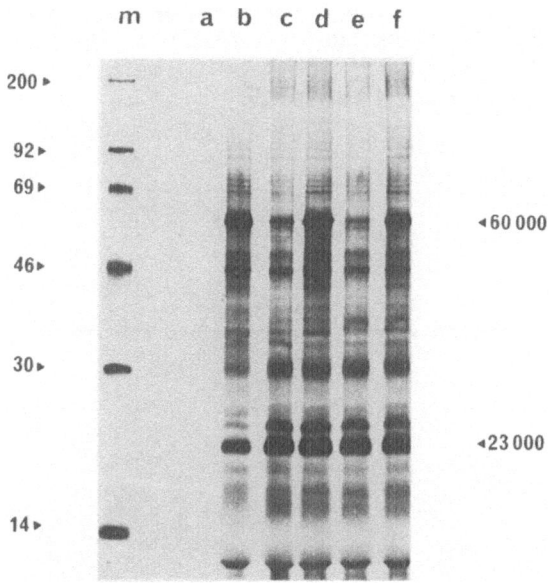

Fig. 1 Hybrid-arrested translation of MHV-JHM mRNA7

Autoradiograph of the ^{35}S-methionine-labelled products synthesized in a rabbit reticulocyte lysate and separated on a 15 % polyacrylamide-SDS gel. The samples translated were: (a) no added RNA, (b-f) 250 ng of polyadenylated, cytoplasmic RNA from cells infected with MHV-JHM, and either 500 ng of the insert DNA (c and d) or 1000 ng of the insert DNA (e and f). Samples (c) and (e) were in the hybrid conformation and samples (d) and (f) were heated to melt the hybrids. The major products of 60,000 and 23,000 mol.wt. have been identified as the nucleocapsid and matrix proteins,respectively. Sample (m) contained ^{14}C-labelled molecular weight markers (CFA626, Amersham Buchler, Braunschweig, F.R.G.).

RESULTS AND DISCUSSION

    JHM-specific cDNA clones were isolated from two independent
cDNA preparations. The largest clone derived from each preparation
(1700 bp in pSS38 and 830 bp in pMS38) were then mapped by partial
digestion with restriction endonucleases. This analysis showed
that the two clones, both of which hybridized to the genomic and
all the subgenomic RNAs of JHM (unpublished results) were overlapping such that the insert from pMS38 carried an extra 40 base
pairs at one end. The 1700 base pair insert (in pSS38) was sufficient to account for most of mRNA7, and hybrid-arrested translation was used to confirm that this insert represented the body
of mRNA7 (Fig.1). Hybridization of the cDNA insert to infected
cell RNA, before translation of the RNA, resulted in specific
inhibition of the translation of a 60,000 mol.wt. polypeptide
that has been identified as the intracellular precursor of the
virion N protein[1]. Melting of the hybrids before translation
restored the synthesis of N protein.

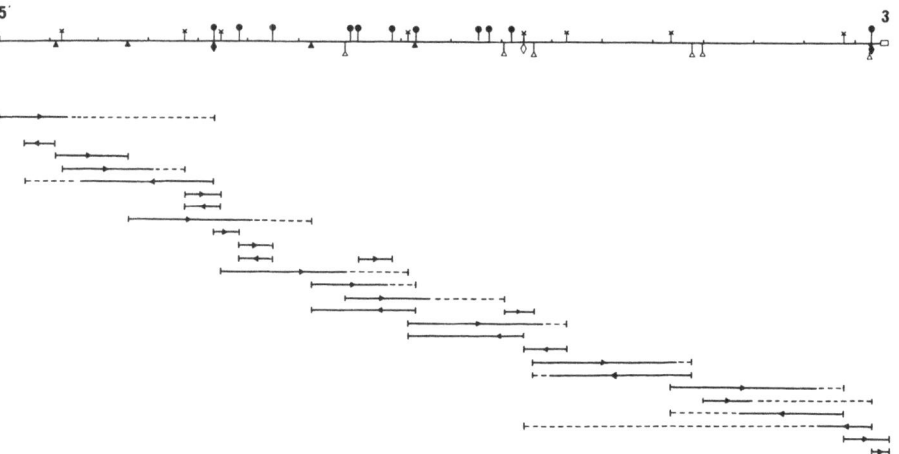

Fig. 2 Diagram showing those restriction endonuclease sites,
        in the DNA copy of MHV-JHM mRNA 7, used for subcloning
        into M13 vectors. Solid arrows show the direction and
        extent of sequence obtained from each clone. Broken
        lines indicate the probable extent of each clone.
        Restriction endonuclease cleavage sites are denoted
        by the symbols: ♀ HaeIII, ▲ MspI, ◆ BalI, ✶ AluI,
        ⏃ Sau3a and ◇ PvuII. The box at the 3' terminus
        represents the poly(A) tract.

On the basis of the restriction enzyme map, fragments of both cDNA inserts were subcloned into M13 vectors and their sequences were determined (Fig.2). The combined sequence of 1767 base pairs (contained between the oligo dC/dG tails made during the process of cloning) is shown in Fig.3. The sequence contains an open-reading frame, beginning at the first possible AUG codon (nucleotide 84) and ending at nucleotide 1449, capable of encoding a basic protein (Table 1) of 455 amino acids with a molecular weight of 49,700. As the N protein is known to be basic and phosphorylated, such a figure is consistent with the apparent molecular weight of 60,000. The only other open-reading frame of greater than 100 nucleotides was from nucleotides 361-771, potentially able to encode 137 amino acids.

The N protein of Semliki Forest Virus has large clusters of lysine and proline residues in the 110 amino acids adjacent to the N terminal[13]. Such a feature is not seen in the predicted amino acid sequence of the JHM nucleocapsid protein (Fig.3) but some regions enriched in basic amino acids are apparent (e.g. arg-43 to lys-50, lys-101 to lys-113, arg-196 to lys-230, arg-264 to arg-290 and lys-392 to lys-405). Such regions may be responsible for binding of the N protein to the RNA. As in the N protein of SFV, the carboxy terminus is acidic. In view of the fact that phosphorylation of the N protein appears to be important in allowing it to associate with membranes (S. Stohlman, unpublished) and that N protein is phosphorylated at serine residues , it is interesting to consider the distribution of serine residues in the predicted sequence. It is striking that the region ser-194 to ser-220 contains 9 serine residues, or 24 % of the total serine

Table 1 Amino acid composition of the predicted
       nucleocapsid protein sequence of MHV-JHM.

Arg	29	Glu	22
Lys	33	Asp	22
His	3		
		Val	29
Ser	38	Ile	12
Thr	23	Leu	25
Tyr	12	Phe	17
Gln	40	Ala	35
Asn	25	Pro	34
Gly	45	Trp	5
Cys	2	Met	4

```
TATAAGAGTGATTGGCGTCCGTACGTACCCTCTCTACTCTAAAACTCTTGTAGTTTAAATCTAATCTAATCTAAACTTTAAGG
```

| | Met Ser Phe Val Pro Gly Gln Glu Asn Ala Gly Ser Arg Ser Ser Ser Gly Asn Arg Ala Gly Asn Gly Ile Leu (25) |
| (84) | ATG TCT TTT GTT CCT GGG CAA GAA AAT GCC GGT AGC AGA AGC TCC TCT GGA AAC CGC GCT GGT AAT GGA ATC CTC |

| | Lys Lys Thr Thr Trp Ala Asp Gln Thr Glu Arg Gly Leu Asn Asn Gln Asn Arg Gly Arg Lys Asn Gln Pro Lys (50) |
| (159) | AAG AAG ACC ACT TGG GCT GAC CAA ACC GAG CGC GGG TTA AAT AAT CAA AAT AGA GGC AGA AAG AAT CAG CCC AAG |

| | Gln Thr Ala Thr Thr Gln Pro Asn Ser Gly Ser Val Val Pro His Tyr Ser Trp Phe Ser Gly Ile Thr Gln Phe (75) |
| (234) | CAG ACT GCA ACT ACT CAA CCC AAT TCC GGG AGT GTG GTT CCC CAT TAC TCT TGG TTT TCG GGC ATT ACC CAA TTC |

| | Gln Lys Gly Lys Glu Phe Gln Phe Ala Gln Gly Gln Gly Val Pro Ile Ala Asn Gly Ile Pro Ala Ser Gln Gln (100) |
| (309) | CAG AAG GGA AAA GAG TTT CAG TTT GCA CAA GGA CAA GGA GTG CCT ATT GCC AAT GGA ATC CCA GCT TCA CAG CAA |

| | Lys Gly Tyr Trp Tyr Arg His Asn Arg Arg Ser Phe Lys Thr Pro Asp Gly Gln Gln Lys Gln Leu Leu Pro Arg (125) |
| (384) | AAG GGA TAT TGG TAC AGA CAC AAC CGA CGT TCC TTT AAA ACA CCT GAT GGC CAG CAG AAG CAG CTA CTG CCC AGA |

| | Trp Tyr Phe Tyr Tyr Leu Gly Thr Gly Pro Tyr Ala Gly Ala Glu Tyr Gly Asp Asp Ile Glu Gly Val Val Trp (150) |
| (459) | TGG TAT TTT TAC TAT CTT GGA ACA GGG CCC TAT GCT GGC GCA GAG TAT GGC GAC GAT ATC GAA GGA GTT GTC TGG |

| | Val Ala Ser Gln Gln Ala Glu Thr Arg Thr Ser Ala Asp Ile Val Glu Arg Asp Pro Ser Ser His Glu Ala Ile (175) |
| (534) | GTC GCA AGC CAA CAG GCC GAG ACT AGG ACC TCT GCC GAT ATT GTT GAA AGG GAC CCA AGT AGC CAT GAG GCT ATT |

| | Pro Thr Arg Phe Ala Pro Gly Thr Val Leu Pro Gln Gly Phe Tyr Val Glu Gly Ser Gly Arg Ser Ala Pro Ala (200) |
| (609) | CCT ACT AGG TTT GCG CCC GGT ACG GTA TTG CCT CAA GGT TTT TAT GTT GAA GGC TCA GGA AGG TCT GCA CCT GCT |

| | Ser Arg Ser Gly Ser Arg Pro Gln Ser Arg Gly Pro Asn Asn Arg Ala Arg Ser Ser Ser Gln Arg Gln Pro (225) |
| (684) | AGT CGA TCT GGT TCG CGG CCA CAA TCC CGT GGG CCA AAT AAT CGC GCT AGA AGC AGT TCC AAC CAG CGC CAG CCT |

| | Ala Ser Thr Val Lys Pro Asp Met Ala Glu Glu Ile Ala Ala Leu Val Leu Ala Lys Leu Gly Lys Asp Ala Gly (250) |
| (759) | GCC TCT ACT GTA AAA CCT GAT ATG GCC GAA GAA ATT GCT GCT CTT GTT TTG GCT AAG CTC GGT AAA GAT GCC GGC |

| | Gln Pro Lys Gln Val Thr Lys Gln Ser Ala Lys Glu Val Arg Gln Lys Ile Leu Asn Lys Pro Arg Gln Lys Arg (275) |
| (834) | CAG CCT AAG CAA GTA ACA AAG CAA AGT GCC AAA GAA GTC AGG CAG AAA ATT TTA AAC AAG CCT CGT CAA AAG AGG |

| | Thr Pro Asn Lys Gln Cys Pro Val Gln Gln Cys Phe Gly Lys Arg Gly Pro Asn Gln Asn Phe Gly Gly Pro Glu (300) |
| (909) | ACT CCA AAC AAG CAG TGC CCA GTG CAG CAG TGT TTT GGA AAG AGA GGC CCC AAT CAG AAT TTT GGA GGC CCT GAA |

| | Met Leu Lys Leu Gly Thr Ser Asp Pro Gln Phe Pro Ile Leu Ala Glu Leu Ala Pro Thr Ala Gly Ala Phe Phe (325) |
| (984) | ATG TTA AAA CTT GGA ACT AGT GAT CCA CAG TTC CCC ATT CTT GCA GAG TTG GCC CCA ACA GCT GGT GCC TTC TTC |

| | Phe Gly Ser Leu Glu Leu Val Lys Lys Asn Ser Gly Ala Asp Gly Pro Thr Lys Asp Val Tyr Glu Leu (350) |
| (1059) | TTT GGA TCT AAA TTA GAA TTG GTC AAA AAG AAC TCT GGT GGT GCT GAT GGA CCC ACC AAA GAT GTG TAT GAG CTG |

| | Gln Tyr Ser Gly Ala Val Arg Phe Asp Ser Thr Leu Pro Gly Phe Glu Thr Ile Met Lys Val Leu Asn Glu Asn (375) |
| (1134) | CAA TAT TCA GGT GCA GTT AGA TTT GAT AGT ACT CTA CCT GGT TTT GAG ACT ATC ATG AAA GTG TTG AAT GAG AAT |

| | Leu Asn Ala Tyr Gln Asn Gln Asp Gly Gly Ala Asp Val Val Ser Pro Lys Pro Gln Arg Lys Arg Gly Thr Lys (400) |
| (1209) | TTG AAT GCC TAC CAG AAT CAA GAT GGT GGT GCA GAT GTA GTG AGC CCT AAG CCT CAG AGA AAG AGA GGG ACA AAG |

| | Gln Lys Ala Gln Lys Asp Glu Val Asp Asn Val Ser Val Ala Lys Pro Lys Ser Ser Val Gln Arg Asn Val Ser (425) |
| (1284) | CAA AAG GCT CAG AAA GAT GAA GTA GAT AAT GTA AGC GTT GCA AAG CCC AAA AGC TCT GTG CAG CGA AAT GTA AGT |

| | Arg Glu Leu Thr Pro Glu Asp Arg Ser Leu Leu Ala Gln Ile Leu Asp Asp Gly Val Val Pro Asp Gly Leu Glu (450) |
| (1359) | AGA GAG TTA ACC CCT GAG GAT CGC AGC CTT CTG GCT CAG ATC CTA GAT GAT GGC GTA GTG CCA GAT GGG TTA GAA |

| | Asp Asp Ser Asn Val |
| (1434) | GAT GAC TCT AAT GTG TAAAGAGAATGAATCCTATGTCGGCACTCGGTGGTAACCCCTCGCGAGAAAGTCGGGATAGGACACTCTCTATCAGAAT |

| (1528) | GGATGTCTTGCTGTCATAACAGATAGAGAAGGTTGTGGCAGACCCTGTATCAATTAGTTGAAAGAGATTGCAAAATAGAGAATGTGTGAGAGAAGTTAG |

| (1627) | CAAGGTCCTACGTCTAACCATAAGAACGGCGATAGGCGCCCCCTGGGAAGAGCTCACATCAGGGTACTATTCCTGCAATGCCCTAGTAAATGAATGAAG |

| (1726) | TTGATCATGGCCAATTGGAAGAATCACAAAAAAAAAAAAAAA |

Fig. 3   Complete nucleotide sequence of the DNA copy of MHV-JHM mRNA7 (1767 nucleotides), including a 15 base long, terminal poly (A) tract. The predicted sequence of the encoded protein is also depicted. Underlined sequences show the RNase T$_1$-resistant oligonucleotides, found in the 5' non-coding sequence, that are considered in the discussion. The triple repeat of the pentamer AATCT is also indicated.

content within just 6 % of the coding sequence. Moreover, this
is a basic region of the protein (Fig. 4). Another 4 serine
residues occur in the five residues from ser-12 to ser-16.

The sequence of the N gene of JHM can also be compared with
the N gene from MHV-A59 (J. Armstrong, this volume). The nucleotide
sequences show 94 % overall homology within the coding sequences
and this is reflected within the predicted amino acid sequences
(93 % homology). Although the homology is high overall, it is not
constant throughout the length of the coding sequence. Between
nucleotides 497-569 the sequence homology falls to 63 % (16 out
of the 24 amino acids are conserved) and in a sequence of 23
bases (nucleotides 1271-1293) only 9 bases are common to both
strains (39 % homology). Although none of the 8 amino acids
are conserved the region retains its basic nature in both strains.
In addition to these differences, the JHM sequence has an extra
glutamine codon at position 1227.

The 5' non-coding region of the JHM sequence has a terminal
RNase T$_1$-resistant oligonucleotide TATAAG, which is very similar [14]
to the sequence found at the 5' end of MHV-A59 RNAs by Lai et al.
(cap-NUAAG). The 301 bases of 3' non-coding sequence are followed
by a 15 base poly (A) tract. Thus it is probable that the sequence
represents a full copy of JHM mRNA7.

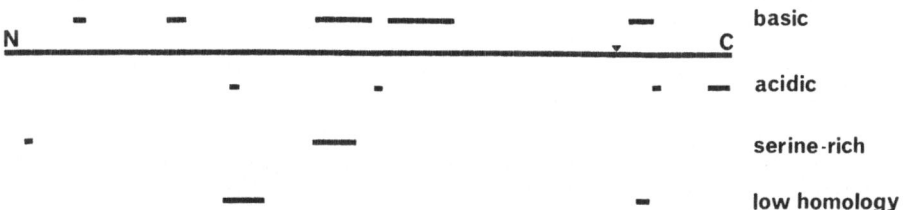

Fig. 4   Illustration to show features of the coding sequence of
         JHM mRNA7: basic and acidic regions, regions of high
         serine content and the two regions where the homology with
         the A59 sequence (J. Armstrong, this volume) is notably
         reduced. The arrowhead indicates the position where the
         extra glutamine codon is found in the JHM sequence.

Within the 5' non-coding sequence, two large RNase T_1-resistant oligonucleotides can be found. Examination reveals that their base compositions are similar to those of oligonucleotides 10 and 19 of A59[14]. It has been suggested[15] that oligonucleotide 10 (equivalent to the JHM oligonucleotide at position 26-50) is contained within a leader sequence derived from the 5' end of the genome and that oligonucleotide 19 (equivalent to the JHM oligonucleotide at position 54-82) is formed by fusion of the leader to the body of mRNA7[14,15]. The relative positions of the two oligonucleotides in the 5' non-coding sequence of JHM mRNA7 are consistent with such a proposal. This matter is considered in more detail by Spaan et al., in this volume. It should be noted, however, that the JHM equivalent of oligonucleotide 19 contains a triple repeat of the pentamer AATCT (or ATCTA), a striking feature which probably plays a significant role in the production of subgenomic mRNAs. The triple repeat was seen in both cDNA clones and so is unlikely to represent a sequence found in only a minor population of mRNA7. Comparison of the 3' non-coding sequences of JHM and A59 reveals that the two are highly conserved in this region (98 % homology). Such a high conservation of sequence in a non-coding region is possibly due to the fact that it must contain the binding site for the RNA polymerase function which synthesises negative-strand template.

Consideration of the protein sequence of the JHM nucleocapsid protein has shown several interesting structural features. It is to be hoped that studies on the interaction of N protein with genomic RNA and with other viral proteins will elucidate the functional role of these features. As might have been expected, the sequences encoding the N protein of MHV have been well conserved even between two strains that show differences in pathogenicity. It will be interesting to determine the level of homology for genes more directly involved in the interaction between the virus and the host.

ACKNOWLEDGEMENTS

We thank Helga Kriesinger for typing the manuscript. This work was supported by the Deutsche Forschungsgmeinschaft.

REFERENCES

1. Siddell, S.G., Wege, H., Barthel, A. and ter Meulen, V. (1980). J. Virol. 33, 10-17.
2. Siddell, S., Wege, H., Barthel, A. and ter Meulen, V. (1981). J. Gen. Virol. 53, 145-155.
3. Stohlman, S.A. and Lai, M.M.C. (1979). J. Virol. 32, 672-675.
4. Siddell, S.G., Barthel, A. and ter Meulen, V. (1981). J. Gen. Virol. 52, 235-243.

5. Land, H., Grez, M., Hauser, H., Lindenmaier, W. and Schütz, G., (1983). In Methods in Enzymology, eds. Wu, R., Grossman, L. and Moldave, K. (Academic Press, New York), Vol. 100, in press.
6. Dagert, M. and Ehrlich, S.D. (1979). Gene 6, 23-28.
7. Holmes, D.S. and Quigley, M. (1981). Anal. Biochem. 114, 193-197.
8. Messing, J. and Vierira, J. (1982). Gene 19, 269-276.
9. Sanger, F., Nicklen, S. and Coulson, A.R. (1977). Proc. Natl. Acad. Sci. USA 74, 5463-5467.
10. Hu, N. and Messing, J. (1982). Gene 17, 271-277.
11. Paterson, B.M., Roberts, B.E. and Kuff, E.L. (1977). Proc. Nat. Acad. Sci. USA 74, 4370-4374.
12. Laemmli, U.K. (1970). Nature (London) 227, 680-685.
13. Garoff, H., Frischauf, A., Simons, K., Lehrach, H. and Delius, H. (1980). Proc. Natl. Acad. Sci. USA 77, 6376-6380.
14. Lai, M.M.C., Patton, C.D. and Stohlman, S.A. (1982). J. Virol. 41, 557-565.
15. Spaan, W.J.M., Rottier, P.J.M., Horzinek, M.C. and van der Zeijst, B.A.M. (1982). J. Virol. 42, 432-439.

TRANSCRIPTION STRATEGY OF CORONAVIRUSES: FUSION OF NON–CONTIGUOUS

SEQUENCES DURING mRNA SYNTHESIS

Willy Spaan[1], Hajo Delius[2], Mike A. Skinner[3], John Armstrong[2],
Peter Rottier[1], Sjef Smeekens[1], Stuart G. Siddell[3] & Bernard
van der Zeijst[1]

[1]Institute of Virology, Veterinary Faculty, State
University, Utrecht, The Netherlands

[2]European Molecular Biology Laboratory, Heidelberg, FRG

[3]Institute of Virology, Wuerzburg, FRG

SUMMARY

MHV replicates in the cell cytoplasm and viral genetic
information is expressed in infected cells as one genomic sized
RNA (mRNA1) and six subgenomic mRNAs. The seven RNAs were assumed
to have common 3' ends of the size of RNA7, the smallest RNA. The
data reported here, show that this model is too simple and that
the mRNAs are composed of a leader and body sequence. Electron
microscopic analysis of hybrids formed between single stranded
cDNA copied from mRNA7 and genomic RNA or mRNA6 shows that
genomic RNA, mRNA6 and mRNA7 have common 5' terminal sequences.
Furthermore, nucleotide sequence analysis shows that the
nucleotide sequence of the 5' end of mRNA7 diverges from the
corresponding region of the genome just upstream from the
initiation codon of the nucleocapsid gene. Because the synthesis
of each mRNA is inactivated by UV irradiation in proportion to its
own length, the subgenomic mRNAs are apparently not produced by
the processing of larger RNAs. The available data have to be
explained by translocation of the polymerase/leader complex to
specific internal positions on the negative strand. In this way
the leader and body sequences are joined together by a mechanism
completely different from conventional RNA splicing but
nevertheless giving the same end result.

INTRODUCTION

Viruses were discovered at the end of the nineteenth century (1,2). In the mean time they have been studied to unravel their structure, replication mechanism and pathogenic properties, but they have also been an extremely valuable tool for the study of gene expression of animal cells. Viruses have played a role in the elucidation of protein processing from larger precursors, capping of mRNAs and gene splicing (3,4,5,6). Another interesting aspect of viruses is, that they are the only group of self replicating organisms using RNA as genetic material. The genes of DNA viruses and even RNA tumour viruses are expressed in a way very similar to their host. RNA viruses on the other hand have developed independent strategies (7), but share many biosynthetic pathways with the host cell making them excellent probes for study of cell processes (8,9,10, Rottier et al., this volume).

Although enormous progress has been made in the study of viruses in the last century, there are still a number of virus families of which the replication strategy is almost, or even completely, unknown. These viruses could have new, undetected, mechanisms of gene expression. Until recently coronaviruses were such a group in spite of their pathogenic properties and resulting economic losses (11). However, in the last few years the basic aspects of coronavirus replication have been elucidated (for reviews see 12,13), and the data presented here demonstrates that their strategy involves mechanisms of viral gene expression which have not been described previously.

Coronaviruses are enveloped positive-stranded RNA viruses. The genome RNA is linear, unsegmented and 15000 to 20000 bases in length. The most studied member of the group is murine hepatitis virus (MHV). MHV replicates in the cell cytoplasm and viral genetic information is expressed in infected cells as one genomic sized and six subgenomic mRNAs. These mRNAs are synthesized in non-equimolar amounts, but in relatively constant proportions throughout infection (14). The template for viral mRNA synthesis is a genomic length negative strand (15).

RNase T1 oligonucleotide analysis of MHV-A59 genomic RNA, size-fractionated 3' coterminal (i.e. poly(A)-selected) fragments of genomic RNA and viral mRNA (14,16,17,18) reveals that the viral mRNAs have a "nested set" structure with 3' coterminal ends and sequences extending for different lengths in a 5' direction. Each subgenomic mRNA is capped and polyadenylated, as is genomic RNA (17), and is translated independently to produce a single protein the size of which corresponds to the coding capacity of the 5' sequences not found in the next smallest mRNA (19,20,21). The T1 oligonucleotide analysis also reveals unique oligonucleotides that do not fit into the "nested set" structure. We have demonstrated

that T1 oligonucleotides 10 and 19 from RNA7 of MHV-A59 (using the
nomenclature of Lai et al., 17) are not present in the
corresponding 3' end of the genome , suggesting that these
oligonucleotides come from a leader sequence which all mRNAs might
share (18). Oligonucleotide 10 is apparently identical for each
mRNA, but mRNA specific electrophoretic mobility differences have
been detected for the second oligonucleotide. It is present as
oligonucleotide 19, 19a and 3a in mRNA7, mRNA6 and mRNA5 ,
respectively. Oligonucleotides 19, 19a and 17 have very similar
base compositions. The latter oligonucleotide is found in mRNA6
and larger mRNAs, but not in mRNA7 (17). Finally, the mRNAs share
at least 5 nucleotides at their 5' end (17). These data can be
interpreted in the model shown in Fig.1. In this model sequences
present at the 5' end of genomic RNA (mRNA1) are also found at the
5' end of each subgenomic mRNA (these sequences will be referred
to as leaders). MHV-A59 oligonucleotide 10 would be entirely
encompassed within these sequences. MHV-A59 oligonucleotides 19
and 19a would only partly be encompassed within the leader. Their
variation would arise from fusion of the leader sequence with the
various bodies of the mRNAs. Oligonucleotide 17 would represent
sequences at the 5' end of the mRNA7 body, part of which would be
lost during the construction of mRNA7 but not for example mRNA6.

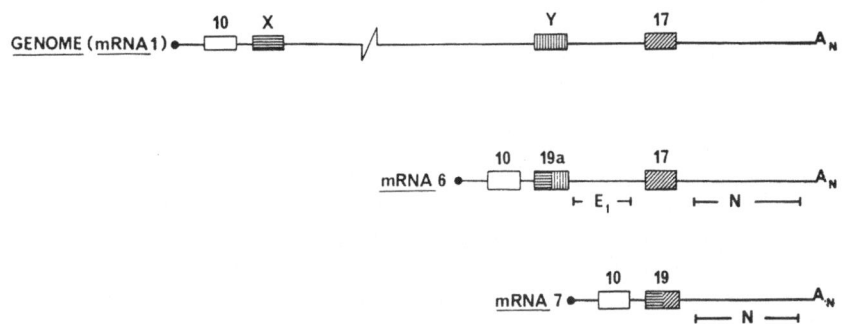

Fig.1. A model for the structural relationships of MHV-A59
        genomic RNA and mRNA6 and 7.
        The symbols ● and (A)n represent 5' terminal cap
        structures and 3' terminal polyadenylate tracts
        respectively. RNase T1 resistant oligonucleotides are
        identified by numbers (17). The sequences X and Y have
        not yet been identified. E1 (matrix protein) and N
        (nucleocapsid protein) are the translation products of
        mRNA6 and mRNA7 respectively. The boxed regions are on a
        larger scale than the other regions of the mRNAs.

This model is consistent with the available data but lacks experimental evidence. We therefore tested the model by electron microscopic analysis of hybrids formed between cDNA to mRNA7 and genomic RNA or mRNA6. In addition the nucleotide sequence at the 5' end of mRNA7 was compared with the corresponding region of the genome to determine at what point both sequences started to diverge. The above experiments were carried out with MHV-A59. Comparison of the A59 and JHM sequences of mRNA7 was also undertaken. The two viruses have unrelated RNase T1 fingerprints (22) but the recognition sites for the fusion of the leader sequence and the mRNA body can be expected to be conserved.

METHODS

Hybrid duplex mapping

cDNA was prepared as described before (23). The cDNA was incubated with RNA at a concentration of about 1 ug/ml in 50% formamide containing 10 mM Tris-HCl, 1 mM EDTA and 0.2 M CsCl for 30 min at 40oC. A 10-fold diluted aliquot was spread from 30% formamide, 0.1 M Tris-HCl, 1 mM EDTA, 0.1 ug/ml PM2 DNA with CNBr-treated cytochrome (24) on a hypophase of distilled water. Samples were picked up on Parlodion-coated grids, stained with uranyl acetate and rotary shadowed with platinum.

RNA sequencing

For the dideoxy reaction, 2 μl of the single stranded synthetic DNA primer (Biolabs New England) (10 ng/ul) 1 μl of RNA7 or genomic RNA (1 mg/ml), 2 μl tenfold concentrated reverse transcriptase buffer (1x buffer is 50 mM Tris-HCl pH 8.3, 50 mM KCl and 8 mM MgCl) 8 μl H_2O, 0.5 μl of 10 mM DTT, and 3 μl reverse trancriptase (2 U/μl; from W.Beard) were mixed. To 4 μl of this primed mRNA 1 μl of one of the following chain-terminating nucleotide stock mixtures were added; ddA mixture: 50 μM dCTP, 50 μM dGTP, 50 μM dTTP and 1 μM ddATP; ddC mixture: 25 μM dCTP, 50 μM dGTP, 50 μM dTTP and 2.5 μM ddCTP; ddG mixture: 50 μM dCTP, 25 μM dGTP, 50 μM dTTP and 2.5 μM ddGTP, ddT mixture: 125 μM dCTP, 125 μM dGTP, 125 μM dTTP and 12.5 μM ddTTP. All these mixtures contained 4 μCi α -^{32}P dATP (400 Ci.mmol-1). Incubation was at 42oC for 30 min and 1 μl of a 0.125 mM solution of unlabeled deoxynucleoside triphosphate was then added and the mixture was chased for an additional 0.5 hr. The reaction products were analyzed on 0.25 mm thick and 40 cm long 6% polyacrylamide gels (25). The sequence procedure for clone S9 has been described (23).

RESULTS

Electron microscopy of hybrids between cDNA to RNA7 and genomic RNA or mRNA6

cDNA was prepared as described before (23). After hydrolysis of the RNA template it was treated with glyoxal and dimethylsulfoxide and analyzed by agarose gel electrophoresis. A main band of approximately the size of the RNA7 was seen (data not shown). This cDNA was annealed to genomic RNA and prepared for electron microscopy by cytochrome spreading. A sequence homology between the 5' end of mRNA7 copied into the cDNA, and the 5' end of the genomic RNA should lead to the formation of a looped hybrid. Indeed such structures were observed. Fig.2A shows such a hybrid molecule accompanied by a tracing outlining the possible arrangement of the RNA and DNA strands. No circles but only linear molecules were observed in preparations of RNA alone prepared in the same way, so that the circularization has to be attributed to the hybrid formation. The length of the hybrid region in these molecules corresponds to 1995± 160 bp, using PM2 DNA as a standard and after correction for the shortened hybrid length (26). The size of the loop was determined as 19.4± 1.0 kb. This value is only an approximation due to lack of a suitable RNA standard of this size. No double strand could be discerned at the point of the re-entry of the genomic RNA into the hybrid near the 5' end. This excludes a double strand region much larger than 50 nucleotides. Fig.2B shows a hybrid between the same cDNA and RNA6. Again, a double-stranded region (1890± 140 bp) caused by the hybridization between the cDNA and the 3'-end of mRNA6, and a single-stranded loop structure (but in this case a much smaller one of 600± 80 nucleotide) were observed. This single stranded loop probably represents the E1 gene. Its size would be sufficient to code for a polypeptide of 22.0± 2.9 K daltons, the approximate size of the non-glycosylated form of polypeptide E1 found in MHV-A59 infected cells (20, Armstrong et al., this volume). Again, the most likely explanation of the loop formation in these hybrids is the presence of common leader sequences in mRNA6 and mRNA7, although again no hybrid stretch on the 5' side of the loop could be detected. The data very strongly support the model given in Fig.1.

Sequence analysis of mRNA7 and the region of the genome between the E1 and N genes

Another prediction of the model is that the nucleotide sequence of the region immediately upstream from the nucleocapsid gene of mRNA7 should diverge from the region upstream from the nucleocapsid gene in the genome. Therefore we determined the nucleotide sequences in these regions.

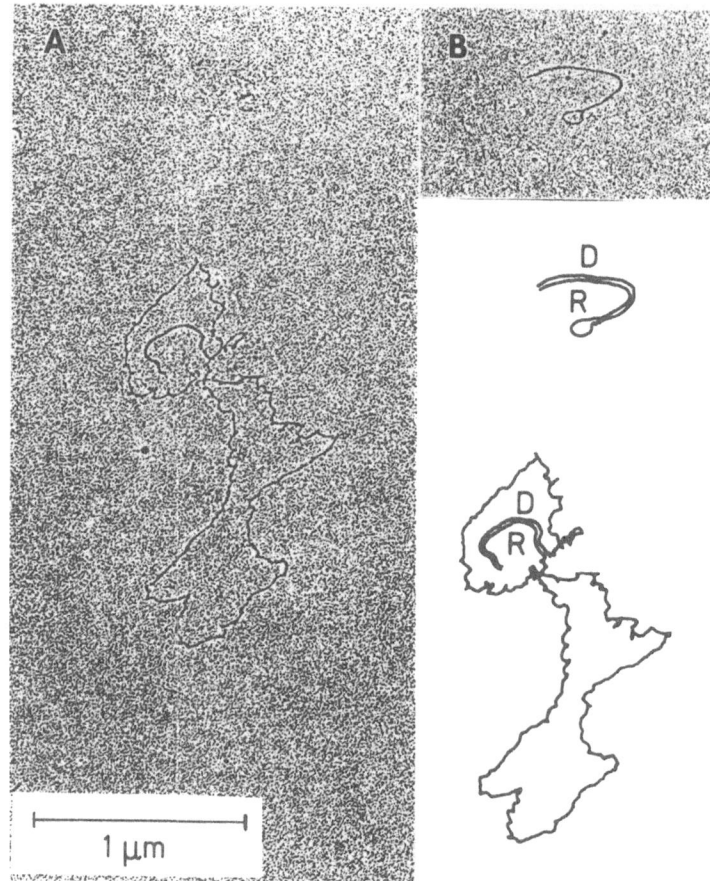

Fig.2. Electron micrographs of hybrids between coronavirus MHV-
        A59 RNAs and cDNA synthesized on RNA7.

        (A) Hybrid between cDNA and the genomic RNA.
        (B) Hybrid between cDNA and RNA6.

        The tracings indicate the hypothetical arrangement of the
        cDNA (D) and the RNA (R). The structure of the joint
        between the 5' end of the RNA loops and the cDNA cannot be
        identified in the electron micrographs. Viral RNAs were
        isolated as described (18).

        Recently we have cloned and sequenced cDNA prepared from MHV-
A59 mRNAs (23). A sequence of 1817 nucleotides of the 3' end of
the genome, including the nucleocapsid gene was determined by
shot-gun sequencing of restriction fragments in phage M13. The
approach we have used here was to sequence directly the 5' end of
mRNA7 and the corresponding region of the genome of MHV-A59 using

a DNA primer and reverse transcriptase for dideoxy sequencing on RNA (27). The primer was complementary to position 11 to 24 of the nucleocapsid gene sequence (23). A sequence of 86 bases could be read on RNA7 (Fig.3A). The following conclusions can be drawn. First, two large T1 oligonucleotides are predicted from this sequence. One oligonucleotide (position -53/-29) would have a base composition very similar to T1 oligonucleotide 10. The other one (position -25/-2) was very similar to oligonucleotide 19. Second, although the extreme end of RNA7 could not be determined the sequence NAAG at the 5' end is almost identical to the sequence found at the 5' end of MHV-A59 RNAs by Lai et al. (cap - NUAAG) (17). Therefore we assume that the 5' noncoding region (including the leader sequence) of mRNA7 is 78 nucleotides long.

The same DNA primer was used for dideoxy sequencing on the genome. This sequence is shown in Fig. 3B. The sequence starting at position -21 until position -2 is very similar to the predicted sequence of T1 oligonucleotide 17. The T1 oligonucleotides 10 and 19 are not present in this sequence, which is to be expected from the model shown in Fig.1. The sequence preceding T1 oligonucleotide 17 represents the 3' end of the E1 gene. This sequence is in good agreement with the sequence of E1 obtained from cDNA clones (Armstrong et al., this volume). Comparison of the sequence of the 5' terminus of RNA7 and the sequence of the genome shows that both sequences are identical until position -22 (Fig.3C). From this position RNA7 and the genome start to diverge. The divergence site is located at the beginning of T1 oligonucleotide 17 and within T1 oligonucleotide 19.

Localization of the fusion site of leader and body sequences of MHV mRNAs

From the above data, summarized in Fig.4, it is clear that the 5' terminus of the MHV-A59 mRNA7 body cannot extend beyond position -21, the site of divergence of mRNA7 and the genome. As mentioned before T1 oligonucleotide 19a, (specific for RNA6) and T1 oligonucleotide 19 (specific for RNA7) have a very similar base composition. By predicting the sequence of 19a from the base composition and by comparing this sequence to the sequence of mRNA7 between -24 and -2 it can be seen that the 3' terminus of the leader sequence fused to mRNA6 cannot extend beyond the first base difference (reading in a 5' to 3' direction) between oligonucleotide 19 and 19a. Thus the data suggest that for MHV-A59 the fusion of leader and body sequences producing oligonucleotides 19 and 19a occurred within the sequence 5' AAUCUAAUCUAAACU 3', a sequence that does not contain the concensus (A/C) AG/G established for splice junctions in viral and cellular mRNAs (6). This sequence contains two copies of the palindromic pentamer AUCUA (or the pentamer AAUCU). It was surprising that the only major difference between A59 and JHM virus was the presence of a

A

```
        -70         -60         -50         -40
     NAAGNGUGAUUGGCGUCCGUACGUACCCUCUCAACUCUN
                                    |—————— T₁ spot —
        -30         -20         -10          1
     AAACUCUUGUNGUUUAAAUCUAAUCUNAACUUUAAGGAUG
     no 10 —————|   |——T₁ spot no 19—————————| M
           10
     UCUUUUGUUCCUGGG
      S  F  V  P  G
```

B

```
     -200                    -180                   -160
     CUUUGUCUGACUUGCCCGCUUAUGUUACAGUUGCUAAGGUGUCAC
                    -140                   -120
     ACCUNUGCACUUAUAAGCGCGNNUUCUUAGACAAGGUAGNNGGUN
                  -100                   -80
     UUAGCGGUUUUGCUGUUUAUGUGAAGUCCAAGGNNGGAAAUUACC
            -60                   -40
     GACUGCCCUCAAACNAACCGAGUGGCGCGGACACCGCAUUGUUGA
     -20                    1
     GAAUCUNAUCUNAACUUUAAGGAUNUNUNUUGUUCCUGGG
     |—T₁ spot no 17—————|  M  S  F  V  P  G
```

C

```
               5'
     GENOME    CCCUCAAACAAACCGAGUGGCGCGGACACCGCAU

     RNA7      GUCCGUACGUACCCUCUCAACUCUNAAACUCUUG


                    |————— T₁ spot no 17—|
                   _____
     UGUUGAGAAUCUNAUCUNAACUUUAAGGAUNUNU   3'

     UNGUUUAAAUCUAAUCUNAACUUUAAGGAUGUCU
                   ‾‾‾‾‾‾‾‾‾‾‾‾‾‾‾‾‾‾‾‾‾‾‾‾‾‾‾‾‾‾‾‾‾‾
                    |——— T₁ spot no 19 —————|  M  S
```

Fig.3. Nucleotide sequence of the 5' end of RNA7 (A) and the homologous part of genome RNA (B); comparison of both sequences (C).

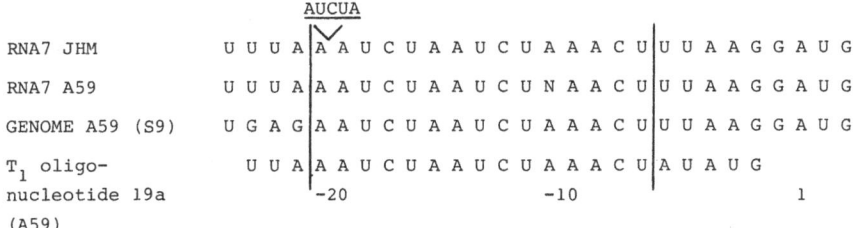

                                    AUCUA
                                     ⌄
RNA7 JHM   U U U A│A A U C U A A U C U A A A C U│U U A A G G A U G

RNA7 A59   U U U A│A A U C U A A U C U N A A C U│U U A A G G A U G

GENOME A59 (S9)   U G A G│A A U C U A A U C U A A A C U│U U A A G G A U G

T₁ oligo-   U U A│A A U C U A A U C U A A A C U│A U A U G
nucleotide 19a   └-20   -10   └   1
(A59)

Fig.4.   Localization of the fusion site between body and leader of
         MHV mRNA. For details see text.

third copy of the pentamer AUCUA (or the sequence AAUCU). Despite
some differences the sequence homology is extended over the
complete noncoding and coding region (Skinner and Siddell, this
volume). The presence of a third copy of the palindromic
pentamer AUCUA (or the sequence AAUCU) in the MHV–JHM sequence may
suggest that it functions as a recognition signal during the
fusion process.

DISCUSSION

How are leader and body of coronaviral mRNAs fused?

There is at present no indication that the replication of MHV
involves a nuclear phase or nuclear factors. MHV is reported to
grow in enucleated cells and its replication is not inhibited by
actinomycin D or alpha–amanitin (28,29,30). Also, the synthesis of
each mRNA is inactivated by UV irradiation in proportion to its
own length (31). Thus the subgenomic mRNAs are apparently not
produced by the processing of larger RNAs. These data exclude that
conventional splicing mechanisms are involved in MHV mRNA
synthesis.

However, the data could be explained by a RNA polymerase jump
or translocation during the synthesis of the positive strands. Two
possible models are shown in Fig.5. Translocation could occur by
formation of stable loop structures in the negative strand
(Fig.5A). When the sequence located just upstream from the fusion
site is also present downstream of the leader sequence at the 5'
end of the genome but in a complementary inverted way a stable
loop structure can be formed. In this way the polymerase would
translocate through intervening sequences on the negative strand
and resume transcription at the beginning of a particular cistron.
In the second model the leader acts as a primer at different sites
on the negative stranded template (Fig.5B). This mechanism would
involve the synthesis of a short RNA transcript from the 3' end of

POLYMERASE JUMP

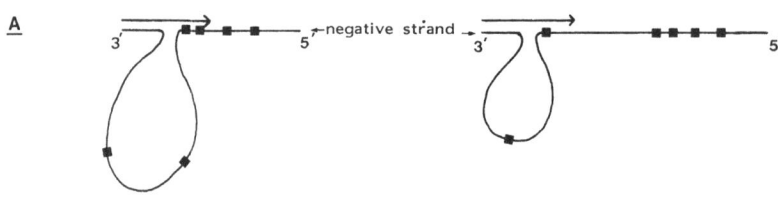

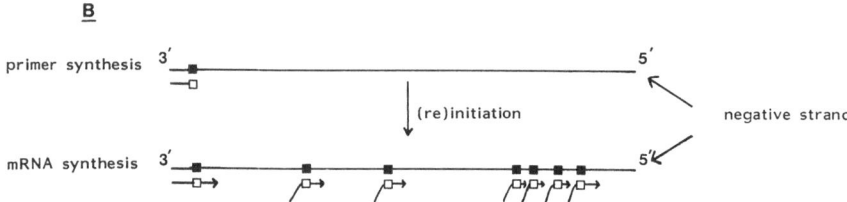

Fig.5. A model for an RNA polymerase jump or translocation
        mechanism during the synthesis of positive stranded MHV-
        A59 RNAs.
        (A) Formation of stable loop structures
        (B) Primed RNA synthesis
        The black boxes represent the beginning of a particular
        cistron.

the negative stranded-template. The leader or polymerase/leader
complex would then be translocated to an internal position on the
negative stranded template where transcription would resume.   This
translocation may or may not involve dissociation of the polyme-
rase/leader complex from the template. Translocation would have to
occur to specific positions and at specific frequencies.   It seems
likely that this specificity would be, at least in part, related
to sequences in the 5' non-coding region of MHV mRNAs. We have
argued that the fusion of leader and body sequences during the
synthesis of mRNA7 and mRNA6 occurs within the sequence
5'AAUCUAAUCUAAACU 3'. This sequence or its 5' end might also be
present within region X of the leader (Fig.1). Although we have
no sequence data of this region X, we assume that T1
oligonucleotide 19, which is also present in a T1 fingerprint of
genomic RNA (17,18), is located at this position. Thus the same
sequence of 15 nucleotides is present at the 5' end of the genome
as at the region just upstream from the nucleocapsid gene. When
the synthesis of the primer would terminate within this 15
nucleotides long repeat, a donor and acceptor site sequence
homology would be created (Fig.6).

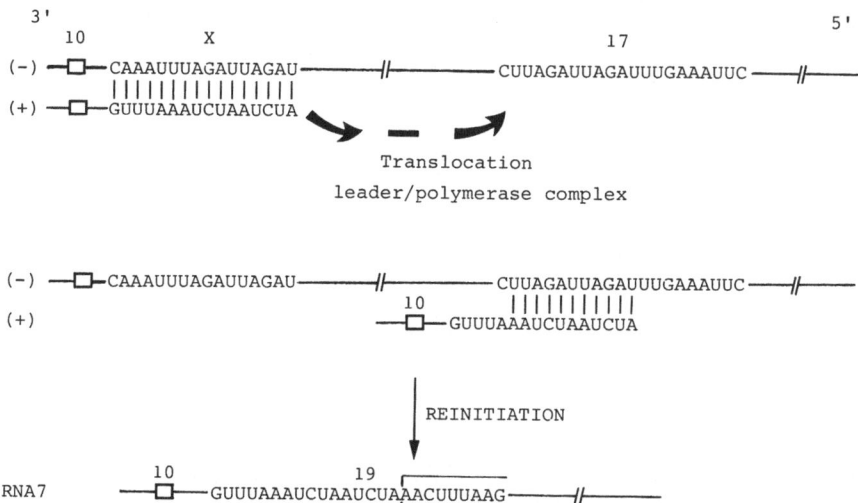

PRIMER BINDING MODEL

Fig.6.   Primer binding model for the synthesis of MHV-A59 mRNA7.
In this model the sequence upstream from the initiating
ATG is also present in region X of the genome. The
synthesis of the leader is terminated in region X and the
leader is translocated to the region just upstream from
the nucleocapsid gene. Because the 3' end of the leader is
complementary to that part of the negative strand
equivalent to T1 oligonucleotide 17 it can bind to this
region. After (re)initiation of RNA synthesis mRNA7 is
made. (The numbers 10, 17 and 19 represent RNase T1
resistant oligonucleotides).

Considering the fact that only one double-stranded replicative
form has been found in infected cells (15, Lai et al., this
volume) we favor the model depicted in Fig.5B and Fig.6. The
mechanism we propose for the generation of coronaviruses would
resemble that observed for the formation of DI influenza virus RNA
(32). Fields and Winter suggest that after the termination of
transcription in a U-rich region of influenza genomic RNA, sequences at the 3' terminus of the nascent chain play a role in the
recognition of reinitiation positions downstream on the template.

A similar mechanism might also explain the high frequency of recombination between aphthovirus RNAs (33).
Primed RNA synthesis is furthermore found during the replication of influenza virus. Newly synthesized cellular mRNA sequences are sequestered and used as primers for mRNA synthesis (34). However, because T1 oligonucleotide 10 is labeled in the presence of actinomycin D, the primer involved in the coronavirus mRNA synthesis must be virus-coded rather than transcribed from a host cell gene.

In addition, translocations caused by leaping of the RNA polymerase are thought to cause the generation of defective interfering (DI) particles of RNA viruses. (35,36). Therefore, it could be argued that the way MHV mRNAs are constructed is not unique to coronaviruses, but rather that it represents a refinement of a mechanism which occurs quite generally, in a haphazard way, in cells infected with RNA viruses.

The transcription process has many interesting features that remain to be resolved. How is the transcription regulated so that the mRNAs are synthesized in non-equimolar amounts? How many proteins are involved in the synthesis of the MHV RNAs and where are the recognition signals located on the RNA template(s)? We have determined the sequence of the 5' end of mRNA7 and because this sequence is derived from the 5' end of the genome we now know the sequence of the 3' end of the negative strand. Comparison of this sequence to the 3' end of the genome (23) shows that there is no sequence homology. This suggests that different enzymes with different recognition signals are involved in the synthesis of negative and positive strands. This is in agreement with the finding of two polymerase activities in MHV-A59 infected cells (37) and the identification of five to six complementation groups in complementation analysis of ts-mutants which were defective in their ability to induce virus-specific RNA synthesis (38, Van der Zeijst manuscript in preparation). Clearly, further sequence analysis of the extreme 5' end of the genome and of more intergenic regions are needed to elucidate the details of this unusual mechanism of RNA synthesis.

ACKNOWLEDGMENTS

We thank Maud Maas Geesteranus for preparation of the manuscript. This investigation was supported by the Foundation for Medical Research (FUNGO) (W.S.) and by the Deutsche Forschungsgemeinschaft (M.S. and S.S.). P.R. was supported at the EMBL by a short-term EMBO fellowship and J.A. by a European Fellowship from the Royal Society.

REFERENCES

1. M.W. Beijerinck, Centralbl. Bacteriol. Parasitenk. Abt. II
   5:27–33 (1899).
2. D.I. Ivanovsky, Sel.'. Khoz. Lêsov. 169:108–121 (1882).
3. B.E. Butterworth, Curr.Top.Microbiol.Immunol. 77:1–41 (1977).
4. A.J. Shatkin, Curr.Top.Microbiol.Immunol. 93:1–4 (1981).
5. A.K. Banerjee, Microbiol. Rev. 44:175–205 (1980).
6. S.J. Flint, Curr.Top.Microbiol.Immunol. 93:47–79 (1981).
7. D. Baltimore, Bacteriol. Rev. 35:235–241 (1971).
8. H. Garoff, C. Kondor–Koch, H. Riedel, Curr.Top.Microbiol.
   Immunol. 99:1–50 (1982).
9. H.F. Lodish, W.A. Braell, A.L. Schwartz, G.J.A.M. Strous, and
   A. Zilberstein, Int.Rev.Cytol.suppl. 12:247–307 (1981).
10. M.F.G.Schmidt, Curr.Top.Microbiol.Immunol. 102:107–129 (1983).
11. B.W.J. Mahy, Nature 288:536–538 (1980).
12. S.G. Siddell, H. Wege, and V. ter Meulen, J.gen.Virol. 64:761–
    776 (1983).
13. L.S. Sturman and K.V. Holmes, Advances in Virus Research, 28:
    in press (1983).
14. J.L. Leibowitz, K.C. Wilhelmsen, and C.W. Bond, Virology
    114:39–51 (1981).
15. M.M.C. Lai, C.D. Patton, and S.A. Stohlman, J.Virol. 44:487–
    492 (1982).
16. M.M.C. Lai, P.R. Brayton, R.C. Armen, C.D. Patton, C. Pugh,
    and S.A. Stohlman, J.Virol. 39:823–834 (1981).
17. M.M.C. Lai, C.D. Patton, and S.A. Stohlman, J.Virol. 41:557–
    565 (1982).
18. W.J.M. Spaan, P.J.M. Rottier, M.C.Horzinek, and B.A.M. Van der
    Zeijst, J.Virol. 42:432–439 (1982).
19. S.G. Siddell, J.gen.Virol. 64:113–125 (1983).
20. P.J.M. Rottier, W.J.M. Spaan, M.C. Horzinek, and B.A.M. Van
    der Zeijst, J.Virol. 38:20–26 (1981).
21. J.L. Leibowitz, S.R. Weiss, E. Paavola and C.W. Bond, J.
    Virol. 43:905–913 (1982).
22. M.M.C. Lai and S.A. Stohlman, J.Virol. 38:661–670 (1981)·.
23. J. Armstrong, S. Smeekens, and P. Rottier, Nucleic Acids Res.
    11:883–891 (1983).
24. H. Delius, H. Westphal, and N. Axelrod, J.Molec.Biol. 74:677–
    687 (1972).
25. H. Garoff and W. Ansorge, Analyt.Biochem. 115:450–457 (1981).
26. H. Priess, B. Koller, B. Hess, and H. Delius, Molec.gen.Genet.
    178:27–34 (1980).
27. D. Zimmern and P. Kaesberg, Proc.natn.Acad.Sci.U.S.A. 75:4257–
    4261 (1978).
28. P.R. Brayton, R.G. Ganges, and S.A. Stohlman, J. gen. Virol.
    56:457–460 (1981).
29. K.C. Wilhemsen, J.L. Leibowitz, C.W. Bond, and J.A. Robb,
    Virology 110:225–230 (1983).

30. B.W.J. Mahy, S. Siddell, H. Wege, and V. Ter Meulen, J.gen.Virol. 64:103–111 (1983).
31. L. Jacobs, W.J.M. Spaan, M.C. Horzinek, and B.A.M. Van der Zeijst, J.Virol. 39:401–406 (1981).
32. S. Fields and G. Winter, Cell 28:303–313 (1982).
33. A.M.W. King, D. McCahon, W.R. Slade, and J.W.I. Newman, Cell 29:921–928 (1982).
34. S.J. Plotch, M. Bouloy, I. Ulmanen, and R. Krug, Cell 23:847–858 (1981).
35. J. Perrault, Curr.Topics Microbiol.Immunol. 93:151–207 (1981).
36. R.D. Lazzarini, J.D. Keene, and M. Schubert, Cell 26:145–154 (1981).
37. P.R. Brayton, M.M.C. Lai, C.D. Patton, and S.A. Stohlman, J.Virol. 42:847–853 (1982).
38. J.L. Leibowitz, J.R. DeVries, and M.V. Haspel, J.Virol. 42:1080–1087 (1982).

STUDIES ON THE MECHANISM OF

RNA SYNTHESIS OF A MURINE CORONAVIRUS

Michael M.C. Lai, Ralph S. Baric, Peter R. Brayton,
and Stephen A. Stohlman

University of Southern California, School of Medicine
2025 Zonal Avenue, Los Angeles, CA 90033

ABSTRACT

   The mechanism of viral RNA replication in mouse hepatitis virus
(MHV)-infected cells was   studied by oligonucleotide mapping of every
mRNA. We discovered that an oligonucleotide, No. 10, was localized at
the 5'-end of every mRNA, and was not colinear with the sequences of the
virion genomic RNA. This result indicates that all of the mRNAs contain
a leader sequence which is joined to the body sequences of the mRNAs.
We have also studied the structure of the replicative intermediate (RI)
RNA in the MHV-infected cells. This RI RNA consists of a single species
corresponding to the MHV genomic RNA. No subgenomic RI structures
were detected. Furthermore, the nascent RNA chains in the RI structure
contained the leader sequences, suggesting that the leader RNA was not
added to the mRNA post-transciptionally, but rather, it was probably
synthesized independently and then used as a primer for the synthesis of
mRNAs. We have also shown that the poly (A) sequences in the MHV
genome were transcribed from the poly (U) sequences present in the
negative-strand template. The RNA polymerases involved in the MHV
RNA synthesis were also characterized. The early polymerase synthesizes
a single negative-stranded, full-length RNA. The late polymerases could
be separated into two activities, one synthesizing positive-stranded
genomic RNA, and the other synthesizing genomic as well as subgenomic
RNAs. Thus, the replication and transcription functions of MHV could
probably be separated.   A plausible model of MHV replication is
presented.

INTRODUCTION

   Murine coronaviruses contain a single-stranded 60 S RNA of 5.4 x
10^6 daltons in molecular weight (Lai and Stohlman, 1978). This RNA has a

187

cap structure at the 5'-end and a stretch of poly (A) at the 3'-end (Lai and Stohlman, 1981). It can be translated in vitro into several proteins in cell-free translation systems (Leibowitz et al., 1982). Therefore, the genomic RNA of murine coronaviruses is positive-stranded. The RNA genome can be divided into at least seven genetic regions (Lai et al., 1981), which encode three structural proteins, pp50, gp25, and gp90/180 (Sturman and Holmes, 1983), and potentially can also code for at least four nonstructural proteins. One or more of these nonstructural proteins could be the RNA-dependent RNA polymerases (Brayton et al., 1982; Mahy et al., 1983), which are responsible for the transcription and replication of viral RNA.

Seven virus-specific mRNA species have been detected in the murine coronavirus-infected cells (Lai et al., 1981; Leibowitz, et al., 1981; Spaan, et al., 1981). These mRNAs, ranging from $0.6 - 5.4 \times 10^6$ daltons, are arranged as a nested set from the 3'-terminus of the genome, so that the sequences of each smaller RNA are conserved at the 3'-end of every larger RNA (Lai et al., 1981). All of the virus-specific mRNAs are capped and polyadenylated, and share at least 5 nucleotides at the 5'-ends (Lai et al., 1982a). Furthermore, some of the mRNAs contain a unique oligonucleotide which is not present in the genomic RNA (Lai et al., 1981, 1982a; Leibowitz et al., 1981). These data suggest that there might be some unusual mechanism of RNA processing involved in the synthesis of mRNAs of murine coronaviruses.

The mechanism of RNA synthesis in murine coronaviruses has only been partially elucidated. We have shown previously that these viruses replicate through a negative-sensed RNA intermediate of full genomic length (Lai et al., 1982b). Consistent with this finding, we have also shown that there is only one single species of double-stranded replicative form (RF) RNA, corresponding to the genomic-sized RNA (Lai et al., 1982b). These results suggest that all of the mRNAs are transcribed from the same genome-sized negative-stranded RNA template. The transcription of both the negative-stranded RNA template and mRNAs appear to be mediated by the virus-coded RNA-dependent RNA polymerases (Brayton et al., 1982). But the detailed mechanism of RNA synthesis is largely unknown. To understand further the replication cycle of murine coronavirus, we have studied the sequences of mRNAs, and the properities of replicative intermediates and RNA polymerases of a murine coronavirus, the A59 strain of mouse hepatitis virus (MHV).

MATERIALS AND METHODS

Virus and cells. The A59 strain of mouse hepatitis virus (MHV-A59) was used throughout this study. DBT cells or Sac (-) cells were used for the growth of virus and preparation of intracellular RNA. The procedures for the growth of virus have been described (Lai et al., 1981). All experiments were performed at $37^{\circ}C$ at a multiplicity of infection of 1-5 and in the presence of actinomycin D (2 ug/ml).

Preparation of intracellular RNA.   The MHV-infected cells were labeled with ^{32}P-orthophosphate at 6 h post-infection (p.i.) for various lenghts of time.   The intracellular RNA was extracted by SDS-phenol as described (Lai et al., 1981).   The ^{32}P-labeled MHV-specific RNA was separated by electrophoresis on 1% agarose gels and each RNA band was eluted out of the gel.

For preparation of replicative intermediate (RI) RNA, the intracellular RNA was adjusted to 2 M NaCl and 0.05% SDS, and incubated at 0-4°C for 24-30 h.   Afterwards, the incubation mixture was centrifuged at 14,500 rpm in a Ti 30 rotor for 60 min.   The precipitate was resuspended in LSB buffer (0.01 M Tris HCl, pH 7.4 and 1 mM EDTA) containing 1% SDS and fractionated by chromatography on a Sepharose 2B-CL column (98x1.5 cm) (Spector and Baltimore, 1975).   The fractions in the void volume consisted of the replicative intermediate RNA.

Oligonucleotide fingerprinting and mapping.   The ^{32}P-labeled RNA prepared from the agarose gels or from the RI was digested exhaustively with RNase T$_1$ and separated by two-dimensional polyacrylamide gel electrophoresis as described (Lai, et al., 1981).   Briefly, the first dimension was performed on 8% polyacrylamide gel slabs (30x10x0.15 cm) at pH 3.3, 700 V for 4 hours.   The second dimension was performed on 22% polyacrylamide gel slabs (40x35x0.075 cm) at pH 8.0, 650 V for 16 hours.

For oligonucleotide mapping, the RNA was partially degraded by boiling at 100°C for 3 min.   The poly (A)-containing RNA fragments were selected by chromatography on oligo (dT)-cellulose.   These RNAs were separated by sucrose gradient sedimentation and each size fraction was studied by oligonucleotide fingerprinting.

Membrane fractionation and RNA polymerase assay.   The MHV-infected cells were disrupted by Dounce homogenization in RSB buffer (0.01 M Tris HCl, pH 7.4, 0.01 M NaCl and 0.0015 M MgCl$_2$).   After removal of the nuclei, the cellular membranes were centrifuged in a 9 to 50% sucrose gradient made in 2xRSB with 40 ug dextran sulfate per ml at 90,000 xg for 1.5 h.   The 0.2ml fractions were collected and each fraction was assayed for RNA polymerase activity according to published procedures (Brayton, et al., 1982).

RESULTS

Presence of Leader RNA Sequences in the mRNAs of mouse hepatitis virus (MHV). Previous studies of the sequences of the MHV mRNAs indicated that the 5'-ends of each mRNA share at least 5 nucleotides, and that several mRNAs contain a T$_1$-oligonucleotide not present in the oligonucleotide fingerprints of the virion genomic RNA (Lai et al., 1981, 1982a).   These data suggest the possible presence of leader RNA sequences in the mRNAs. To identify such RNA sequences, we studied all of the large T$_1$-oligonucleotides in every mRNA with respect to their map locations on the respective mRNA. This study was designed to determine whether all of the sequences in the mRNAs are colinear with those in the genomic RNA. The ^{32}P-labeled mRNAs were separated by gel electrophoresis, eluted and then partially degraded by boiling. The poly (A)-containing fractions of such partially degraded mRNAs were selected by oligo (dT)-cellulose chromatography and separated by sucrose gradient sedimentation. The different size fractions separated under such conditions represent the 3'-RNA fragments of different sizes derived from each mRNA. These mRNA fragments were studied by T_1-oligonucleotide fingerprinting. Some of these fingerprints are shown in Fig. 1. Examination of these oligonucleotides showed that all of the oligonucleotides in the different mRNAs and genomic RNA are mapped at the corresponding positions, i.e. they are colinear in all of the mRNAs and genomic RNA. However, closer examination revealed an oligonucleotide, No. 10, which is not present at the same position in each mRNA species. It is located at the 5'-ends of every mRNA (Fig. 2). Since the oligonucleotide No. 10 is present only once in the genomic RNA, this result indicates that this oligonucleotide represents a leader RNA segment which is joined to the body sequences of every mRNA of MHV. Since this oligonucleotide has 23 bases, and the first 5 nucleotides at the 5'-ends of mRNAs are identical for all of the mRNAs (Lai et al., 1982a), the leader RNA sequences must be at least 28 nucleotides long. These results provided the strongest evidence so far for the presence of leader RNA sequences in MHV mRNAs. Thus, the unique oligonucleotides which are present only in the mRNAs could represent the junction oligonucleotides between the leader and the body sequences of mRNAs. This is consistent with the base sequences of these oligonucleotides, which showed that they are identical at the 5'-half, but differ at the 3'-half, sequences of the oligonucleotides (Lai et al., 1982a). The 5'-half presumably is derived from the leader and the 3'-half from the body sequences of the mRNAs.

Models of mRNA Synthesis in MHV. The presence of the leader RNA sequences in the MHV mRNAs suggest that RNA splicing might be involved in the synthesis of mRNA. However, UV transcriptional mapping studies suggest that the mRNAs are not derived from the cleavage of precursor RNAs (Jacobs et al., 1981). These two pieces of data indicate that the leader RNA and the body suquences of MHV mRNAs must be joined by a novel nucleus-independent mechanism. We propose three possible mechanisms for the synthesis of such mRNAs (Fig. 3): In the first model, the RNA polymerase "jumps" from the leader RNA region to various initiation sites for different mRNAs, probably as a result of "looping out" of the RNA template. The second model proposes that the leader RNA is synthesized independently and falls off the negative-stranded RNA template. This free leader RNA then binds to RNA polymerase or a short complementary region at the initiation sites for different mRNAs. In this fashion, the leader RNA serves as a primer for mRNA synthesis. The third model proposes that the leader RNA and the body sequences of MHV mRNAs are synthesized independently and then linked together post-transcriptionally by an unknown mechanism.

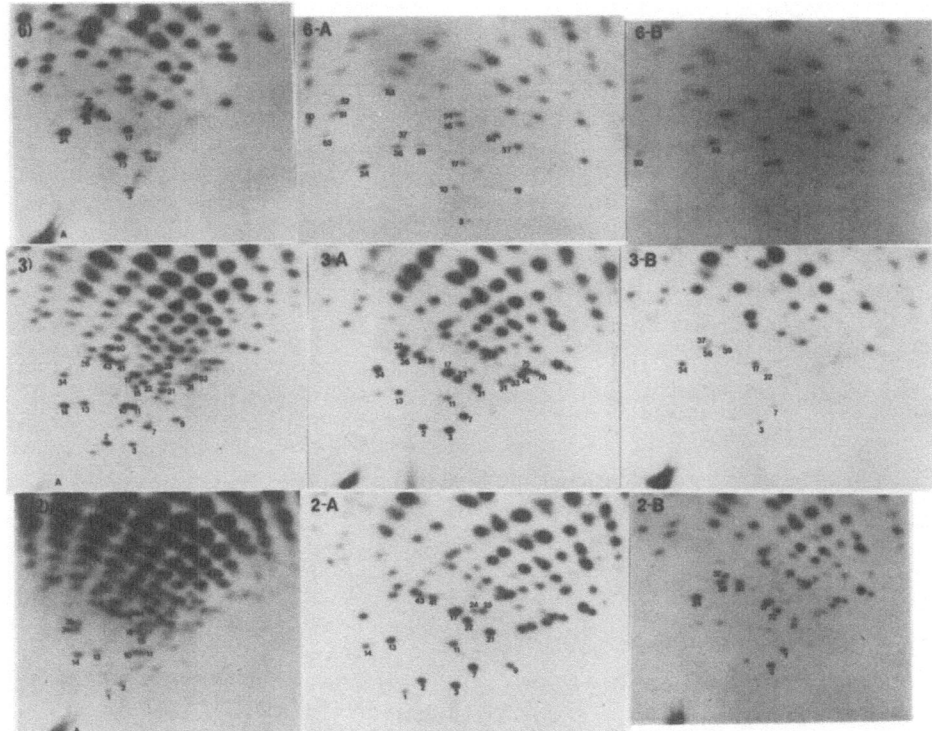

Fig. 1.   Oligonucleotide maps of mRNAs #6, 3 and 2.   The poly (A)-containing RNA fragments derived from different mRNAs were digested with RNase T$_1$ and fingerprinted. (6) (3) and (2) represent full-length mRNAs. The other panels represent the fragments derived from the 3'-ends of different mRNAs.   Note that the oligonucleotide No. 10 was detected only in the full-length mRNA.

$$(\underline{10},\underline{19},57,56,55,51,36,34,52)\,50\,(53,54) \; \#7$$

$$(\underline{10}(?),\underline{19a},3,17,37,39,63)(57,56,55,51,36,34,52)\,50\,(53,54) \; \#6$$

$$(\underline{10}(?),\underline{3a},75,76,74,22)(3,17,37,39,63)(57,56,55,51,36,34,52)\,50\,(53,54) \; \#5$$

$$(\underline{10},43)(9,41,50,25,11,14)(21,13,2,33,31,7,75,76,74,22)(3,17,37,39,63)(57,56,55,51,36,34,52)\,50\,(53,54) \; \#3$$

$$(\underline{10},16,15,44,35)(24,1,43)(9,41,50,25,11,14)(21,13,2,33,31,7,75,76,74,22)(3,17,37,39,63)(57,56,55,51,36,34,52)\,50\,(53,54) \; \#2$$

Fig. 2.   Schematic drawing of oligonucleotide maps of MHV mRNAs.
The oligonucleotides were arranged in the order of 5' 3' ends. The order of the oligonucleotides within each bracket is not certain.

MODEL 1: "LOOP OUT"

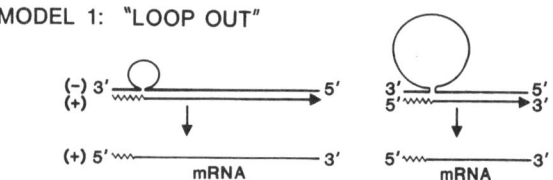

MODEL 2: LEADER-PRIMED TRANSCRIPTION

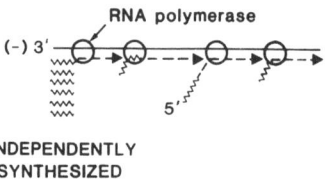

INDEPENDENTLY
SYNTHESIZED
LEADER RNA

MODEL 3: POST-TRANSCRIPTIONAL PROCESSING

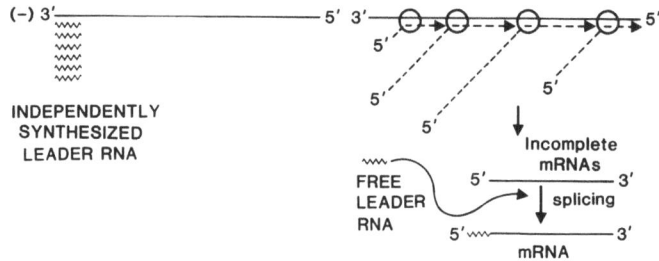

INDEPENDENTLY
SYNTHESIZED
LEADER RNA

Fig. 3.   Proposed models for the mechanism of transcription of
MHV mRNAs.

To distinguish these three transcriptional models for MHV, we have
performed several types of experiments. The first experiment is the
identification of the replicative-form (RF) RNA species derived from
RNase digestion of the intracellular MHV-specific RNAs.   If MHV
replication utilizes the mechanism as proposed in the first model, there
should be seven RF RNA species of different sizes, corresponding to the
seven mRNA species. But only one RF RNA of genomic size was detected
(Fig. 4). This result makes the first model quite unlikely.   To decide
between the second and the third model, we studied the replicative
intermediate (RI) RNA, which should represent the RNA structure
actively involved in MHV RNA replication.   The leader RNA should be
present in the RI if the second model is correct. The properties of such
RI is described in the next section.

Fig. 4.   Agarose gel electrophoresis of replicative form (RF) RNA. The RF RNA was isolated from the supernatant of the 2M NaCl precipitation of the intracellular RNA followed by RNase A digestion. The electrophoresis was performed in 1% agarose gels.

Studies of Replicative Intermediate RNA of MHV. The RI RNA was prepared from the intracellular MHV-specific RNA by precipitation with 2M NaCl followed by gel filtration chromatography on Sepharose 2B-CL. The RI RNA was collected from the void volume (the first peak in Fig 5A) and was found to be 38% RNase A-resistant. This result indicates that this RNA structure is partially double-stranded and partially single-stranded as predicted from the structure of replicative intermediates.   The RI RNA was further analyzed by agarose gel electrophoresis and found to migrate as a single band with an electrophoretic mobility very closely resembling that of the single-stranded genomic RNA (Fig. 5B). The RI RNA was heat-denatured into a heterogeneous collection of RNAs ranging from the genomic size to RNAs smaller than the mRNA #7.   This result is consistent with the interpretation that the RI structure consists of a genome-length negative-stranded RNA, hydrogen-bonded to multiple growing nascent (+)-strand RNAs. RNase digestion of this RI structure produced a single species of double-stranded RF RNA (data not shown). This result again demonstrated that the mechanism depicted by the first model is not applicable to the transcription of MHV RNA.

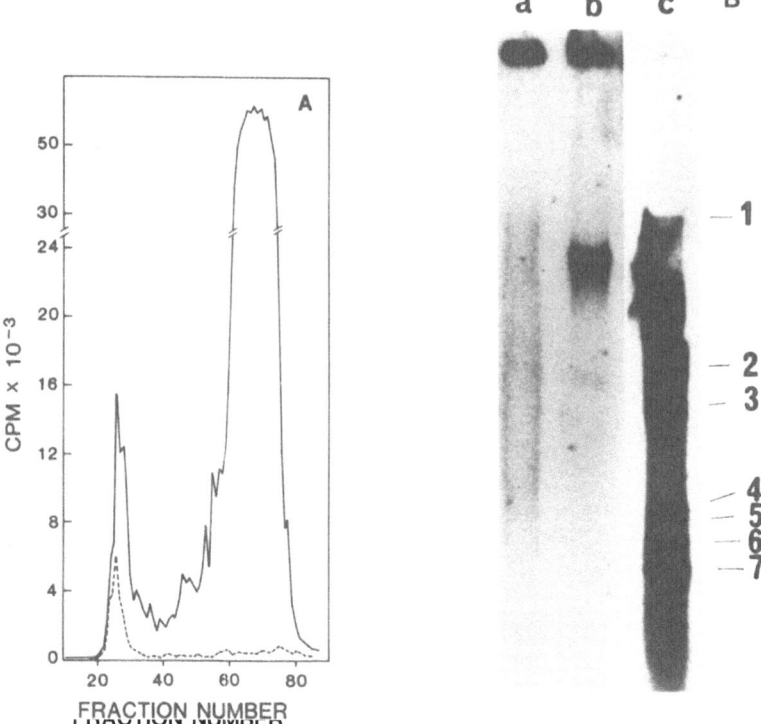

Fig. 5   Characterization of replicative intermediate (RI) RNA.   (A)
Chromatography on Sepharose 2B-CL column of the 2M NaCl
precipitate of the ^{32}P-labeled intracellular RNA. (B) Agarose gel
electrophoresis of the first peak in (A).   (a) heat-denatured RI; (b)
native RI; and (c) total mRNAs as molecular weight markers.

To further distiguish the second from the third models of RNA
transcription, we studied the oligonucleotide fingerprints of the RI RNA.
If the second model is correct, the nascent (+)-strand RNAs are expected
to contain the leader RNA sequences.   On the other hand, if the third
model is correct, the leader RNA sequences will not be present in the RI
structure,   since   the   leader   RNA   is   added   to   the   mRNA
post-transcriptionally. We performed the oligonucleotide fingerprinting
of the RI without heat-denaturation. This approach will identify only the
newly synthesized nascent (+) RNA strands which have become the
single-stranded RNA tails in the RI structure (see Fig. 9 for the possible
structure of RI). As shown in Fig. 6, the "leader"-specific oligonucleotide,
No. 10, was present in the RI. This result indicates that the leader RNA
sequneces are joined to the mRNAs during transcription, rather than
post-transcriptionally.   Thus the second model is the most likely
mechanism of MHV RNA transcription.

Additional information concerning the mechanism of RNA synthesis was obtained from the oligonucleotide fingerprints of the heat-denatured RI. This reflects the sequences represented in the double-stranded portion as well as the single-stranded tails, of RI. Fig. 6B shows that the oligonucleotide fingerprint of the heat-denatured RI is essentially identical to that of the undenatured RI. However, the former contains a prominent poly (A) spot. This result suggests that the poly (A) sequences are transcribed from the poly (U) sequences present on the negative-stranded RNA templates, rather than added post-transcriptionally. This mechanism is similar to that observed during the replication of poliovirus (Spector and Baltimore, 1975).

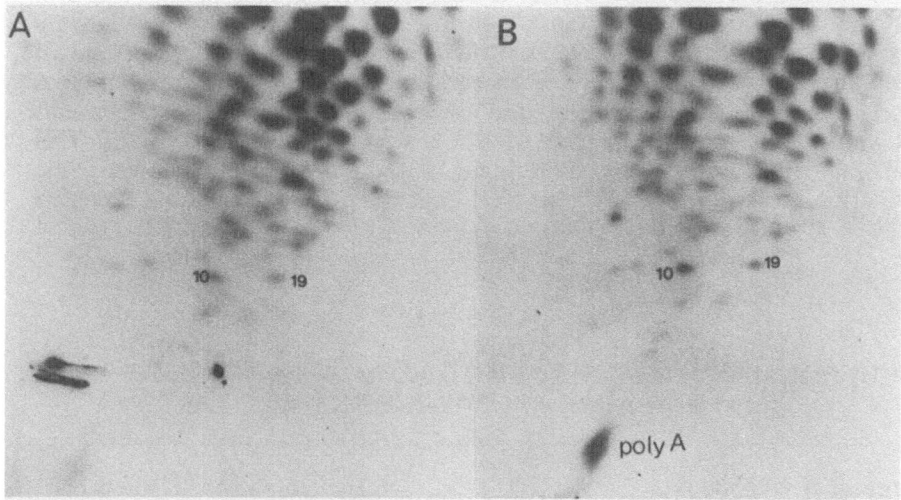

Fig. 6.   Oligonucleotide fingerprints of the RI RNA.   (a) native; (b) heat-denatured.

Studies of MHV-specific RNA polymerases. The studies described in the previous sections suggest that a very unique mechanism of RNA synthesis is employed in the synthesis of MHV RNA. Therefore, the RNA polymerases of MHV might possess very unique biochemical properties. Previous studies in our laboratories have indicated that two different RNA polymerases, one early (1 hour post-infection) and the other late (6 hour post-infection), can be detected in MHV-infected cells. We further studied the properties of these two polymerases in order to understand the mechanism of MHV RNA synthesis. We first attempted to fractionate the membrane complexes containing the RNA polymerase activities in MHV-infected cells. We subjected the cellular membranes, excluding the nuclei, from the MHV-infected cells to sucrose gradient sedimentation analysis. As shown in Fig. 7, the early RNA polymerase activity was contained in a single membrane complex, while the late RNA polymerase activity was divided into two separate membrane complexes. The functions of the polymerases contained in these membrane complexes were examined by studying the sense and size of the RNA species made by these membrane complexes in vitro. As shown in Table 1, the early RNA polymerase synthesizes RNA of negative sense which was completely hybridized by virion genomic RNA. Furthermore, the RNA synthesized consisted of a single RNA species of genomic size (Fig. 8). This is consistent with the properties of the MHV-specific RNA made in the infected cells early in the infection (Lai, et al, 1982). The RNA made in vitro by the two membrane complexes at 6 h p.i., on the other hand, was positive-stranded, since they were completely hybridized by the representative cDNA of the MHV genome but not the genomic RNA itself (Table 1). The heavy (H) fraction of the late membrane complexes synthesized genomic as well as most, if not all, of the subgenomic mRNAs similar to those found in the MHV-infected cells. These results indicate that the RNA polymerase contained in this fraction is the enzyme responsible for the synthesis of mRNAs in vivo. Therefore, this membrane complex can be considered as the transcription complex. Surprisingly, the light (L) fraction of the late membrane complexes synthesized only a single species of RNA, which is of genome size. This result indicates that this fraction might be the enzyme responsible for the replication of the viral RNA genome. Therefore, this membrane complex might be a replication complex.

Table 1

Hybridization of the in vitro RNA products of the early and late polymerase peaks with MHV-A59 RNA or cDNA

Source of RNA products	% Hybridization to the probe	
	genomic RNA	cDNA
Early polymerase (1 h. p.i.)	102	9
Late polymerase (L) (p h. p.i.)	8	125
Late polymerase (H) (6 h. p.i.)	12	115
^{3}H uridine-labeled genomic RNA	4	99

The membrane fractions separated by sucrose grandients as shown in Fig. 7 were assayed for RNA polymerase activities. The RNA products obtained from the activity peaks were phenol-extracted and used for hybridization with excess (at least 100 fold) of genomic RNA or cDNA made with genomic RNA. Hybridization was perfomed in the presence of 0.75M NaCl at 68°C for 12-16 hours as described elsewhere (Lai et al., 1979).

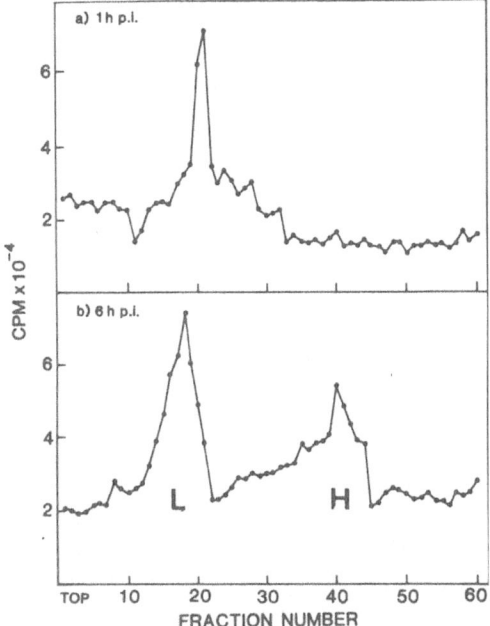

Fig. 7. <u>Sucrose gradient sedimentation of the polymerase-containing membrane complexes.</u> Sedimentation was performed on a 9–50%sucrose gradient in an SW27 rotor at 25K for 1.5 hour. Each fraction was assayed for RNA polymerase activity as measured by incoporation of the ³H-UTP.

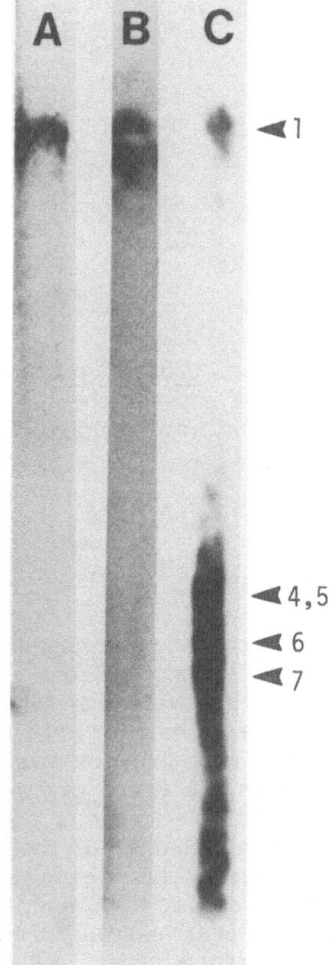

Fig. 8. <u>Agarose gel electrophoresis of the RNA products of the in vitro RNA polymerase activities.</u> (a) 1 hr p.i.; (b) 6 hr. p.i. L fraction; and (c) 6 hr. p.i. H fraction.

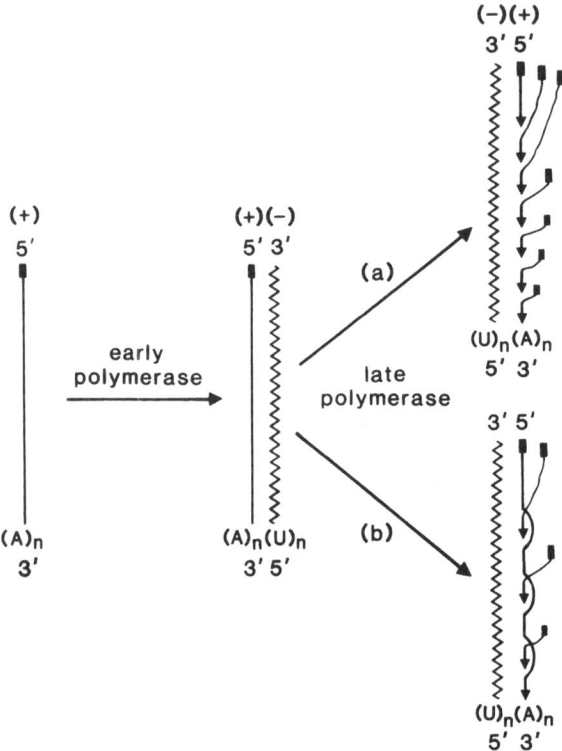

Fig. 9.   Proposed models of the replication of MHV. The solid boxes at the ends of the (+) strands represent the leader sequences.   (a) semiconservation; (b) conservation mechanisms.

DISCUSSION

From the studies published elsewhere (Lai et al., 1982a,b; Brayton et al., 1982; Jacobs et al., 1981) and presented in this communication, the replication cycle of murine coronaviruses can be summarized as in Fig. 9. It is clear that the RNA synthesis, particularly the mRNA synthesis, of murine coronaviruses involves a very complex and unique mechanism. It involves the fusion of two noncontiguous RNA segments, one of which serves as the leader or primer for the synthesis of every mRNA species. It appears that all of the mRNAs contain the same kind of leader RNA sequences. These leader sequences are also present at the 5'-end of the virion genomic RNA, and, therefore, might be transcribed from the 3'-end of the negative-stranded full-length RNA intermediate. The mechanisms by which the leader RNA is synthesized and joined to the body sequences of the mRNAs are still poorly understood. But, it is most likely, as proposed by the model 2 (Fig. 3) that the leader RNA is synthesized independently and then serves as the primer for the synthesis of the body sequences of mRNAs. Therefore, this process is entirely different from the conventional post-transcriptional RNA splicing. It is, in some aspects, similar to the RNA synthesis of influenza virus (Krug, 1981). But, in the case of coronavirus, the primer RNA is more likely viral RNA rather than cellular mRNA. The presence of leader RNA is also reminiscent of vesicular stomatitis virus (Colonno and Banerjee, 1976). But, these two viruses are again different, since the leader RNA in VSV is not joined to the mRNAs. Therefore, the mechanism of mRNA synthesis in MHV is unique among all of animal viruses.

There are still many unanswered and puzzling questions in the mechanism of RNA synthesis for murine coronaviruses: First of all, the mechanism by which the leader RNA is synthesized and then used as a primer is unknown. So far, no free leader RNA has been detected in the MHV-infected cells. Secondly, the structure of the replicative intermediate poses a very difficult problem. This RI must be simultaneously synthesizing 7 mRNAs at different rates. The entire sequences of every negative-strand RNA template probably are used for transcription. Furthermore, there must be a mechanism by which the rate of initiation for different mRNAs are regulated. The exact details of the structure of this kind of RI remains to be studied.

The RNA polymerases involved in the synthesis of the negative-stranded RNA template early in the infection and the positive-stranded RNA later in the infection are probably different (Brayton et al, 1982). However, it is not clear whether they are two different enzymes or a modification of the same enzyme. If the latter is the case, modification could be caused by a viral gene product of by a host cell factor. It is not yet possible to distinguish between these two possibilities.

The possible separation of the transcription and replication complexes raises an interesting question. Is there a structural difference between the genomic RNA destined for packaging into viral particles and that used for mRNAs? Such a difference could conceivably be achieved by the way the leader RNA is joined to the viral RNA. Such issue requires further studies.

ACKNOWLEDGMENT

We thank Chris Patton, Todd Kennell and Mahmood Kafaii for excellent technical assistance, and Cathy Wung, Raymond Mitchell and Alisa Young for editorial assistance in manuscript preparation.

This work was supported by Public Health Service research grant AI 19244 from the National Institutes of Health, grant PCM-4507 from the National Science Foundation, and grant RG 1449-A from the National Multiple Sclerosis Society.

REFERENCES

- Brayton, P.R., Lai, M.M.C., Patton, C.D and Stohlman, S.A. 1982. Characterization of two RNA polymerase activities induced by mouse hepatitis virus. J. Virol. 42:847-853.
- Colonno, R.J. and A.K. Banerjee. 1976. A unique RNA species involved in initiation of vesicular stomatitis virus RNA transcription. Cell 8:197-204.
- Jacobs, L., W.J.M. Spaan, M.C. Horzinek and B.A.M. Van der Zeijst. 1981. Synthesis of subgenomic mRNAs of mouse hepatitis virus is initiated independently:evidence from UV transcription mapping. J. Virol. 39:401-406.
- Krug, R.M. 1981. Priming of influenza viral RNA transcription by capped heterologous RNAs. Curr. Topics in Microb. Immunol. 93:125-149.
- Lai, M.M.C., Brayton, P.R., Armen, R.C., Patton, C.D., Pugh, C., and S.A. Stohlman. 1981. Mouse hepatitis virus A59: Messenger RNA structure and genetic localization of the sequence divergence from a hepatotropic strain MHV-3. J. Virol. 39:823-834.
- Lai, M.M.C., S.S.F. Hu and P.K. Vogt. 1979. Avian erythroblastosis virus: Transformation-specific sequences form a contiguous segment of 3.25 kb located in the middle of the 6-kb genome. Virology 97:366-377.
- Lai, M.M.C., Patton, C.D., and S.A. Stohlman. 1982a. Further characterization of mRNAs of mouse hepatitis virus: presence of common 5'-end nucleotides. J. Virol. 41:557-565.
- Lai, M.M.C., C.D. Patton and S.A. Stohlman. 1982b. Replication of mouse hepatitis virus: negative-stranded RNA and replicative form RNA are of genome length. J. Virol. 44:487-492.
- Lai, M.M.C. and S.A. Stohlman. 1978. The RNA of mouse hepatitis virus. J. Virol. 271:236-242.
- Lai, M.M.C. and Stohlman, S.A. 1981. Comparative analysis of RNA genome of mouse hepatitis virus. J. Virol. 38:661-670.
- Leibowitz, J.L., S.R. Weiss, E. Paavola and C.L. Bond. 1982. Cell-free translation of murine coronavirus RNA. J. Virol. 43:905-913.
- Leibowitz, J.L., K.C. Wilhelmsen and C.W. Bond. 1981. The virus-specific intracellular RNA species of two murine coronaviruses: MHV-A59 and MHV-JHM. Virology 114:29-51.
- Mahy, B.W.J., S. Siddell, H. Wege and V. ter Meulen. 1983. RNA-dependent RNA polymerase activity in murine coronavirus-infected cell. J. Gen. Virol. 64:103-111.
- Spaan, W.J.M., P.J.M. Rottier, M.C. Horzinek and B.A.M. van der Zeijst. 1981. Isolation and identification of virus-specific mRNAs in cells infected with mouse hepatitis virus (MHV-A59). Virology 108:424-434.
- Spector, D.H. and D. Baltimore. 1975. Polyadenylic acid on poliovirus RNA. II. Poly A on intracellular RNAs. J. Virol. 15:1418-1431.
- Sturman, L.S. and K.V. Homes. 1983. The molecular biology of coronaviruses. Adv. in Virus Research (in press).

GLYCOPROTEIN E1 OF MHV-A59: STRUCTURE OF THE O-LINKED CARBOHYDRA-
TES AND CONSTRUCTION OF FULL LENGTH RECOMBINANT cDNA CLONES

Heiner Niemann[1], Gudrun Heisterberg-Moutsis[2], Rudolf
Geyer[3], Hans-Dieter Klenk[1], and Manfred Wirth[1]

[1] Institut für Virologie, Fachbereich Humanmedizin
    Frankfurter Str. 107, D-6300 Giessen
[2] Gesellschaft für Biotechnologische Forschung
    Mascheroder Weg, D-3301 Stöckheim-Braunschweig
[3] Biochemisches Institut am Klinikum der JLU, Fried-
    richstr. 24, D-6300 Giessen

INTRODUCTION

The murine coronaviruses contain two different classes of
glycoproteins (for review see [1]). The envelope glycoprotein E2
resembles in its composition and biosynthetic processing the
classical type of viral glycoprotein: E2 acquires N-glycosidically linked carbohydrate side chains in a cotranslational event
at the rough endoplasmic reticulum (RER) [2] and in addition, it
contains covalently linked fatty acids [3]. The 180K species of E2
is processed posttranslationally by proteolytic cleavage into two
90K species [2,4]. The second type of coronavirus envelope glycoprotein which was designated the matrix glycoprotein E1 is unique
in many ways:
1. The transmembranal nature of E1 allows it to interact with the
viral nucleocapsid like a matrix protein of other viruses [5]. The
intracellular distribution of E1 in perinuclear regions of the infected cell (GERL) determines the budding site of coronaviruses [6].
2. The intramembranal hydrophobic domain of glycoprotein E1 has a
capability for auto-aggregation [7].
3. In the murine and bovine coronaviruses E1 has exclusively O-
linked carbohydrate side chains which are only added posttranslationally after transfer of the E1 polypeptide from the site of
its biosynthesis (RER) to the trans-cisternae of the Golgi complex
[2,3].
With these two classes of glycoprotein, mouse hepatitis virus A59
offers an ideal system to study the potential functions of N- versus O-glycosylation as well as the biosynthesis and intracellular

transport of these two different molecules. Therefore, we are interested in studying the expression of the E1 gene using recombinant DNA techniques and appling site specific mutagenesis to alter
the glycosylation sites of E1. We present here the structures of
the carbohydrates of E1 and describe the construction of full
length clones of glycoprotein E1 with the help of a synthetic
oligodeoxyribonucleotide primer.

MATERIALS AND METHODS

Virus and cells. MHV-A59 was grown in 17C11 cells and purified as previously described [8].

Isolation of Q-linked carbohydrate side chains. Glycoprotein
E1 was metabolically labelled with ^{3}H-galactose, purified by preparative gel electrophoresis and subjected to ß-elimination using
$NaBH_4$ as a reducing agent[3]. The released oligosaccharides were
desalted by passage over a Biogel P2 column (35 x 1 cm) and separated by high performance liquid chromatography (HPLC) as indicated in the legend to Figure 1.

Permethylation analyses and combined gas chromatography-mass-
spectrometry. Purified oligosaccharides were permethylated, hydrolyzed, reduced with $NaBD_4$ and analyzed as partially methylated
alditol acetates by combined gas chromatography mass-spectrometry
as detailed elsewhere [9].

Vibro-cholerae-neuraminidase treatment of purified oligosaccharides was carried out as described earlier [3].

Synthesis of the oligodeoxynucleotide primer. A pentadeca-
deoxyribonucleotide was synthesized on the polydimethylacrylamide-
Kieselguhr support (C-resin, 75 µMole dC/g) following the phosphotriester method as described by Gait et al. [10]. The partially deprotected, 5'-dimethyoxytrityl-substituted oligomer was purified
by reversed phase HPLC as outlined in the legend to Figure 1a.
Detritylation was performed in 5 ml acetic acid:water (8:2) for
30 min at room temperature (yield after lyophilisation and ether
extraction: 95 OD). Part of the material was 5'-^{32}P-labelled using
T4-polynucleotide kinase (Boeheringer, Mannheim) and analyzed on
a 20 % acrylamide gel (Figure 1b) using oligo(dA)$_{3-n}$ and oligo(dT)$_{3-m}$
as length markers. Radioactive length markers were prepared by
elongation of oligo(dA)$_3$ or oligo(dT)$_3$ with terminal deoxynucleotidyl transferase and 5'-^{32}P-labelled [11].

Isolation of total poly-A$^+$-RNA. Poly-A$^+$-RNA was isolated
from infected 17C11 cells (m.o.i. = 50 PFU/cell) 16 hrs post infection, purified by oligo-dT-cellulose (P.L. Biochemicals) and
assayed by in vitro translation [2].

Construction of full length E1-cDNA. First strand cDNA was
synthesized in a mixture containing poly-A$^+$-RNA (10 µg), pentadeca
oligodeoxyribonucleotide (20 ng), Tris/HCl, pH 8.3 (50 mM), KCl
(30 mM), $MgCl_2$ (10 mM), sodium pyrophosphate (2 mM), RNasin (Bol-
ton Biological), dithiothreitol (1 mM), dATP, dGTP, dTTP (1 mM

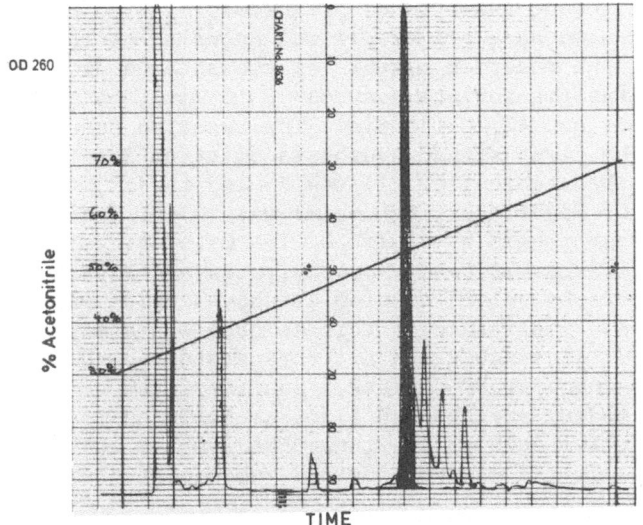 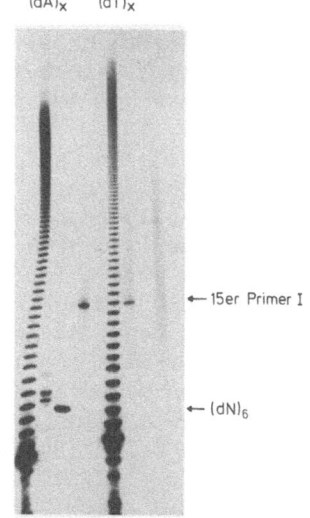

Fig. 1a:
  HPLC of the partially deprotected pentadeca-
  oligodeoxy-ribonucleotide 5'dTTCTTGCCCAGGAAC$^{3'}$
  before detritylation. Column: 5 μ Lichrosorb
  RP18 (Merck); Elution: linear gradient of
  0.1 M ammonium acetate (A) and 0.1 M ammonium acetate/acetonitrile (2:8 v/v) (B).

Fig. 1b:
  Polyacrylamide gel
  electrophoresis of the
  5'-^{32}P-labelled deprotected oligonucle-
  otide. The primer was
  5' labelled with poly-
  nucleotide kinase and
  analyzed on a 20% acry-
  lamide gel prepared
  according to Frank
  et al.[11].

each), dCTP (0.2 mM), α-^{32}P-dCTP (50 μCi; Amersham 410 Ci/mM) and
AMV reverse transcriptase (200 U, Life Sciences) in a total volume
of 250 μl. Prior to the addition of dithiothreitol, dNTP's, and
enzyme, the primer was annealed by incubation at 55° C for 5 min,
50° C for 10 min and 42° C for 15 minutes. The reaction was carried
out at 42° C for 60 min and stopped by adjusting the mixture to
0.5 N NaCl, 20 mM EDTA pH 7.5, and 0.5 % SDS. The mixture was extracted with chloroform/isoamylalcohol (24:1), the organic phase
was re-extracted with one volume of water. The dried material was
taken up in 40 μl of freshly prepared 0.4 N NaOH and left for 7
hrs at room temperature to degrade the RNA. Free nucleotides were
removed by passage over a Sephadex G-100 column in 10 mM NaOH
(siliconized Pasteur pipette, bed volume 2 ml). The radioactive
material in the void volume was collected, neutralized with HCl
and precipitated with ethanol after the addition of 1/10 volume
of 3.0 M potassium acetate. The addition of homopolymeric dC-
tails to the 3'end of the single stranded cDNA was carried out
for 10 min as described by Land et al. [12]).

To synthesize the second DNA-strand, oligo(dG)$_{12-18}$ (30 μg/ml,
P.L.-Biochemicals) was used as a primer. It was annealed to the
template by incubating the reaction mixture in the absence of nucleotides and AMV reverse transcriptase at 65° C (5 min), 55° C
(5 min), 50° C (10 min), and 42° C (15 min). The reaction conditions
were the same as for the first strand synthesis omitting RNasin.
After 60 min at 42° C the sample (100 μl) was cooled to 15° C and
Klenow polymerase (20 U, Boehringer, Mannheim) was added. The mixture was incubated for another 8 hr at 15° C. The material was extracted with chloroform/isoamylalcohol, precipitated and separated from free nucleotides by gel filtration as above, using water
as an eluent. S1 nuclease resistance of this ds-cDNA was assayed
together with an aliquot of ss-cDNA and nick-translated λ-DNA in
reaction mixtures containing 10.000 Cerenkov counts of the respective DNA in 50 mM sodium acetate (pH 4.5), NaCl (0.2 M), ZnSO$_4$
(1 mM), 0.5 % glycerol. For each of the three DNA samples control
values were determined after 3 min boiling and subsequent quenching
on ice.
A second tailing reaction was performed on ds-cDNA, adding an
average of 15 dC-residues per 3'end.

Bacterial transformation with hybrid plasmid DNA. Vector
pUR 250 [13]) (kindly provided by Ulrich Rüther, Köln), was restricted with AccI in the presence of alkaline phosphatase. After the
addition of an average of 15 dG-residues per 3'end with terminal
nucleotidyl transferase the tailed vector was purified by electrophoresis through a preparative 1 % agarose gel and recovered by
electroelution. dG-Tailed pUR250 and dC-tailed cDNA were mixed in
a molar ratio with a final concentration of 200 ng vector/ml in
Tris-HCl, pH 7.5, 100 mM NaCl and 1 mM EDTA. The mixture was first
heated to 68° C for 5 min and then kept at 43° C for 2 hrs and
allowed to cool to room temperature over a 1 hr period. 10 μl of
annealing solution (2.0 ng vector) was added to 100 μl of competent RRI cells. Transformation was carried out as described by
Dagert and Ehrlich [14]).

Screening for plasmids containing E1 sequences. Colony hybridization of lac⁻ colonies was performed as described by Grunstein and Hogness [15]) using an E1 specific probe obtained by reverse transcription of purified viral RNA with the synthetic primer. Plasmid DNA was prepared from chloramphenicol amplified 100
ml-cultures by lysis with alkali and purified by chromatography
over a NACS 52 column (Bethesda Research Laboratories) as detailed
by the manufacturer.

Subcloning and sequencing in pEMBL8 (in collaboration with
J. Armstrong, EMBL.) E1-specific DNA was released from cloned
p42-DNA by double digestion with HindIII and EcoRI and ligated
into pEMBL8 which had been cleaved with the same restriction nu-

cleases. Dideoxy-sequencing was performed on ss-pEMBL8-DNA, obtained after superinfection of the pEMBL8-culture with wild type
f1 as described by Dente et al. [16] using a 15-base synthetic
single stranded universal primer (P.L.-Biochemicals). Reaction
products were analyzed on thermostated 6 % acrylamide gels [17].

RESULTS AND DISCUSSIONS

Structure of the O-linked carbohydrate side chains of glycoprotein E1. Glycoprotein E1 of MHV-A59 contains exclusively O-
linked carbohydrate side chains. They could be released from the
protein backbone in an intact form by ß-elimination in the presence of $NaBH_4$ to avoid peeling of the carbohydrate chain [3]. Two
peak fractions designated A and B were separated by HPLC (Fig.2,
upper panel). By removal of sialic acid residues fraction A and B
were converted into an identical product which eluted in the position of an aminosugar-containing disaccharide alditol (Fig. 2,
lower panel).

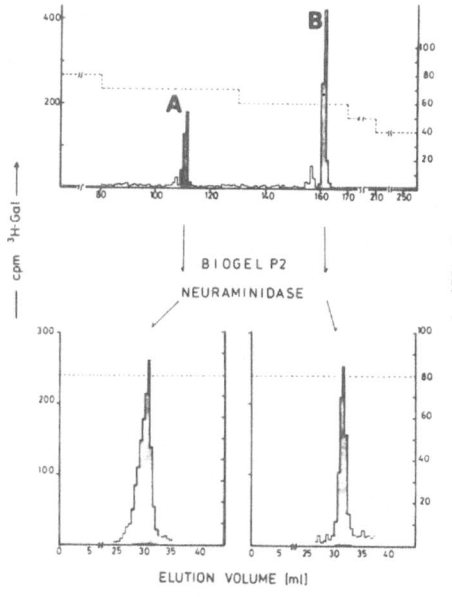

Fig. 2: HPLC of reduced carbohydrate side chains obtained
from E1 by ß-elimination
column: 5 µ Lichrosorb-NH_2
(Merck, Darmstadt)
flow rate: 0.5 ml/min
elution: Acetonitrile/15 mM
KH_2PO_4, pH 5.5, in a stepwise
gradient.
(peak fraction A: 70 % acetoni-
trile/30 % KH_2PO_4
peak fraction B: 60 % acetoni-
trile/40 % KH_2PO_4)

Part of fractions A and B (about 5 µg each) were permethylated,
hydrolyzed, reduced and analyzed as partially methylated alditol
acetates by gas-chromatography-mass-spectrometry. Figure 3 shows
the gaschromatogram obtained from peak fraction B. The two major
peaks were in an equimolar ratio and the underlying compounds
were identified by mass-spectrometry to be derived from a 3-sub-

stituted galactose (2,4,6,-Gal) and a 3,6-di-substituted N-acetyl-
galactosaminitol (1,2,4,5-GalNAc). None of the other peaks in
Figure 3 showed a sugar-specific fragmentation pattern in mass-
spectrometric analysis.

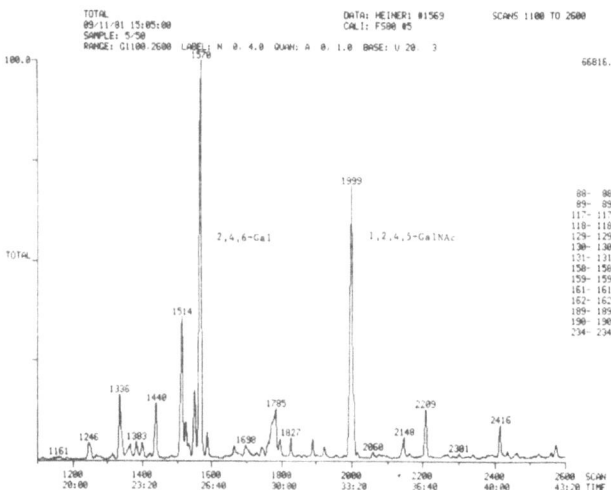

Fig. 3: Gas-chroma-
togram of partially
methylated alditol
acetates derived from
oligosaccharide B.
column: 25 m fused
silica capillary
column; OV101 statio-
nary phase
temperature: 100 –
240° C, 3°/min

2,4,6-Gal =
2,4,6-tri-O-methyl-
1,3,5-tri-O-acetyl-
galactitol

Permethylation analysis of material from peak A (Fig. 2) indicated that this oligosaccharide also contained galactose and N-
acetylgalactosamine in a 1:1 ratio. By mass-spectrometry it was
shown that the N-acetyl-galactosamine derivative present in A
was only mono-substituted in position 3 (data not shown). In both
structures, however, the galactosamine residue had to be the
innermost sugar linked to the protein backbone. The combined data
lead to the following structures for oligosaccharides A and B:

A
$$\text{NeuNAc } 2 \xrightarrow{\alpha} 3 \text{ Gal } 1 \xrightarrow{\beta} 3 \text{ GalNAcOH}$$

$$
\begin{array}{c}
\text{NeuNAc} \\
2 \downarrow \alpha \\
6
\end{array}
$$
$$\text{NeuNAc } 2 \xrightarrow{\alpha} 3 \text{ Gal } 1 \xrightarrow{\beta} 3 \text{ GalNAcOH}$$

B

Similar carbohydrate structures have been reported for mucin type
glycoproteins (for review see [18]), but this is the first time
that any O-linked carbohydrate structure has been elucidated from

viral glycoproteins. The comparison of the molecular weight of the non-glycosylated precursor of E1 and the fully glycosylated E1 species suggests that about 3 carbohydrate side chains are attached per molecule of E1.

When this work was begun, very little was known about the structure and the function of the glycosylated portion of E1 extending on the outside of the virus particle [1]. Studies with monensin have shown that glycosylation of E1 is inhibited in the presence of this ionophore while virus particle formation continues into the lumen of the RER [2]. The amino-terminal part of E1 may also contain specific signals for the intracellular transport, defining the characteristic budding sites of coronaviruses in the RER and the Golgi [6]. The O-linked carbohydrates of E1 could contribute to the rigidity of the viral membrane as was proposed for the anti-freeze glycoprotein from polar fish [19].

Construction of full length E1 clones. To study possible functional interactions at a molecular level, full-length recombinant DNA of E1 was constructed in order to eventually express this gene in eucaryotic cells using an appropriate vector. Cloning of the E1 gene was facilitated after the structure of mRNA 7 (encoding the nucleocapsid protein) had been elucidated [20]. A pentadeca-oligodeoxyribonucleotide d(TTCTTGCCCAGGAAC) complementary to nucleotides 10 to 24 of the 5'coding region of mRNA 7 was synthesized following the phosphotriester method and applied as a primer in first strand cDNA synthesis as shown in Figure 4. The primer sequence contains restriction sites for EcoRII, TagX1, BstN1. The computer search for further base sequence complementary between the primer and the mRNA 7 sequence showed that the primer should bind specifically only in the desired position. The method outlined in Fig. 4 was originally described by H. Land et al. [12]. The C-tailing of the single-stranded cDNA and the application of the oligo(dG)$_{12-18}$ as a primer for second strand synthesis protects the extreme 3'terminal region of the ss-cDNA (corresponding to the 5'terminus of the mRNA and thus to the N-terminus of the protein). Part of these sequences would have been lost, if self-primed second strand synthesis and S1 nuclease digestion of the hair pin loop had been employed. The products of the first strand synthesis were analyzed together with those of the first C-tailing reaction on a 2 % alkaline agarose gel (Fig. 5, lanes 1, 2). The presence of discrete bands in the expected molecular weight range showed that primer synthesis had been successfull. When oligo(dT)$_{12-18}$, was used as a primer, the bands appeared to be less discrete and they corresponded as to be expected to products of higher molecular weight, indicating that the synthetic primer had primed cDNA-synthesis internally (Fig. 5, lane 3).
Synthesis of the second strand was followed by determination of the amount of radioactive cDNA that was rendered S1 nuclease resistant. 85 % of the cDNA was resistant indicating that the C-

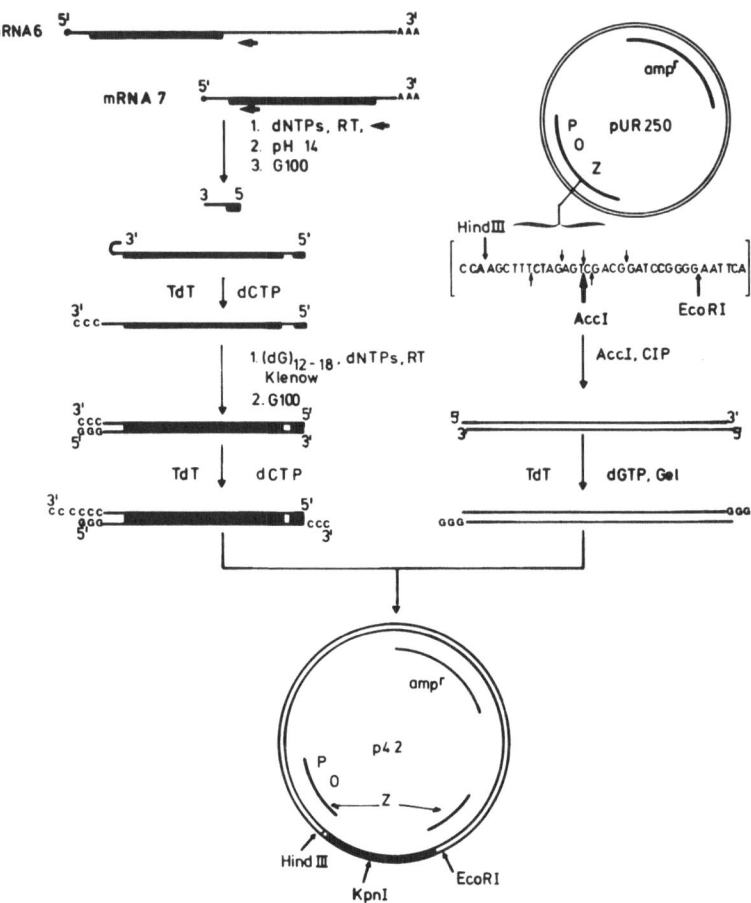

Fig. 4:   Construction of full length E1 clones.

In A59-infected cells a nested set of 7 mRNA molecules
is produced, which extend from a common 3'-end towards
the 5'-end of the genome [21]. Each mRNA functions mono-
cistronically.
Only mRNA 7 (encoding the nucleocapsid protein) and
mRNA 6 (encoding E1) are shown. Thick strands illustrate
the coding regions. The arrow indicates the synthetic
primer. For further details see Materials and Methods.

tailing and oligo(dG)$_{12-18}$-priming had been efficient. In comparison second strand synthesis with non-tailed cDNA as template yielded only 45 % nuclease resistance (data not shown).

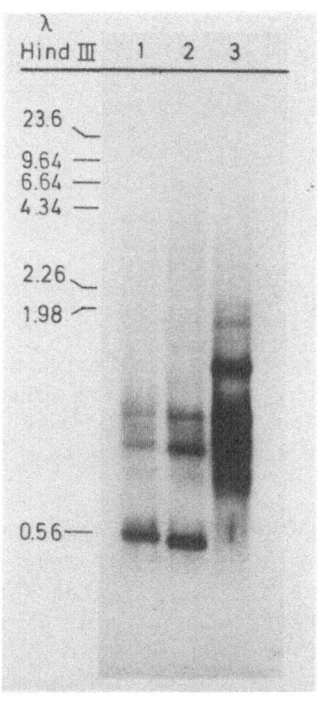

Fig. 5: Analysis of single-stranded cDNA on a 2 % horizontal alkaline agarose gel.

lane 1: dC-tailed cDNA obtained with the synthetic primer.

lane 2: cDNA obtained with the synthetic primer.

lane 3: cDNA obtained with oligo (dT)$_{12-18}$ as a primer.

λ-HindIII: molecular weight markers in Kb.

The pUR250 vector [13]) was chosen as a cloning vehicle (Fig. 4), because any GC-tailed material cloned into six of the eight unique restriction sites of the 36 base polylinker region could easily be recovered by cleavage at adjacent restriction sites. In addition, the presence of similar polylinker regions in the pUC-M13-,or pEMBL-families allowed an easy conversion from ds-DNA to ss-DNA in any desired orientation. The AccI site (Fig.5) was chosen as the cloning site, because GC-tailed inserts could eventually be sequenced according to Maxam and Gilbert [22]) without time consuming strand separation [13]).

Characterization of recombinant clones. A total of 70 recombinant clones were obtained with material corresponding to 1 µg of starting poly-A$^+$-RNA. These clones were assayed by colony hybridization and in part characterized by restriction mapping. Figure 6 shows the results obtained with clone p42. As expected, it could be linearized with either HindIII or EcoRI yielding identical cleavage products of 3.5 Kb (as compared to 2.7 Kb for pUR250). The 800 bp insert contained restriction sites for KpnI (Figure 6) and BglII (data not shown).

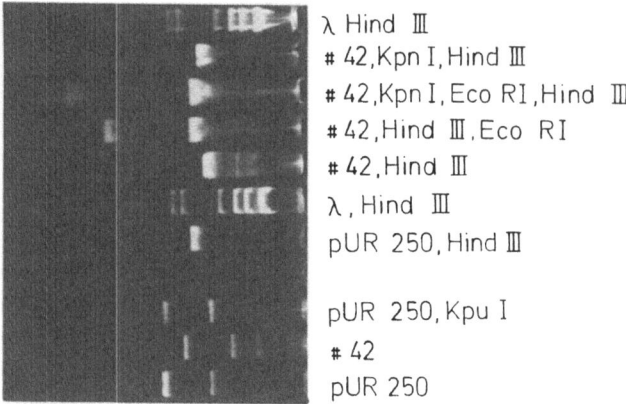

λ Hind Ⅲ
42,Kpn I,Hind Ⅲ
42,Kpn I,Eco RI,Hind Ⅲ
42,Hind Ⅲ,Eco RI
42,Hind Ⅲ
λ,Hind Ⅲ
pUR 250,Hind Ⅲ

pUR 250,Kpu I
42
pUR 250

Fig. 6: Restriction digestion of p42. Plasmid DNA was isolated from
         clone 42, purified by chromatography over a NACS52 column
         and restricted as indicated. λ-HindIII-fragments were used
         as molecular weight markers on the 1.6% agarose gel.
         Staining: ethidium bromide.

The position of these sites was in agreement with the sequence of
E1 as determined by J. Armstrong by shotgun cloning. The EcorRI-
HindIII fragment, containing the recombinant DNA, was ligated into
pEMBL8, and ss-DNA was sequenced to characterize the termini of the
insert. The insert is flanked on either end by homopolymeric GC-tails
(21, 25 bp in length) which are followed at the one end by the synthetic primer sequence and the E1 carboxy terminus. At the end corresponding to the 5'end of mRNA 6, a 76 base pair-noncoding leader sequence is present (Fig. 7).

-76   -70   -60   -50   -40   -30
CCTATA AGAGTGATTG GCGTCCGTAC GTACCCTCTC AACTCTAAA CTCTTGTAGT

-20   -10   -1 +1   30
TTAAATCTAA TCCAAACATT ATG AGT AGT ACT ACT CAG GCC CCA GAG CCC GTC
                       Met Ser*Ser*Thr*Thr*Gln Ala Pro Glu Pro Val
                                        60
TAT CAA TGG ACG GCC GAC GAG GCA GTT CAA TTC CTT AAG GAA TGG
Tyr Gln Trp Thr*Ala Asp Glu Ala Val Gln Phe Leu Lys Glu Trp
             90
AAC TTC TCG TTG GGC ATT ATA CTA CTC TTT...
Asn Phe Ser Leu Gly Ile Ile Leu Leu Phe...
===========

Fig. 7:   Sequence of the 5'region of mRNA 6. A76 nucleotide non-
          coding leader sequence precedes the coding region. Note
          the cluster of four hydroxy amino acids in series at the
          NH$_2$-terminus of E1 as potential attachment sites for O-link-
          ed carbohydrate side chains.

While the sequence of this leader may be interesting with respect to the splicing mechanism which leads to the formation of the nested set, the amino acid sequence of the E1 NH_2-terminus is quite unique for several reasons: i) There is no hydrophobic signal sequence as commonly present in viral glycoproteins. ii) The cluster of four hydroxy-amino acids adjacent to the initial methionine are presumably the attachment site of the O-linked carbohydrate side chains (marked with an asterix in Figure 7). iii) The potential N-glycosylation site involving Asn(27) (underlined in Figure 7) is just at the beginning of one of the three hydrophobic domains which presumably span the membrane. Our present studies focus at the expression of the E1 gene and the construction of primers in order to alter or delete the O-glycosylation sites.

ACKNOWLEDGEMENT

We thank J. Armstrong, EMBL Heidelberg, for making the sequence of the MHV-A59 nucleocapsid protein available to us prior to publication. In addition, we thank him for teaching us the skills of dideoxy sequencing.

The constructive discussions of the members of the DNA synthesis group at the Gesellschaft für Biotechnologische Forschung (Stöckheim) is gratefully acknowledged.

This work was supported by the Deutsche Forschungsgemeinsc. .ft (SFV 47, Virologie).

REFERENCES

1. L. S. Sturman and K. V. Holmes (1983) The molecular biology of coronaviruses, in: Adv. in Virus Research 28, in press.
2. H. Niemann, B. Boschek, D. Evans, M. Rosing, T. Tamura, and H.-D. Klenk (1982) Post-translational glycosylation of coronavirus glycoprotein E1: inhibition by monensin. The EMBO J. 1, 1499-1504.
3. H. Niemann and H.-D. Klenk (1981) Coronavirus glycoprotein E1, a new type of viral glycoprotein. J. Mol. Biol. 153, 993-1010.
4. K. V. Holmes, E. W. Doller and J. N. Behnke (1981) Analysis of the functions of coronavirus glycoproteins by differential inhibition of synthesis with tunicamycin, in: Biochemistry and Biology of Coronaviruses, Adv. in Exp. Med. and Biol. Vol. 142, pp.133-142, V. ter Meulen, S. Siddell, and H. Wege,

eds., Plenum-Press, New York, London.

5. L. S. Sturman (1981) The structure and behavior of Coronavirus
   A59 glycoproteins, in: Biochemistry and Biology of Corona-
   viruses. Adv. in Exp. Med. and Biology Vol. 142, p. 1., V. ter
   Meulen, S. Siddell, and H. Wege, eds., Plenum-Press, New York.

6. E.W. Doller and K. V. Holmes (1980) Different intracellular
   transportation of the envelope glycoproteins E1 and E2 of
   coronavirus MHV. Abstracts of the American Society of Microbiology, p. 267.

7. L. S. Sturman (1977) Characterization of a coronavirus. I. Structural proteins: effects of preparative conditions on the migration of protein in polyacrylamide gels. Virology 77, 637.

8. L. S. Sturman, K. V. Holmes and J. Behnke (1980) Isolation of
   coronavirus envelope glycoproteins and interaction with the
   viral nucleocapsid. J. Virol. 33, 449.

9. R. Geyer, H. Geyer, S. Kühnhardt, W. Mink and S. Stirm (1983)
   Methylation analysis of complex carbohydrates in small amounts:
   Capillary gas chromatography-mass fragmentography of methyl-
   alditol acetates obtained from N-glycosidically linked glycoprotein oligosaccharides. Anal. Biochem. 133, in press.

10. M. J. Gait, H. W. D. Matthes, M. Singh, B. S. Sproat and R.
    Titmas (1982) Rapid synthesis of oligodeoxynucleotides VII.
    Solid phase synthesis of oligodeoxyribonucleotides by a con-
    tinous flow phosphotriester method on Kieselguhr-polyamide
    support. Nucl. Acids Res. 10, 6243.

11. R. Frank, D. Müller, and C. Wolff (1981) Identification and
    suppression of secondary structures formed from deoxynucleo-
    tides during electrophoresis in denaturing polyacrylamide
    gels. Nucl. Acids Res. 9, 4967.

12. H. Land, M. Grez, H. Hauser, W. Lindenmaier and G. Schütz (1981)
    5'-Terminal sequences of eucaryotic mRNA can be cloned with
    high efficiency. Nucl. Acids Res. 9, 2251.

13. U. Rüther (1982) pUR250 allows rapid chemical sequencing of
    both DNA strands of its inserts. Nucl. Acids Res. 10, 5765.

14. M. Dagert and S. D. Ehrlich (1979) Prolonged incubation in
    calcium chloride improves the competence of Escherichia coli
    cells. Gene 6, 23.

15. M. Grunstein and H. Hogness (1975) Colony hybridization: A
    method for the isolation of cloned DNAs that contain a speci-
    fic gene. Proc. Natl. Acad. Sci. USA 72, 3961.

16. L. Dente, G. Cesareni and R. Cortese (1983) pEMBL: a new family
    of single stranded plasmids. Nucl. Acids Res. 11, 1645.

17. H. Garoff and W. Ansorge (1981) Improvement of DNA-sequencing
    gels. Anal. Biochem. 115, 450-457.

18. R. Kornfeld and S. Kornfeld (1980) Structure of glycoproteins
    and their oligosaccharide units, in: The Biochemistry of
    Glycoproteins and Proteoglycans, W. J. Lennarz, ed., Plenum-
    Press, New York, London, p. 1-34.

19. R. E. Feaney and Y. Yeh (1978) Advances in protein Chemistry
       32, 192-282.
20. J. Armstrong, S. Smeekens and P. Rottier (1983) Sequence of
       the nucleocapsid gene from murine coronavirus MHV-A59.
       Nucl. Acids Res. 11, 883-891.
21. M. M. C. Lai, C. D. Patton and S. A. Stohlman (1982) Further
       characterization of mouse hepatisis virus: presence of
       common 5'end nucleotides. J. Virol. 41, 557-565.
22. A. M. Maxam and W. Gilbert (1980) Sequencing end-labelled DNA
       with base-specific chemical cleavages. Methods Enzymol.
       65, 499.

DNA SEQUENCING STUDIES OF GENOMIC cDNA CLONES OF AVIAN INFECTIOUS

BRONCHITIS VIRUS

M.E.G. Boursnell and T.D.K. Brown

Houghton Poultry Research Station
Houghton, Huntingdon
Cambridgeshire, England

INTRODUCTION

Avian infectious bronchitis virus (IBV) has a positive stranded
RNA genome about 20 kilobases in length. The virus particle
contains three major structural proteins, the nucleocapsid protein
(which is associated with the RNA genome), the matrix or membrane
protein and the spike or surface projection protein [1]. Infection
with IBV results in the synthesis of six major polyadenylated
messenger RNAs [2]. One of these is equal in size to the genomic RNA
and the other five form a 3' coterminal ('nested') set, with the
sequences from each RNA present in all the larger RNA species [3].
These mRNAs have been named A,B,C,D,E and F, RNA A being the
smallest. In vitro translation studies [4], have shown that RNA A
directs the synthesis of the viral nucleocapsid protein and RNA C
directs the synthesis of the viral matrix polypeptide. Unpublished
results of Stern and Sefton show that an unglycosylated form of the
viral spike precursor can be synthesised by in vitro translation of
RNA E.

Work on murine hepatitis viruses has shown that sequences from
the 5' end of the genomic RNA are fused to the 5' end of each
messenger RNA [5,6]. It is thought that the RNA polymerase may
transcribe a short sequence from the 3' end of the negative
stranded template and then jump to specific recognition sequences
in the main part of the template which would then form the start of
each messenger RNA. Thus each messenger RNA consists of 'leader'

and 'body' sequences which originate from non-contiguous regions of
the genomic RNA. The protein-coding region of each mRNA is thought
to consist of that part of the 'body' of the message which is not
present in smaller mRNAs. At the moment it is not clear whether
the same mechanism operates in IBV. Analysis of RNase T_1
oligonucleotides[3], gives no indication of leader sequences, but
this evidence is not conclusive.

DNA sequencing of clones complementary to genomic IBV RNA has
been undertaken to determine the sequence of the viral RNA at the
point corresponding to the 5' ends of messenger RNAs A and B.
Combined with S1 mapping data to locate the boundaries of the
'bodies' of the messenger RNAs it should be possible to find out if
there are any recognition signals in the genomic RNA which might
direct the fusion process.

METHODS

Isolation and analysis of cDNA clones

Double-stranded cDNA was synthesised from viral[+] genomic RNA
using an oligo-dT primer and AMV reverse transcriptase for the
first strand and reverse transcriptase again for the second strand.
This was treated with S1 nuclease and tailed with dC residues. The
tailed cDNA was annealed to dG-tailed PstI digest pAT153 and
used to transform E.coli HB101 to tetracycline resistance.
Ampicillin-sensitive colonies were picked and grown, the plasmid
DNA isolated and analysed by restriction endonuclease digestion.
Restriction sites were mapped in 25 of the clones and this enabled
them to be fitted together into a continuous map, 3.3kb in length.

Orientation and confirmation of viral origin

Clones were digested with PstI and run on agarose gels and the
DNA was transferred to nitrocellulose by the Southern blot method[7].
Duplicate blots were hybridised with a) polynucleotide
kinase-labelled IBV genomic RNA fragments, b) nick-translated
pAT153 and c) kinase-labelled poly-U. The IBV probe was to confirm
that the DNA inserted into the PstI site of the plasmid is a copy
of viral sequences. The pAT153 probe was to confirm that no
plasmid sequences were present in the putative 'viral' band. The
poly-U probe was to identify which clones had a copy of the poly-A
sequences present on the 3' end of the viral genome. This last
blot was repeated with other restriction digests of the appropriate
clones to identify which end of the inserted DNA had the poly-A
sequences.

[+] IBV Beaudette strain

S1 mapping

   The PstI/PvuII fragment (see figure 1b) of the cDNA clone used
for DNA sequencing (C5.136) was purified on a polyacrylamide gel
and 5' labelled using 32PγATP and polynucleotide kinase. Total
cytoplasmic RNA was prepared from IBV infected chick kidney cells
using an NP40 lysis procedure. S1 mapping was carried out using
essentially the modification of the Berk and Sharp procedure,[8] as
described by Weaver and Weissman [9]. Protected 32P-labelled DNA
fragments were analysed on 5% non-denaturing polyacrylamide gels.
Sizes of the protected fragments were estimated from their
positions relative to those of end-labelled Hae III fragments of
ϕX174 RF DNA.

DNA sequence determination

   Plasmid DNA was prepared from E.coli by a modification of the
method of Holmes and Quigley [10]. DNA restriction fragments, 3'
end-labelled with 32P-dNTP using Klenow polymerase, were sequenced
essentially as described by Maxam and Gilbert[11]. The depurination
reaction was carried out in 2% diphenylamine, 66% formic acid, 1mM
EDTA for 10 minutes at 20°C, followed by 3-fold dilution in water,
three ether extractions and lyophilisation. Piperidine hydrolysis
was done as described[11]. For sequencing some regions of the DNA,
restriction digests of the 'viral' insert were recloned into the
plasmid pUC9, which contains the cloning sites corresponding to
those in the M13 vector M13mp9. Sequence data were stored and
analysed on an Apple IIe microcomputer using the programs of
Larson and Messing[12].

RESULTS

   One clone, C5.136, which represented from 1kb to 3.3kb from the
3' end of the viral genome was chosen for DNA sequencing. A
preliminary sequence from only one DNA strand has been obtained
from 1600 bases in this region. This sequence is located as shown
in figure 1a. In figure 1b the arrows indicate the direction and
amount of sequence information obtained from individual restriction
enzyme cleavages. The DNA sequence from this region is shown in
figure 2. Figure 3 shows the positions of stop and start codons in
the three reading frames, the positions of the main open reading
frames and the estimated positions of the ends of messenger RNAs A
and B that were obtained from S1 mapping experiments using cDNA
clones derived from genomic RNA.

   The results of an S1 mapping experiment in which varying
quantities of total cytoplasmic RNA from IBV infected chick kidney

a

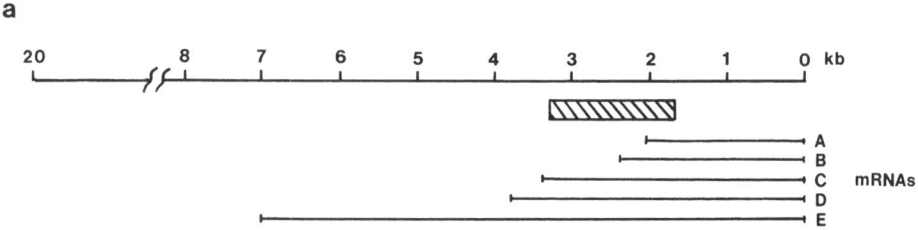

b

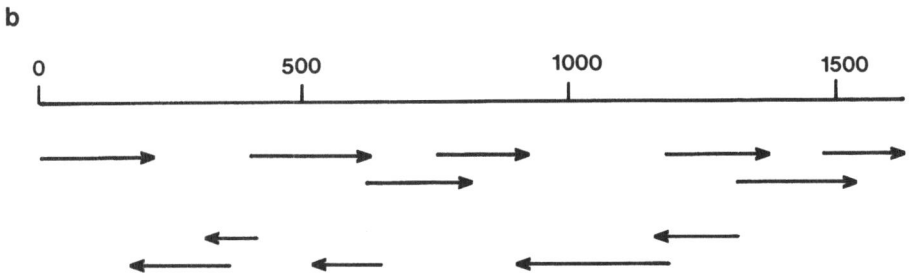

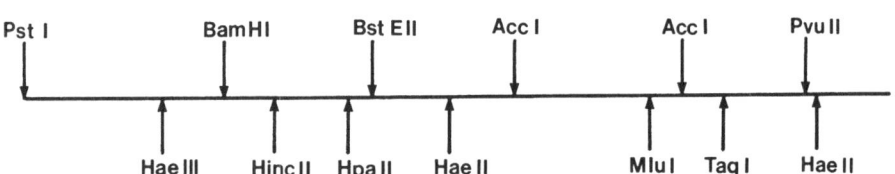

Figure 1.   a)   Map showing the region of IBV for which cDNA clones
have been sequenced (hatched box). b) Restriction map
of the 1600 base region which has been sequenced.
Arrows indicate direction and extent of sequence
information from individual restriction sites.

cells were annealed with a 5' labelled Pst I/Pvu II fragment (see
figure 1b) are shown in figure 4.   Three DNA fragments are
protected by the RNA.   The sequence organisation of the genomic
clone C5.136 has been demonstrated to correspond to the 3' nested
set shown for IBV mRNAs by Stern and Kennedy[3].   Labelled
restriction fragments of the clone were used to probe IBV mRNAs

```
                                                50
GGGGGGGGGGGGGGGGGGGGGGGGGGGGGGGGGGGGGGGGGGGGGAAGAA

                                   ¦--->       100  First ATG codon
CGGTTGGAATAATAAAAATCCAGCAAATTTTCAAGATGCCCAACGAGACA  in Matrix ORF

                                               150
AATTGTACTCTTGACTTTGAACAGTCAGTTCAGCTTTTTAAAGAGTATAA

                                               200
TTTATTTATAACTGCATTCTTGTTGTTCTTAACCATAATACTTCAGTATG

                                               250
GCTATGCAACAAGAAGTAAGGTTATTTATACACTGAAAATGATAGTGTTA

                                               300
TGGTGCTTTTGGCCCCTTAACATTGCAGTAGGTGTAATTTCATGTACATA

                                               350
CCCACCAAACACAGGAGGTCTTGTCGCAGCGATAATACTTACAGTGTTTG

                                               400
CGTGTCTGTCTTTTGTAGGTTATTGGATCCAGAGTATTAGACTCTTTAAG

                                               450
CGGTGTAGGTCATGGTGGTCATTTAATCCAGAATCTAATGCCGTAGGTTC

                                               500
AATACTCCTAACTAATGGTCAACAATGTAATTTTGCTATAGAGAGTGTGC

                                               550
CAATGGTGCTTTCTCCAATTATAAAGAATGGTGTTCTTTATTGTGAGGGT

                                               600
CAGTGGCTTGCTAAGTGTGAACCAGACCACTTGCCTAAAGATATATTTGT

                                               650
TTGTACACCGGATAGACGTAATATCTACCGTATGGTGCAGAAATATACTG

                                               700
GTGACCAAAGCGTAAATAATAAAAGGTTTGCTACGTCTATGCAAAGCAGT

 <---¦ ORF1                                    750  UAG stop codon
CAGTAGATACTGGCTAGCTATAAAGTGTAGCAACAGTAGTAAGTAGTCTT  at the end of
                                                    the Matrix gene
                                               800
TACACATAAATGTGTGTGTGTATATAGTATTTAAAATTATTCTTTAATAG
```

Figure 2. DNA sequence of the cDNA clone C5.136. The positions of the open reading frames (ORFs) are shown. Asterisks indicate the end of the mRNAs as measured by S1 mapping. Lines over the sequence show regions of homology at the messenger termini. (continued on next page)

```
                                                   850
CGCCTCTGTTTTAAGAGCGCATAAGAGTATTTATTTTGAGGATACTAATA

                                                   900
TAAATCCTCTTTGTTTTATACTCTCCTTTCAAGAGCTATTAACGGTGTTA

                                                   950
CCTTTCAAGATAATGGAAAGTCTACTACGAAGGAACACCAGTTTTACAAA

                                                  1000
AAGGTTGTTGTAGGATGTGGTCCAATTATAAGAAAGAATAATTGAACCAC

                                   *
CTACTACACTTATTTTTATAAGAGGTGTTTTACTTAACAAAAACTTAACA    * indicates end
                                   *                  of RNA B
        |---> ORF2                                1100   Start codon for
AATACGGACGATGAAATGGCTGACTAGTTTTGGAAGAGCAGTTATTTCTT      ORF2

                                                  1150
GTTATAAATCCCTACTATTAACTCAACTTAGAGTGTTAGATAGGTTAATT

                                                  1200
TTAGATCACGGACTACTACGCGTTTTAACGTGTAGTAGGCGCGTGCTTTT

                                                  1250
AGTTCAATTAGATTTAGTTTATAGGTTGGCGTATACGCCCACCCAATCGC

     |---> ORF3                                   1300   Start codon for
TGGCATGAATAATAGTAAAGATAATCCTTTTCGCGGAGCAATAGCAAGAA      ORF3
     <--| ORF2                                          UGA stop codon
                              *                         for ORF2
AAGCTCGAATTTATCTGAGAGAAGGATTAGATTGTGTTTACTTTCTTAAC    * indicates end
                              *                         of RNA A
                                                  1400
AAAGCAGGACAAGCAGAGCCTTGTCCCGCGTGTACCTCTCTAGTATTCCA

                              ORF4 |--->             Start codon for
AGGGAAAACTTGTGAGGAACACATACATAATAATAATCTTTTGTCATGGC      ORF4
                                                        (Nucleocapsid?)
                                                  1500
AAGCGGTAAAGCAGCTGGAAAAACAGACGCCCCAGCGCCAGTCATTAAAC

<-| ORF3                                          1550   UAG stop codon
TAGGAGGACCAAAACCACCTAAAGTCGGTTCTTCTGGAAATGCATCTTGG      for ORF3

                                                  1600
TTTCAAGCAATAAAAGCCAAGAAGTTAAATACACCTCCGCCCAAGTTTGA

AGGTAGCGGTGTTCCTGATAAC
```

Figure 2. (continued) See caption on previous page.

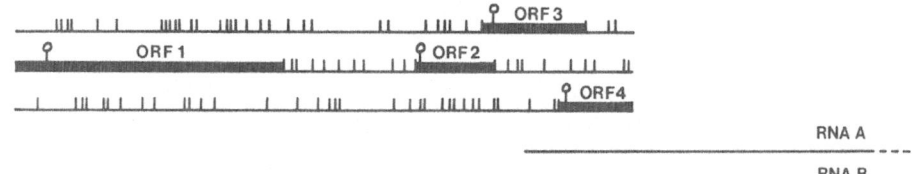

Figure 3. Positions of termination codons (vertical bars) and
potential initiation codons (bars with open circles on
top) in the three reading frames. The heavy black
lines show the positions of the main open reading frames
(ORFs). The lines underneath show the positions of the
mRNAs as determined by S1 mapping.

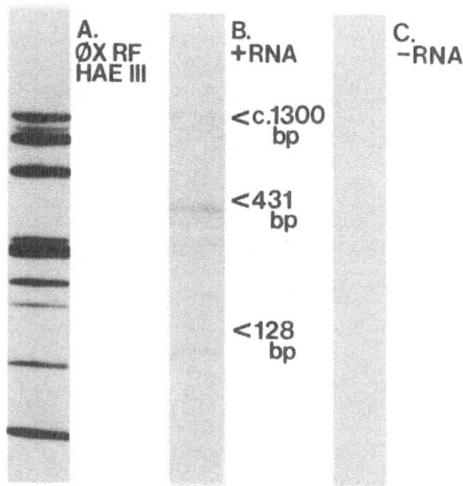

Figure 4. S1 mapping of the non-leader 5' termini of mRNAs A and B
on cDNA clone C5.136 using a 5' ^{32}P-labelled Pst1/Pvu II
fragment.

separated on formaldehyde gels (Brown & Boursnell, unpublished results). Given these data on sequence organisation the protected bands can be interpreted as mapping the distances of the 5' termini of the mRNAs A and B from the PvuII site in C5.136, excluding any leader sequences which may be joined to the mRNAs. The presence of a band at essentially the same length as the PstI/PvuII fragment also indicates that the terminus of the non-leader sequences of mRNA C is either at or lies beyond the 3.3kb covered by clone C5.136. The latter idea is supported by the observation in primer extension experiments using mRNAs of a major band which maps approximately 350 bases beyond the 5' end of clone C5.136 (Brown & Boursnell, unpublished results).

Knowledge of the positions of the 5' termini of the non-leader sequences of the mRNAs A and B prompted a search for homologies between the two boundary regions. Extensive sequence homologies were indeed observed (see figure 5). In particular a nine base stretch of sequence is common between the two regions, and is present twice at the end of mRNA B.

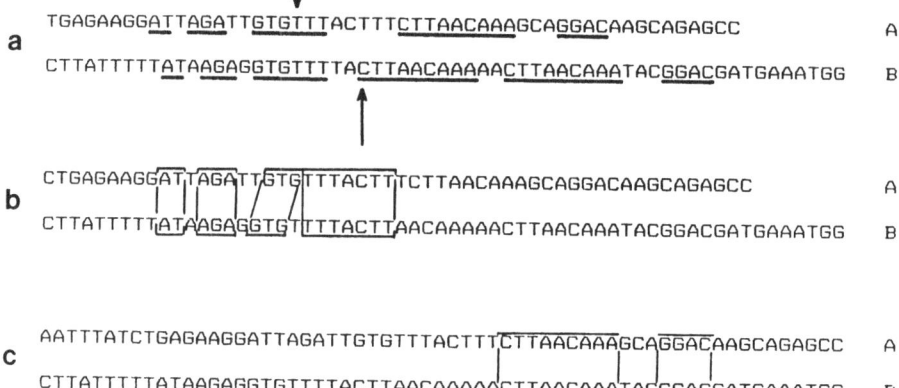

Figure 5.   Sequences of cDNA at the 5' ends of the non-leader sequences of mRNAs A and B. a) The arrows show the position of the ends of the non leader sequences. The underlined regions show homologies between the two regions. b) and c) show two possible alignments of the two regions which give high degrees of homology.

DISCUSSION

As can be seen from figure 1b, approximately 80% of the sequence presented here has not been verified by sequencing the complementary strand. As a result therefore it is in some ways only a preliminary sequence. More work is at present under way in order to obtain sequence information from both strands of the DNA throughout this region.

There are four open reading frames (ORFs) longer than 150 bases and these are shown in figure 3. ORF1 appears to be the protein coding region of messenger RNA C, which has been reported to direct the synthesis of the viral matrix protein [4]. Because the cDNA clone only extends 3.3kb from the 3' end of the virus, it is not possible to tell whether the first AUG codon in this stretch of sequence is in fact the initiation codon for the matrix gene. However, if this sequence were to be translated, it would code for a protein of molecular weight 23,500 daltons which is very similar to the molecular weight of the unglycosylated form of the matrix protein (23,000 daltons) as obtained by polyacrylamide gel electrophoresis [13, 14]. ORF2 corresponds to the part of messenger RNA B which is not present in RNA A and probably represents that region of RNA B which is translated. If it were translated it would code for a hydrophobic polypeptide of molecular weight 7,500 daltons. ORF4 starts within mRNA A and continues to the boundary of the region which has been sequenced. Since it has been reported that RNA A directs the synthesis of the viral nucleocapsid protein it is probable that this open reading frame represents the start of the nucleocapsid gene. ORF3 is more difficult to assign. Current thinking in the coronavirus field suggests that only the part of each messenger RNA which is not present in the next smallest RNA is translated. If this is true then ORF4 would represent a chance open reading frame which is not translated in vivo. This may be the case, and indeed it can be seen that other smaller open reading frames are present at various points in this sequence.

The significance of the sequence homologies found at the 5' termini of the non-leader sequences of mRNAs A and B represented in the genomic RNA clone remains unclear at the present time. It does however seem probable that they have a role in mRNA synthesis and that they might possibly act as recognition sites for the enzymes involved in generating the messenger RNAs. More detailed consideration of their role will however only become possible when the 5' termini of the messenger RNAs have been sequenced.

REFERENCES

1. D. Cavanagh. Structural polypeptides of coronavirus IBV.
   J. Gen. Virol. 53: 93 (1981).
2. D. F. Stern and S. I. T. Kennedy. Coronavirus multiplication
   strategy. I. Identification and characterisation of
   virus-specified RNA. J. Virol. 34: 665 (1980)
3. D. F. Stern and S. I. T. Kennedy. Coronavirus multiplication
   strategy. II. Mapping the avian infectious bronchitis
   virus intracellular RNA species to the genome. J. Virol.
   36: 440 (1980).
4. D. F. Stern, L. Burgess and B. M. Sefton. Structural analysis
   of virion proteins of the avian coronavirus infectious
   bronchitis virus. J. Virol. 42: 208 (1982).
5. M. M. C. Lai, C. D. Patton and S. A. Stohlman. Further
   characterisation of mRNAs of Mouse Hepatitis Virus:
   presence of common 5'-end nucleotides. J. Virol. 41:
   557 (1982).
6. W. J. M. Spaan, P. J. M. Rottier, M. C. Horzinek and B. A. M.
   van der Zeijst. Sequence relationships between the
   genome and the intracellular species 1, 3, 6, and 7 of
   mouse hepatitis strain A59. J. Virol. 42: 432 (1982).
7. E. Southern. Detection of specific sequences among DNA
   fragments separated by gel electrophoresis. J. Mol.
   Biol. 98: 503 (1975).
8. A. J. Berk and P. A. Sharp. Sizing and mapping of early
   adenovirus mRNAs by gel electrophoresis of S1 endonuclease digested hybrids. Cell 12: 721 (1977).
9. R. F. Weaver and C. Weissman. Mapping of RNA by a modification
   of the Berk-Sharp procedure: the 5' termini of $15S\beta$-globin
   mRNA precursor and mature $10S \beta$-globin mRNA have identical
   map coordinates. N. Acids Res. 7: 1175 (1979).
10. D.S. Holmes and M. Quigley. A rapid boiling method for the
    preparation of bacterial plasmids. Anal. Biochem.
    114: 193 (1981).
11. A. M. Maxam and W. Gilbert. Sequencing end-labelled DNA with
    base-specific chemical cleavages. Meth. Enzymol.
    65: 499 (1980).
12. R. Larson and J. Messing. Apple II software for M13 shotgun
    sequencing. N. Acids Res. 10: 39 (1982).
13. D. Cavanagh. Coronavirus IBV polypeptides: size of their
    polypeptide moieties and nature of their oligosaccharides.
    J. Gen. Virol. 64: 1187 (1983)
14. D. F. Stern and B. M. Sefton. Coronavirus proteins: structure
    and function of the oligosaccharides of the Avian Infect-
    ious Bronchitis Virus Glycoproteins. J. Virol.44: 804
    (1982)

THE GENOME OF TRANSMISSIBLE GASTROENTERITIS VIRUS (TGEV)

Lynne Bountiff, David J. Garwes, Geoffrey C. Millson
and G. David Baird

ARC Institute for Research on Animal Diseases
Compton, Nr. Newbury, Berkshire, U.K.

Lysis of isolated TGE virions with sodium dodecyl sulphate (SDS) at room temperature followed by electrophoresis, yields predominantly a single band of RNA running at about molecular weight 6.8×10^6. Heating the SDS lysate at 80°C for 15 min prior to electrophoresis results in a cluster of bands of between $0.2-6.8 \times 10^6$. Electrophoresis of nucleic acids isolated from the SDS lysate using phenol, at room temperature, also gave several discrete bands some of which co-migrated with TGEV subgenomic mRNA species isolated from infected cells.

Single gene lengths of TGEV RNA would be valuable in recombinant nuclei acid technology aimed at antigen production in vitro. Thus experiments were designed to determine whether the instability of TGEV genomic RNA could be manipulated to produce single gene lengths. The factors controlling the break-down of TGEV genomic RNA into discrete fragments were sought by varying virus growth and purification conditions, and also varying the methods used for isolating RNA from virions. Of all the studies where growth and virion purification conditions were varied, only increasing the harvest time from 15 h to 18 h had significant effect showing an increased degradation of genomic RNA. However this was not into the discrete bands observed earlier, but rather into smaller pieces of less than 3×10^5. Varying the methods of isolating virion RNA all had some effect on instability. In general the greater the chaotropic potential of the method the greater the degree of break-down into discrete RNA species (see photograph). Adding nuclease inhibitors to virions before phenol extraction of the RNA did not decrease the degree of break-down. Similar break-down was observed when genomic RNA was extracted from a low melting point gel and re-electrophoresed.

The instability of TGEV genomic RNA appears to be inherent in
its structure, and break-down of the RNA into specific bands can be
manipulated to some extent by controlling the conditions of nucleic
acid purification. The possibilities of using this manipulation
to produce pieces of RNA for cloning are being explored. The
advantages of this approach over isolating TGEV subgenomic mRNA
species from infected cells are:

1.   Contamination with host cell RNA should be minimal

2.   The subgenomic mRNAs consist of a nested set having common
     3' end sequences. It is possible that if break-down of TGEV
     genomic RNA is a reflection of its structure, some of the
     pieces produced may contain the messages required without
     the common 3' ends which may be undesirable for in vitro
     expression via cloning techniques.

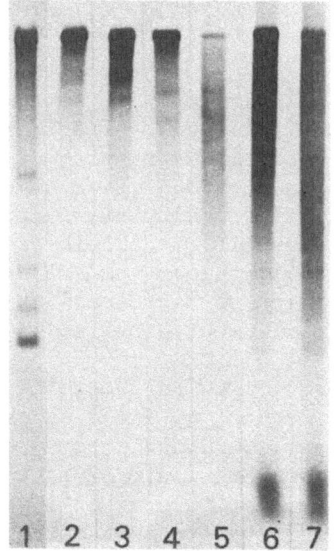

Figure 1

Channel 1)   sub-genomic messenger preparation from infected cells
   "   2)   SDS lysis at room temp
   "   3)   SDS lysis + proteinase K at room temp
   "   4)   SDS lysis + proteinase K at 60°C
   "   5)   SDS lysis + proteinase K at 80°C
   "   6)   SDS lysis ⟶ 1 M sodium perchlorate ⟶ chloroform/
             isoamyl alcohol
   "   7)   SDS lysis ⟶ phenol

BIOLOGY OF CORONAVIRUSES 1983

Volker ter Meulen

Institute of Virology and Immunobiology
University of Würzburg
D - 8700 Würzburg, F.R.G.

INTRODUCTION

At the first international symposion of coronaviruses held in Würzburg in 1980, studies on the biology of coronaviruses were mainly concerned with two subjects: coronavirus persistent infections in tissue cultures and the description of different disease models, in a variety of hosts, with the particular emphasise on subacute or chronic conditions. Much of the discussion centered around the possible mechanisms of persistence and the pathogenic factors playing a role in the development of the different disease types. However, due to the lack of basic information on the molecular biology of coronaviruses the majority of studies reported three years ago were of a more descriptive nature, and in the animal studies immunological and genetic aspects were mainly analysed. In the intervening period, although surprisingly little virological information has been obtained on coronavirus persistent infections in vitro and in vivo, the animal work has been concentrated on two virus groups, namely the murine and feline coronaviruses. Obviously, the involvement of multiple organs in different diseases associated with infections of the two virus groups has turned out to be the most interesting basis for the study of virus-cell and virus-host interactions and the analyses of viral and host factors involved in the development of different disease processes.

MURINE CORONAVIRUS INFECTIONS IN MICE AND RATS

The mouse hepatitis viruses (MHV) cause a broad spectrum of diseases in their natural hosts including hepatitis, pneumonitis, nephritis, enteritis and encephalitis. These different disease types are influenced by the age and genetic backgrounds of the animals, the route of infection and the biological properties of the MHV serotypes used in the experiments. Of particular interest have been subacute and chronic CNS diseases associated with the development of demyelination. Demyelination is a neuropathological hallmark of many CNS disorders in animal and man which can occur in association with virus infection. However, the exact mechanisms by which these lesions develop are unknown. In general, it has been suggested that a direct virus effect on oligodendroglia cells, in the course of a lytic or persistent infection, can be followed by the destruction of myelin (1). Oligodendroglia cells support myelination and their dysfunction has severe consequences. On the other hand, it has been shown that an immune response against myelin also causes demyelination as demonstrated in experimental allergic encephalomyelitis (EAE) (2). In addition, in the event of a virus infection of oligodendroglia cells it is conceivable that an immune response either directed to the infectious agent, or to modified host antigens located on infected oligodendroglia cells, may be another way by which demyelination occurs. Yet, these hypotheses are only based on circumstantial evidence (3). In the case of MHV infections of mice and rats, the different types of demyelinating encephalomyelitides provide for the first time an experimental basis to test these different hypotheses.

The CNS disease models based on coronavirus infection (MHV or SD) presented at this meeting revealed certain similarities. In all instances, a subacute or chronic CNS infection with demyelination was dependent, up to a certain extent, on the neurotropic properties of the virus strain used for infection, on the route of infection as well as on the age and genetic background of the animals. Moreover, in A59 infection of C57 Bl/6 mice the virus dose applied was an additional determining factor (Lavi et al., this volume) in contrast, in JHM infection of rats the type of CNS disease was dose independent (Wege et al., this volume). Of interest is the observation that after MHV inoculation in the majority of animals a biphasic disease process develops (Lavi et al., Wege et al., Jankovski et al., Sörensen et al., this volume). It seems that first of all an acute CNS infection occurs which may or may not be clinically silent. This acute infection is survived by a different proportion of animals, but later some of the survivors come down with a second disease course after varying incubation times. This disease is of a more subacute or chronic nature and differs in the degree of inflammatory demyelinating lesions. This second disease develops as a result of a persistent infection. Viral antigen can be found in glia cells and reisolation of infectious virus is possible at least in JHM infection in rats (Wege et al., this volume). However, persistence also occurs in brain tissue without the detection of antigen. In A59 infection in mice (Lavi et al., this volume) and in JHM infection in Wistar Furth rats (Sörensen et al., this volume) coronavirus RNA can be found by in situ hybridization with specific cDNA in the absence of viral antigens in diseased brain areas. Moreover, under certain conditions an immunosuppressive treatment leads to reactivation of the virus infection (Sörensen et al., this volume) indicating that different forms of persistent infection with and without the production of infectious virus or antigens develop after coronavirus infection in brain tissue in association with subacute or chronic demyelinating encephalomyelitides.

The preliminary data presented on the coronavirus persistence in mice or rat brains resembles to some extent those seen in morbillivirus infections in animal and man (4). These viruses induce in their host acute, subacute and chronic CNS diseases with demyelination and establish with some ease persistent infections in tissue cultures. So far, no common mechanism for the establishment and/or maintenance of morbillivirus persistence has been found. Persistency varies greatly from infections where progeny virus is continually shed to those in which no virus is released and only a small percentage of cells are found to express viral antigens. Factors such as defective interfering particles, interferon or temperature sensitive mutants have been suggested to play a regulative role in these infections. In addition, translational defects of specific viral mRNAs have been detected which prevent assembly of virus particles (5). However, viral antibodies also modify morbillivirus infection changing a lytic infection to a persistent one or causing antigenic modulations on cell membranes as studies in tissue cultures have revealed. It is conceivable that similar mechanisms are operative during the infection of an organism. In general, any factor which promotes cell survival of an initial lytic infection, or diminishes the virulence of a carried virus, will contribute towards morbillivirus persistence and disease. Similar events may also be of importance in coronavirus infection of CNS tissue.

It has been shown at this meeting that host factors also contribute to a disease process in coronavirus infections and to virus persistence. Viral antibodies are capable of modifying a lytic, acute infection to a subacute-chronic, persistent infection or even prevent formation of a chronic disease (Levy et al., this volume) (6). The effectiveness of humoral immunity seems to depend on the titre, the avidity and the neutralising capacity of the antibody. Such antibodies were effective as maternal antibodies or in passive transfer experiments. Of particular interest is the observation of specific cell-mediated immune reactions developing in the course of coronavirus infection in rats. It could be shown that spleen cells of diseased animals not only proliferate in the presence of basic myelin protein (BMP) in vitro but that adoptive transfer of such cells is followed by the occurrence of EAE-like lesions in CNS tissue (Wege et al., this volume) (7). Moreover, animals which recovered from JHM virus infection revealed a reduced susceptibility to the induction of EAE when challenged with BMP in combination with Freund's complete adjuvants suggesting the presence of specific T suppressor cells. These findings are similar to that seen in EAE, where the induction of an acute or chronic form of an inflammatory demyelinating CNS process is pathogenically linked to the presence of T lymphocytes sensitized against basic myelin protein (8). However, it has to be stressed that this auto-immune disease of the CNS can only be induced when immunization against brain antigen is carried out in the presence of Freund's complete adjuvants. In nature, such an immunepathological phenomenon does not develop by itself, since basic myelin protein alone is immunologically inactive, yet, JHM virus infection of brain cells overcomes this immunological barrier. How this phenomenon is achieved is at present unknown but it is conceivable that JHM replication in CNS tissue may lead to alterations of myelin, to cell membrane changes by insertion of viral proteins which trigger an immune response against CNS tissue or antigenic crossreactivity exists between JHM structural proteins and BMP. Certainly, JHM virus infection of CNS tissue not only directly destroys the infected host cell, but also initiates an autoimmune reaction which could perpetuate CNS damage. Whether sensitization of T-lymphocytes against JHM viral antigens also plays a pathogenic role is unknown, but such cells have been found after coronavirus infection in rats and mice (Wege et al., Stohlman, this volume).

It is generally agreed, that the neurotropic MHV strains which cause a subacute or chronic CNS disease process show a distinct cell tropism. In each model discussed at this meeting, the viral mutant used infected oligodendroglia cells predominantly. This selective vulnerability of oligodendroglia cells to coronaviruses explains the marked lesions of demyelination, since viral replication interferes with cell function. In in vitro studies it could be shown for example that the RN2 Schwannoma cell line has the unique ability to discriminate between non-neurotropic MHV3 and neurotropic JHM strains (Flintoff, this volume). These results suggest that the host cells have a profound influence in regulating replication of these agents which certainly not only takes place in vitro but also in brain infections. These experiments underline the importance of viral and host factors which determine the fate and the outcome of a viral infection.

FELINE CORONAVIRUS INFECTIONS OF CATS

Coronavirus infection of cats is another interesting disease model of great complexity. Several organs of these animals are infected resulting in different disease forms. At the present time little pathogenic information is available. It has been proposed that the immune response to the virus infection especially the cell-mediated immune reactions (CMI) play a crucial role for the disease form developing (Pedersen et al., this volume). In animals without a detectable cell-mediated immune reaction to the virus infection the "effusive" form of disease develops. These animals reveal a swelling of the abdomen as a result of peritonitis. Fibrin is deposited on abdominal organs and granulomatous inflammatory reactions, vasculitis, and plaques of focal necrosis are scattered through the panenchyma of the liver, kidneys, lung, spleen and lymph organs. In contrast, cats developing a partial cell-mediated immunity to feline coronaviruses come down with the "non-effusive" form of the disease. Here localized granulomatous lesions are found without ascites which also involve the eye and the central nervous system. However, in animals which are capable of mounting a humoral and complete cell-mediated immune response probably no disease is observed. In such animals the virus is either eliminated or a latent infection is established which can be reactivated when such animals are infected by feline leukaemia virus. It is believed that the feline leukemia viruses have an immune suppressive effect leading to reactivation of feline coronaviruses. Such a reactivation may then be followed by either the effusive or non-effusive form of the disease depending on the state of CMI reaction. Of interest is also the observation that high levels of coronavirus antibodies do not prevent disease (9). Experimentally infected seronegative kittens survive significantly longer and develop a less fulimant disease than seropositive kittens. Moreover, treatment of seronegative kittens with purified anti FIPV-IgG results in an aggravation of the disease. In such animals viral immune complexes can be found in renal glomeruli tissue.

It is unknown whether the impaired cell-mediated immune response observed in the course of feline coronavirus infection results from the coronavirus infection itself, or existed already in a subclinical form before infection. Certainly, this model reveals pathogenically certain similarities to other acquired immuno-deficiency-syndromes in association with an infectious agent. Further analyses of the interaction between feline coronaviruses and the immune system will provide important answers to these disease processes.

OUTLOOK

The studies on the pathogenesis of coronavirus infections presented and discussed at this meeting present only parts of the disease spectrum which this large virus group can induce. The majority of studies has concentrated on the murine coronavirus group because of the interesting diseases associated with these agents and the detailed virological and molecular biological information available concerning these viruses which is a prerequisite for further analysis. In my judgement, future research in this field has to concentrate on the following three topics.

Firstly, it is of great importance that the molecular biologists define the virus-cell interactions in the different diseases observed, in particular in those which are based on a persistent infection. Since the development of a clinical disease is a result of an organ dysfunction it is necessary to learn in what way persistence is established in brain tissue, whether full viral replication occurs, or whether transcriptional or translational defects exist as shown for CNS persistent infections with other virus groups. With the methodology available to search for viral nucleic acids it is possible to identify the infected host cells and to determine the state of infection. The central nervous system reveals anatomical and physiological pecularities which may permit persistence and inhibit virus elimination. Brain tissue consists of a highly differentiated cell population with complex, functionally integrated cell to cell connections and highly specialised cytoplasmic membranes which probably result in great variability in virus receptor sites and cellular capacity to support virus replication (10). Little is known about the spread of viruses within the CNS and in what way host factors may influence viral replication.

Secondly, the impact of a persistent infection on CNS cells has to be evaluated. In vitro studies with different viruses on neuronal cells in culture revealed the development of cellular dysfunctions in the course of infection. It could be demonstrated that persistent lymphocytic choriomeningitis, measles or rabies virus infection influence luxury functions such as production of acetylcholine, acetyltransferase or acetylcholinesterase without effect on cell morphology, growth rate or protein synthesis (11-13). However, in the case of measles persistence in a particular cell line the presence of measles antibodies in the supernatant can overcome a specific virus-induced cellular dysfunction (14). In C6 rat glioma cells, measles virus persistence interferes substantially with the synthesis of catecholamine-dependent β-adrenergic receptor-stimulated cAMP which can be restored when virus-specific proteins inserted into the membrane of infected cells are removed by viral antibodies in a capping process. It is conceivable, that such interactions occurring in infected CNS tissue stabilise the balance between virus and host cells and may explain prolonged incubation periods until a disease with a defined clinical symptomatology eventually develops.

Thirdly, the immune responses are one of the most important host factors in the complex virus host interactions. As it became obvious at this meeting we are just at the beginning of realising how important immune responses are for both murine or feline coronavirus infections. The immune system does not have easy access to the brain which may account for a failure to control infection in this compartment. There is little information on the flux of antibodies, macrophages, antigens or antigen-antibody complexes in and out of the central nervous system and the pathogenetic role of the local immune response is still unknown. Moreover, the effect of the viral infection on the immune system itself could also be a crucial disease determining factor as studies with feline coronaviruses in cats suggest. In the past studies have shown that viruses can alter immune functions (15). Quite often viruses suppress cellular and humoral immune reactivity, whereas enhancement of the immune reactions is uncommon. In this connection, suppression of delayed type hypersensitivity, prolonged allocraft survival or reduced in vitro lymphocyte reactivity have been noticed. Also suppression of antibody formation with a variety of viruses has been observed. Destruction of lymphocytes, abnormalities in macrophage functions, inhibition of lymphocyte activation and proliferation or alteration of lymphocyte traffic have been discussed as possible mechanisms of viral induced immune dysfunctions. Certainly, the diversity of effects which viruses have on immune functions in the course of infections suggest more than one mechanism by which the alteration of the immune system is achieved. In coronavirus infection an additional immune effect has to be understood. The observation of an autoimmune reaction to CNS tissue as a consequence of viral replication in oligodendroglia cells suggests that a CNS disease process could also be maintained by these mechanisms even after the virus infection has waned. It is conceivable that the analysis of this phenomenon will provide information which is relevant to other chronic demyelinating diseases of animal and man including multiple sclerosis.

This meeting has demonstrated the complexity involved in coronavirus infections. Like the meeting in Würzburg, it was of great value to bring together scientists, from different disciplines, involved in the study of coronavirus infections. Certainly, a multi-disciplinary approach is needed in the attempts to elucidate the nature of the different diseases associated with this virus group.

I think, all participants are grateful to Drs. Peter Rottier, Ben van der Zeijst, Willy Spaan and Professor Marian Horzinek for organising this meeting and providing the atmosphere in which scientific and personal discussions as well as friendship could grow for the benefit of coronavirus research.

ACKNOWLEDGMENT
I thank Helga Kriesinger for typing this manuscript.

REFERENCES

1. Weiner, L.P., R.T. Johnson, R.M. Herndon. Viral infections
    and demyelinating diseases. N. Engl. J. Med. 288: 1103-1110
    (1973).

2. Paterson, P.Y. Transfer of allergic encephalomyelitis in rats
    by means of lymphnode cells. J. Exp. Med. 111: 119-136
    (1960).

3. Dal Canto, M.C., Rabinowitz, S.G. and T.C. Johnson. Virus-in-
    duced demyelination. J. Neurol. Sci. 42: 155-168 (1979).

4. ter Meulen, V. and M.J. Carter. Morbillivirus persistent in-
    fections in animals and man. In: "Virus persistence" (B.W.J.
    Mahy, A.C. Minson and G.K. Darby, eds). Cambridge University
    Press 97-132 (1982).

5. Carter, M.J., Willcocks, M.M. and V. ter Meulen. Defective
    translation of measles virus matrix protein in a SSPE line.
    Nature, in press.

6. Wege, H., Koga, M., Wege H. and V. ter Meulen. JHM infection
    in rats as a model for acute and subacute demyelinating dis-
    ease. In: "Biochemistry and Biology of Coronaviruses" (V. ter
    Meulen, S. Siddell, H. Wege, eds). Adv. Exp. Med. Biol. 142:
    327-340 (1981).

7. Watanabe, R., Wege, H. and V. ter Meulen. Adoptive transfer
    of EAE-like lesions from rats with coronavirus-induced de-
    myelinating encephalomyelitis. Nature, in press.

8. Gonatas, N.K. and J.C. Howard. Inhibition of experimental
    allergic encephalomyelitis in rats severely depleted of
    T-cells. Science 212: 672-675 (1974).

9. Horzinek, M.C. and A.D. Osterhaus. The virology and patho-
    genesis of feline infectious peritonitis. Arch. Virol. 59:
    1-15 (1979).

10. ter Meulen, V. and S.G. Siddell. Virus infections of the
    nervous system: molecular, biological and pathogenetic con-
    siderations. In: "The Molecular Basis of Neuropathology"
    (A.N. Davison and R.H.S. Thompson, eds), Edward Arnold Publ.
    150-187 (1981).

11. Oldstone, M.B.A., Holmstoen, J. and R.M. Weese. Alterations
    of acetylcholine enzymes in neuroblastoma cells persistently
    infected with lymphocytic choriomeningitis virus. J. Cell
    Physiol. 91: 459-472 (1977).

12. Halbach, M. and K. Koschel. Impairment of hormone dependent signal transfer by chronic SSPE virus infection. J. gen. Virol. 42: 615-619 (1979).

13. Koschel, K. and M. Halbach. Rabies virus infection selectively impairs membrane receptor functions in neuronal model cells. J. gen. Virol. 42: 627-632 (1979).

14. Barrett, P.N. and K. Koschel. Effect of antibody-induced modulation of measles (SSPE) virus membrane proteins on ß-adrenergic receptor-mediated adenylate cyclase activity. Virology. 127: in press.

15. Woodruff, J.F. and J.J. Woodruff. The effect of viral infections on the function of the immune system. In: "Viral Immunology and Immunopathology" (A.L. Notkins, ed), Academic Press, New York, San Francisco, London 393-418 (1975).

MHV-A59 PATHOGENESIS IN MICE

Ehud Lavi, Donald H. Gilden, Maureen K. Highkin, and
Susan R. Weiss

The Multiple Sclerosis Research Center of the Wistar
Institute of Anatomy and Biology and the Departments
of Neurology and Microbiology, University of Pennsylvania
School of Medicine, Philadelphia, PA 19104 USA

INTRODUCTION

Coronaviruses produce both acute and chronic diseases in various animal species. A recent review summarizes the biology and pathogenesis of coronaviruses.[1] Of special interest is the chronic demyelinating disease produced by mouse hepatitis virus (MHV) in rodents. This model has been used to study the mechanisms of virus-induced demyelination. Information acquired from such an experimental system may shed light on the pathogenesis of human demyelinating disease.

Experimental infection of weanling mice with wild-type MHV-JHM produces an acute panencephalitis with 20-50% mortality; demyelinating disease is found in the survivors.[2] In older mice (12 weeks old) there is no mortality and 46% develop chronic demyelinating disease.[3] Experimental inoculation of 4-5 week old mice with a temperature-sensitive mutant of JHM (ts-8) results in decreased mortality and increased demyelination.[4,5] Why JHM-ts8 preferentially produces chronic demyelination is not known. This may be due to the predilection of ts-8 for growth in non-neuronal central nervous system (CNS) cells in vitro.[6] In the same study another strain of MHV (A59) was also shown to replicate better in non-neuronal cells than in neurons.

MHV-A59 was first discovered in 1961 when mice, inoculated with mouse leukemia virus, developed an unexpected hepatitis.[7] MHV-A59 that was isolated from the liver of these mice produced hepatitis in various mouse strains of different ages. When inoculated intracerebrally (i.c.) into suckling rats, MHV-A59 produced acute necrotizing encephalitis and hydrocephalus.[8] Only recently has the ability of this hepatotropic strain to produce demyelination been appreciated.[9,10] We describe here a detailed study of MHV-A59 pathogenesis in 4-6 week old C57BL/6 mice.

MATERIALS AND METHODS

Virus and Animals

MHV-A59, originally supplied by Dr. J. Leibowitz, was plaque-purified three times in mouse 17CL-1 cells. Stock virus contained 2×10^7 plaque-forming units (pfu)/ml. Certified MHV-free 4-6-week-old C57BL/6 mice (Jackson laboratories) were used. The absence of antibodies against MHV was confirmed by an indirect immunofluore-scence (IF) assay of randomly sampled sera (see below). Mice were inoculated (i.c.) with 0.03ml of different amounts of the stock virus diluted in PBS containing 0.75% BSA. For intraperitoneal (i.p.) inoculation, 0.5 ml of diluted virus was used. For intra-nasal inoculation (i.n.), 0.2 ml of the virus was applied to the nostril of lightly anesthetized mice which were observed until the virus was inhaled. Intragastric (i.g.) inoculation was performed by injection of 0.2 ml of the virus through an oral-gastric tube. Clinical, virological, histological and IF studies were performed as previously described.[11,12] In addition, some mice were perfused with 0.1M PBS (pH 7.4) containing 1% each of glutaraldehyde and formaldehyde. Spinal cords were post-fixed in osmium tetroxide, dehydrated and embedded in Epon. One μm sections were stained with toluidine blue for light microscopy.[13] Thin sections for EM were stained with uranyl acetate and lead citrate.

Growth of MHV-A59 in Infected Tissue and Blood

Serial ten-fold dilutions of homogenized brain, spinal cord, liver or heparinized blood were prepared in Dulbeccos modified Eagle medium supplemented with 2% fetal calf serum and were titrated by plaque assay in 17CL-1 cells.[14]

Immunofluorescence

The indirect IF antibody method[15] was used, as previously described for infected mouse tissue[12] with a 1:10 dilution of mouse anti-A59 hyperimmune serum and a 1:10 dilution of fluorescein isothiocyanate-conjugated goat anti-mouse immunoglobulin G (Cappel, Downingtown, PA). Controls were provided by the substitution of normal mouse serum for hyperimmune serum; uninfected mouse cells and tissue were also stained with hyperimmune anti-MHV-A59 serum.

Serology

    Anti-MHV-A59 antibodies in sera of infected mice were deter-
mined by indirect IF on MHV-A59 infected 17CL-1 cells. Uninfected
cells were stained with the same sera. Sera from infected mice
were also tested for neutralization by the constant-virus-varying-
serum method for plaque reduction.[16]

RESULTS

Intracerebral Inoculation

    Mice that were inoculated with 1.2×10^3 pfu developed mild hind
limb paralysis and ataxia 2-6 weeks post infection (PI); peak
disease occurred at 3-4 weeks. None of the mice died. Histological
examination revealed acute mild meningoencephalitis during the
second week PI but no evidence of acute hepatitis. However, all
the mice had chronic demyelinating lesions in the brain and spinal
cord 25-60 days PI (Table 1).

    Inoculation with 3×10^3 pfu produced a biphasic disease (Table
1). During the second week PI, all the mice developed a hunched
position, ruffled fur and became lethargic. The clinical condition
of the mice improved during the third week PI. A second phase
started during the fourth week PI with neurological signs of hind
limb or four limb spastic paralysis and ataxic gait. The peak of
the second phase was during the second month PI and most of the mice
had continued mild hind limb paralysis for the remainder of the
ten month observation period. Mice died both during the acute
phase (35%) and also at the beginning of the second phase (15%).
During the acute phase histological examination revealed mild
meningoencephalitis and acute massive hepatitis with multiple
necrotic foci in the liver. Occasionally acute myelitis was seen.
Late disease was characterized by lesions confined to the white
matter in the brain and spinal cord (Fig. 1). Primary demyelination was revealed by ballooning and stripping of myelin sheaths
from otherwise preserved axons and by phagocytosis of myelin by
macrophages. This resulted in numerous demyelinated bare axons
(Fig. 2). A short period of viremia developed during the second
and third days PI. Virus could be recovered from the brain 2-25
days PI, from the spinal cord 3-11 days PI and from the liver on
day 5 PI. MHV-A59 antigen was initially detected by IF in the
meninges and ependyma 2-3 days PI, and in the parenchyma from 3
days to 3 months PI. Serum IF and neutralizing antibodies against
MHV-A59 were first detected 7 days PI and reached peak titers
(1:80-1:160) 2-8 weeks PI. Antibodies were still detected at 1:40
5 months PI.

    A dose of 3×10^4 pfu produced severe acute disease with
ruffled fur, hunched position and lethargy. All the mice died by

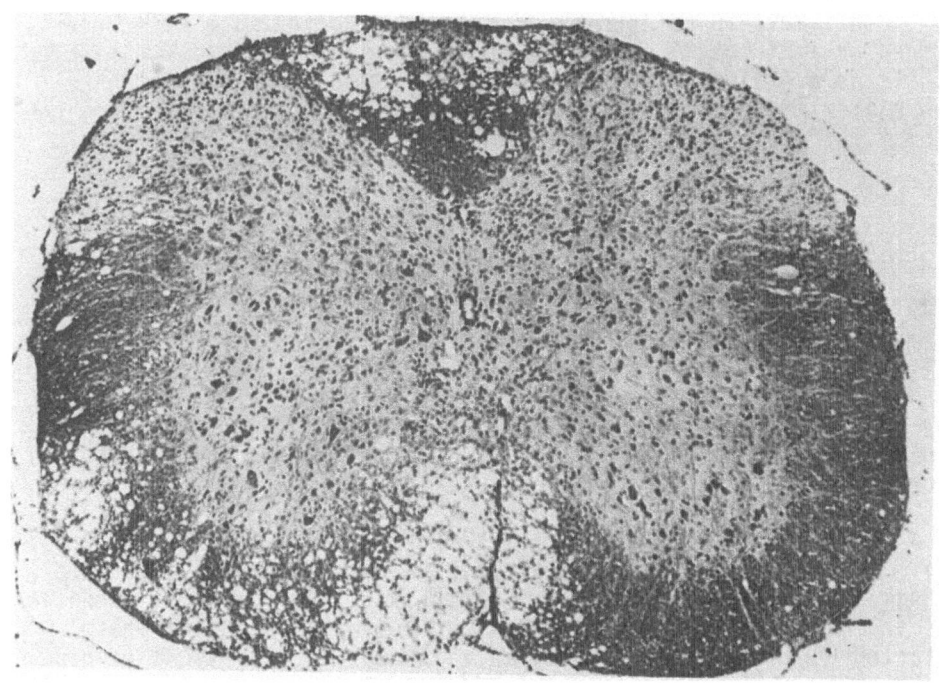

Fig. 1.   Transverse section of mouse spinal cord 60 days after intracerebral inoculation with 3x10^3 pfu MHV-A59. Note primary
damage to white matter. Hematoxylin and Eosin.   x200

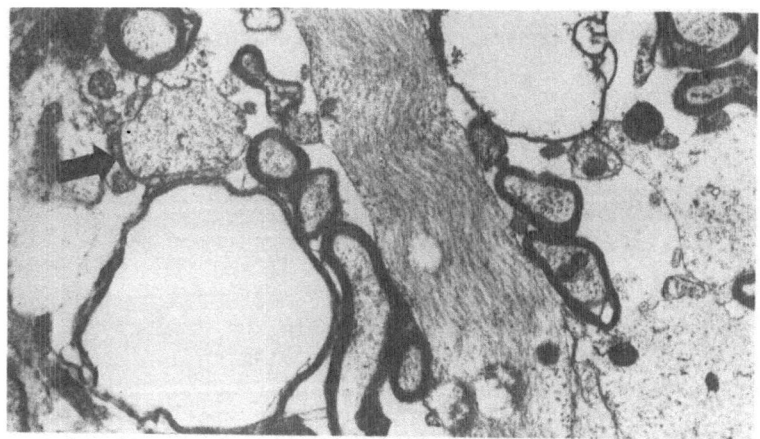

Fig. 2.   Electron micrograph of spinal cord white matter from a mouse
60 days after intracerebral inoculation with 3x10^3 pfu of MHV-
A59. This field contains normal myelinated fibers, a single ba-
are axon (arrow) and a vertically oriented glial fiber.   x7000

the end of the second week PI. Histological examination showed
severe acute hepatitis and moderate meningoencephalitis (Table 1).

Intraperitoneal Inoculation

A dose of $3x10^3$ pfu did not kill or produce any clinical
disease or pathological changes during the two month PI observation
period.

A dose of $3x10^4$ pfu also did not kill or produce clinical
signs; however, discrete foci of hepatic necrosis were found in
the absence of CNS involvement. IF antibodies against MHV-A59
were found at a titer of 1:80 in the serum of mice 30 days PI.

A dose of $3x10^5$ pfu produced moderate to severe acute disease.
The majority of the mice developed hunched position and ruffled fur;
20% died. IF antibodies against MHV-A59 were detected at a titer
of 1:160 in the serum of mice 30 days PI. Virus was recovered from
the liver of mice ($1.2x10^4$ pfu/gr) at day 5 PI, but could not be
recovered from the blood.

A dose of $3x10^6$ pfu led to severe acute disease with 100%
mortality. Histological examination showed severe hepatitis with
massive diffuse necrotic lesions in the liver. There was no CNS
involvement.

Intranasal Inoculation

A dose of $3x10^6$ produced mild clinical disease during the
second week PI characterized by mildly hunched position and ruffled
fur in some of the mice; 1/20 died (Table 1). Histological examination revealed inflammatory infiltration in the livers, lungs and
meninges 4 days PI. By 7 days PI all the mice developed mild
hepatitis and severe meningoencephalitis. Mononuclear infiltration
and perivascular cuffing were seen in the meninges, choroid plexus
and in the brain. Microglial proliferation was also observed
diffusely. Necrotic lesions were pronounced in cortical and
thalamic areas. By 30 days PI, lesions were found only in the
cerebral (50%) and spinal cord (70%) white matter. The white
matter lesions were similar to those produced by the i:c. inoculation. By 60 days PI only one mouse out of ten showed white matter
lesions in the spinal cord. IF anti-MHV-A59 antibodies were
detected from 7-60 days PI (1:20-1:40).

Intragastric Inoculation

Mice did not get sick or die, however 50% of the mice developed
a few circumscribed areas of inflammation in the liver adjacent to
portal veins. In one of 6 mice, acute meningoencephalitis was

found. None of the mice developed chronic white matter lesions
(Table 1). IF anti-MHV-A59 antibodies were detected 10-30 days PI
(1:20-1:40).

DISCUSSION

The relevance of coronaviruses to human demyelinating diseases
has been investigated because of the following findings: the
detection of coronavirus-like particles by EM in the brain of one
MS patient[17]; the isolation of two coronaviruses in mice and from
mouse cell lines inoculated with MS brain tissue[18]; and the
detection of intrathecal synthesis of antibodies against coronaviruses in MS patient[19]. We present here a model system of MHV-A59
infection in mice in which to study the relationship between coronaviruses and demyelination

MHV-A59 is considered mainly hepatotropic and only weakly
neurotropic[7,9]. We show here for the first time that by i.c.
inoculation of 4-6-week-old C57BL/6 mice with 1.2×10^3 pfu of MHV-A59
it is possible to produce disease that is exclusively in the CNS.
Moreover, by the i.n. route of inoculation, which may mimic natural
infection, we produced a nonfatal disease mainly in the CNS, with
only mild liver involvement.

The clinical and pathological findings after i.c. inoculation
with MHV-A59 were dose dependent. An amount of 3×10^4 pfu caused
acute panencephalitis and hepatitis that killed 100% mice. A dose
of 3×10^3 pfu caused biphasic disease. Mice that survived the acute
phase developed chronic demyelinating disease. A dose of 1.2×10^3
pfu led to subacute demyelinating disease without involvement of
the liver.

I.P. inoculation of MHV-A59 produced only hepatitis without
involvement of the CNS. It is of interest that the dose required
for production of severe liver disease by i.c. inoculation (3×10^3
pfu) did not produce any pathological changes when inoculated i.p.
The amounts that were used for the production of liver disease by
i.p. inoculation were markedly higher than the doses that were used
for the induction of liver disease by i.c. inoculation. A possible
explanation for this phenomenon lies in the fact that peritoneal
macrophages from different mouse strains (including C57BL/6) are
capable of suppressing MHV replication[20]. These cells provide
the first defense mechanism against the invasion of MHV into the
peritoneal cavity. Because the brain is a lymphoid-free organ,
macrophages are not present to suppress MHV replication after it
is inoculated intracerebrally.

Table 1. The Pathogenesis of MHV-A59 in C57BL/6 Mice by Different Routes of Inoculation

Route of Inoc. [a]	Number of Mice	Dose of Inoc. [b]	Mortality [c]	Histology [d]			Clinical Signs [e]
				HEPAT.	AC.ME.	CHR.DEMY.	
I.C.	30	1.2×10^3	0	0	100	100	Mild chronic disease.
	30	3×10^3	50	100	100	100	Biphasic disease: moderate-severe acute disease, moderate-severe chronic disease.
	10	3×10^4	100	100	100	—	Severe acute disease.
I.P.	10	3×10^3	0	0	0	0	None
	10	3×10^4	0	100	0	0	None
	10	3×10^5	20	100	0	0	Moderate-severe acute disease.
	5	3×10^6	100	100	0	0	Severe acute disease.
I.N.	30	3×10^6	5	100	100	70	Mild acute disease.
I.G.	10	3×10^6	0	50	10	0	None

a – Route of inoculation: i.c. – intracerebral, i.p. – intraperitoneal, i.n. – intranasal, i.g. – intragastric.
b – Dose of inoculation as expressed in pfu/inoculum.
c – Mortality and histological findings are expressed in percentage of mice out of total in that category.
d – Hepat. – hepatitis, Ac.Me. – acute meningoencephalitis, Chr.Demy. – chronic demyelination.
e – Acute disease: hunched position, ruffled fur, lethargy. Chronic disease: hind limb or 4 limb spastic paralysis and/or ataxic gait.

The i.n. inoculation resulted in invasion of MHV-A59 not only into the lung and liver but also into the CNS, indicating that MHV-A59 is neurotropic as well as hepatotropic. Whether virus enters the brain via the olfactory nerves or via the blood is not yet clear. The weak response to intragastric inoculation suggests that it may be less important than intranasal-acquired infection of MHV-A59 in mouse colonies.

In conclusion, we demonstrated that the ability of the A59 strain of MHV to produce demyelination is dependent both on dose and route of inoculation. These biological properties of MHV-A59 provide a useful model system for further study of the mechanism of virus-induced demyelination.

ACKNOWLEDGEMENTS

The authors wish to thank Dr. Lucy B. Rorke for assistance with the pathological work. This work was supported by grants RG-1421-A-1 and RG-894-C3 from the National Multiple Sclerosis Society and grants AI 17418 and NS 11037 from the National Institutes of Health. E. Lavi was the recipient of a Penn-Israel Wexler Fellowship award and was supported in part by the Kroc Foundation.

REFERENCES

1. H. Wege, S. Siddell, V. ter-Meulen, The Biology and pathogenesis of coronaviruses, Advances in Virology and Immunology, 99:165-200 (1982).
2. L. P. Weiner, Pathogenesis of demyelination induced by mouse hepatitis virus (JHM), Arch. Neurol., 28:298-303 (1973).
3. S. A. Stohlman, L. P. Weiner, Chronic central nervous system demyelination in mice after JHM virus infection, Neurology, 31:38-44 (1981).
4. M. V. Haspel, P. W. Lampert, M. B. A. Oldstone, Temperature-sensitive mutants of mouse hepatitis virus produce a high incidence of demyelination, Proc. Natl. Acad. Sci. USA, 75:4033-4036 (1978).
5. R. L. Knobler, P. W. Lampert, M. B. A. Oldstone, Virus persistence and recurring demyelination produced by a temperature-sensitive mutant of MHV-4, Nature, 298:279-280 (1982).
6. M. E. Dubois-Dalcq, E. W. Doller, M. V. Haspel, K. V. Holmes, Cell tropism and expression of mouse hepatitis virus in mouse spinal cord cultures, Virology, 119:317-331 (1982).
7. R. A. Manaker, C. V. Piczak, A. A. Miller, M. F. Stanton, A hepatitis virus complicating studies with mouse leukemia, J. Nat. Cancer Inst., 27:29-51 (1961).

8. N. Hirano, N. Goto, T. Ogawa, K. Ono, T. Murakami, K. Fujiwara,
    Hydrocephalus in suckling rats infected intracerebrally with
    mouse hepatitis virus MHV-A59, Microbiol. Immunol., 24:825-
    834 (1980).

9. J. A. Robb, C. W. Bond, J. L. Leibowitz, Pathogenic murine
    coronaviruses III. Biological and biochemical characteriza-
    tion of temperature-sensitive mutants of JHMV, Virology,
    94:385-399 (1979).

10. E. Lavi, D. H. Gilden, Z. Wroblewska, L. B. Rorke, S. W. Weiss,
    Experimental demyelination produced by the A59 strain of
    mouse hepatitis virus, (abs), Neurol., (Suppl.), 33:106 (1983)

11. L. B. Rorke, D. H. Gilden, Z. Wroblewska, J. S. Wolinsky,
    Experimental panencephalitis induced in suckling mice by
    parainfluenza type I (6/96) virus. I. Clinical and patho-
    logical features, J. Neuropath. Exp. Neurol., 35:247-258
    (1976).

12. D. H. Gilden, Z. Wroblewska, M. Chesler, M. Wellish, F. S. Lief,
    J. S. Wolinsky, L. B. Rorke, Experimental panencephalitis
    induced in suckling mice by parainfluenza 1 (6/94) virus.
    II. Virologic studies, J. Neuropath. Exp. Neurol., 35:259-
    270 (1976).

13. J. R. Martin, Spinal cord and optic nerve demyelination in
    experimental herpes simplex virus type 2 infection, J.
    Neuropath. Exp. Neurol., 41:253-265 (1982).

14. S. R. Weiss, J. L. Leibowitz, Comparison of the RNAs of murine
    and human coronaviruses, in: "Biochemistry and Biology of
    Coronaviruses," V. ter Meulen,   S. Siddell and H. Wege,
    eds., Plenum Press, New York, 245-259 (1981).

15. M. Goldman, Fluorescent antibody methods, Academic Press, New
    York, 157-158 (1969).

16. E. H. Lennette, N. J. Schmidt, Diagnostic procedures for viral
    and rickettsial infections, American Public Health Assc.,
    New York, 446, (1969).

17. R. Tanaka, Y. Iwasaki, H. Koprowski, Intracisternal virus-like
    particles in brain of a multiple sclerosis patient, J.
    Neurol. Sci., 128:121-126 (1976).

18. J. S. Burks, B. L. Devald, L. D. Jankovsky, J. C. Gerdes, Two
    coronaviruses isolated from central nervous system tissue
    of two multiple sclerosis patients, Science, 209:933-934
    (1980).

19. A. Salmi, B. Ziola, T. Hovi, M. Reunanen, Antibodies to corona-
    viruses OC43 and 229E in multiple sclerosis patients,
    Neurology, 32:292-295 (1982).

20. S. A. Stohlman, J. F. Frelinger, Macrophages and Resistence to
    JHM virus CNS infection, in: "Biochemistry and Biology of
    Coronaviruses," V. ter Meulen,   S. Siddell and H. Wege,
    eds., Plenum Press, New York, 387-398 (1981).

DETECTION OF MHV-A59 RNA BY IN SITU HYBRIDIZATION

Ehud Lavi, Donald H. Gilden, Maureen K. Highkin, and
Susan R. Weiss

The Multiple Sclerosis Research Center of the Wistar
Institute of Anatomy and Biology and the Departments
of Neurology and Microbiology, University of Pennsylvania
School of Medicine, Philadelphia, PA 19104 USA

INTRODUCTION

We have shown that MHV-A59 causes a chronic demyelinating
disease in C57BL/6 mice.[1] Although active demyelination can be
detected as long as five months post inoculation, it has been
difficult to detect viral antigens by immunofluorescence and thus
far impossible to demonstrate replication of infectious virus in
chronically infected mice. Thus we have used in situ hybridization
of CNS and liver samples with radiolabeled virus-specific DNA
probes to investigate the state of the genome in these tissues.
In this paper we report experiments in which we start to address
the question of whether or not viral RNA can be detected in the
CNS and liver of these chronically infected mice and, if so, how
much and in which cell types.

MATERIALS AND METHODS

Virus and Animals

MHV-A59, obtained from Dr. J. Leibowitz, was plaque purified
three times in mouse 17CL-1 cells and grown at a low multiplicity
of infection (m.o.i.). Stock virus contained 2×10^7 plaque forming
units (pfu)/ml. Certified MHV-free 4-6 week old C57BL/6 mice
(Jackson Laboratories) were inoculated intracerebrally (i.c.) with
3×10^3 pfu of virus in 0.03 ml. of PBS containing 0.75% BSA. At
different intervals post infection (PI) mice were anesthetized with
ether and perfused with 20 ml. of PBS followed by 20 ml. of
periodate-lysin-paraformaldehyde (PLP) solution.[2] Brain, spinal

247

cord and liver were removed and immersed in PLP overnight at 4°C, dehydrated and embedded in paraffin. Ten um sections were cut and collected on microscope slides which had been previously coated with Denhardt's solution and acetylated as previously described.[3] Infected and uninfected 17CL-1 mouse cells were harvested approximately 16 hours after infection with MHV-A59 (m.o.i.=1) when a maximum cytopathic effect (CPE) was observed and deposited by cytocentrifugation on microscope slides which had been previously treated as described for tissues above.

Preparation of MHV-A59 Probe

MHV-A59 DNA sequences, cloned into the bacterial plasmid pBR322, were used as probes for viral nucleic acids. cDNA was synthesized using as template either purified genome RNA or poly(A)-containing intracellular RNA from MHV-A59 infected cells, using oligo(dT)$_{12-18}$ as primer and reverse transcriptase as previously described except that all four nucleotide triphosphates were at 0.2mM concentrations.[4] After denaturation, the cDNA was copied into double-stranded DNA with E. coli polymerase I, the duplex was treated with S1 nuclease and deoxycytidine tails were added to the 3' ends with terminal transferase. This tailed DNA was hybridized with deoxyguanosine tailed, Pst-1 cleaved pBR322 and these hybrids were used to transform HB101 all essentially as described by Gough et al.[5] Colonies containing viral inserts were selected by two rounds of hybridization with virus-specific cDNA.[6] The sizes of viral inserts as estimated by migration in agarose gels of Pst-1 digested plasmid DNAs were from 400-1800 base pairs with the majority in the 400-600 base pair range. Clones synthesized from genome RNA were named pBRg1, etc., and those from intracellular RNA were named pBRc1, etc. The plasmid DNAs pBRg344 and pBRc8 were tritium-labeled by nick translation with DNA polymerase I at 14°C for two hours.[7] The specific activity of these probes was approximately 3×10^7 cpm/ugDNA.

In Situ Hybridization

The probe was applied onto MHV-infected and uninfected mouse tissue sections and tissue culture cells at a concentration of $1-1.5 \times 10^5$ cpm/1.13 cm^2 and processed as described for detection RNA[3]. The hybridization mixture contained mouse 17CL-1 cell nucleic acids which was necessary to eliminate non-specific binding of probes to tissue samples.

RESULTS

Characterization of Virus-Specific Cloned DNAs

In order to detect viral nucleic acids in mouse CNS samples, we wanted to use cloned probes representing as much of the viral

genome as possible. The MHV-A59-specific clones that we obtained
(as described in Materials and Methods) were synthesized using
oligo(dT) as a primer and thus would be expected to represent the
3' end of the genome RNA. However, we wanted to map them more
precisely against the genome. Since the MHV intracellular virus-
specific RNAs form a nested set, all overlapping at the 3' end, we
used these RNAs for mapping of the cloned DNAs. Thus, plasmid
DNAs from selected clones were nick translated with ^{32}P-dCTP[7] and
hybridized to Northern blots containing intracellular RNA from
uninfected and MHV-infected 17CL-1 cells. All cloned DNAs tested
hybridized only with RNA from infected cells and to all seven
virus-specific subgenomic RNAs (data not shown). This shows that
all clones must map at least partially within the 3' nucleocapsid (N)
gene which is encoded by the smallest RNA. All cloned DNAs cross-
hybridized with each other except for pBRg344 (data not shown).
Since clone pBRg334 is too long to map to the 3' side of the other
clones, it probably maps to the 5' side and encompasses the El gene
as well as part of N. We have used these data to generate a tenta-
tive map of these clones as shown in Figure 1. The sequences
represented in pBRg344 and pBRc8 together represent approximately
12% of the MHV-A59 genome. We used DNA from both of these clones
as a virus-specific probe.

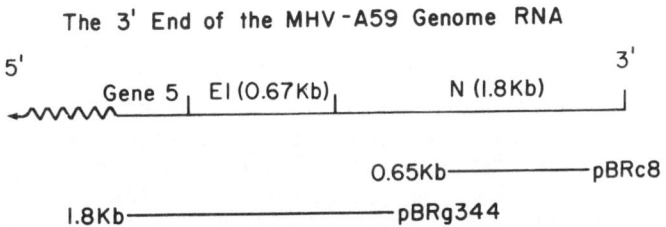

Fig. 1. The 3' end of the MHV-A59 genome RNA. The genes at the
3' end are designated N for nucleocapsid and El for the
small MHV plycoprotein. The positions of two cloned DNA
fragments are shown below.

Detection of MHV-A59 in 17CL-1 Infected Cells

As a positive control for the specificity of the probe in the detection of MHV-A59 RNA by in situ hybridization, we used infected 17CL-1 cells. MHV-A59 RNA was detected at maximal CPE (Figure 2A) in the cytoplasm of all cells, especially in giant syncytia. Uninfected 17CL-1 cells did not hybridize with the probe (Figure 2B).

Detection of MHV-A59 During Acute Infection in Mice

MHV-A59 RNA was detected in all three mice that were inoculated (i.c.) with $3x10^3$ pfu and sacrificed 5 days PI. In the liver, viral RNA was detected mostly in the cytoplasm of hepatocytes (Figure 3A) at the periphery of foci of inflammation and necrosis. The histological findings were compatible with acute hepatitis.

In the brain, viral genome was found at day 5 PI mostly in the white matter, but also in the meninges, cerebral cortex, thalamus and brain stem (data not shown). The histological findings were compatible with mild meningoencephalitis.

In the spinal cord, viral RNA was found at day 5 PI within the cytoplasm of cells (Figure 4A) in both the white and gray matter. The number of infected cells was smaller than in the brain. The histological finding was mild inflammation of spinal meninges and parenchyma.

Liver, brain and spinal cord sections from mock infected mice that were processed for in situ hybridization in parallel did not hybridize with the probe (Figures 3C and 4C).

Detection of MHV-A59 in Chronically Infected Mice

In the search for MHV-A59 RNA in chronically infected mice three mice were sacrificed 10 months PI and the organs were processed for in situ hybridization. MHV-A59 RNA was detected in the liver of one mouse in small foci of 3-4 hepatocytes each (Figure 3B). In spinal cord sections of two mice, viral genome was also detected within the cytoplasm of a few small round cells in the white matter (Figure 4B). It is impossible on the basis of morphology alone to classify the infected cells. It is also difficult to say whether the infected area also has pathological changes since the fixation procedure for in situ hybridization produces some myelin destruction. In both liver and CNS samples there were less foci of cells containing viral sequences during chronic infection

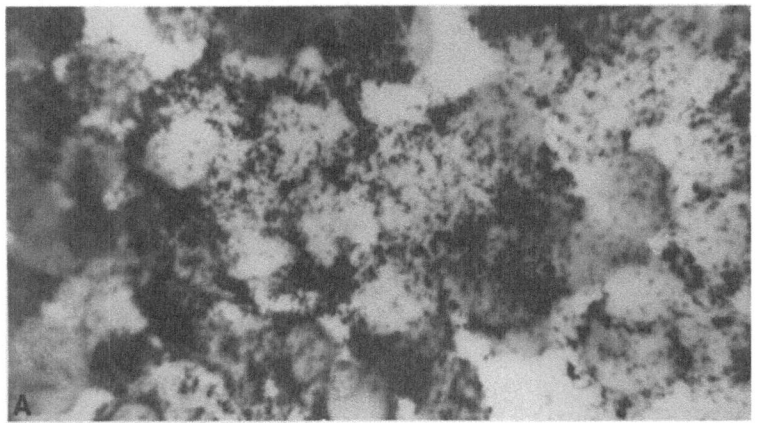

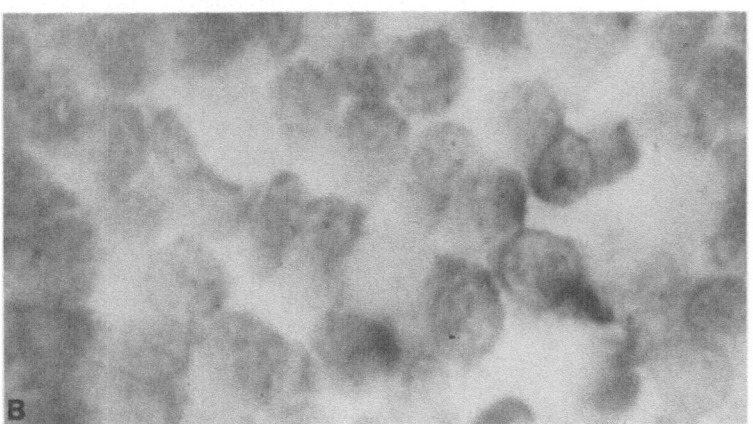

Fig. 2.   MHV-A59 RNA detected by in situ hybridization with an
          H3-labeled specific probe and autoradiographically exposed
          for one week. H&E x385.
          A) MHV-A59 infected 17CL-1 cells (m.o.i.=1), harvested and
              fixed 16 hours PI at maximal cytopathic effect. Silver
              grains of positive hybridization are seen in the cyto-
              plasm of all cells.
          B) Uninfected 17CL-1 cells processed in paralled. No hybri-
              dization is seen.

as compared to acute infection. MHV-A59 could not be found in the
liver, brain or spinal cord of control mock infected mice (Figures
3C and 4C).

Fig. 3. MHV-A59 RNA detected by <u>in situ</u> hybridization with an
         H^3-labeled specific probe and autoradiographically ex-
         posed for one week. H&E   x385

    A) Liver section from a mouse 5 days after i.c. inocula-
        tion with 3 x10^3 pfu MHV-A59. Viral RNA is seen in
        the cytoplasm of hepatocytes adjacent to a portal vein.
    B) Liver section from a mouse 10 months after i.c. ino-
        culation with 3x10^3 pfu of MHV-A59. Viral RNA is
        seen in the cytoplasm of hepatocytes.
    C) Liver section from a mock infected mouse processed in
        parallel. No hybridization is seen.

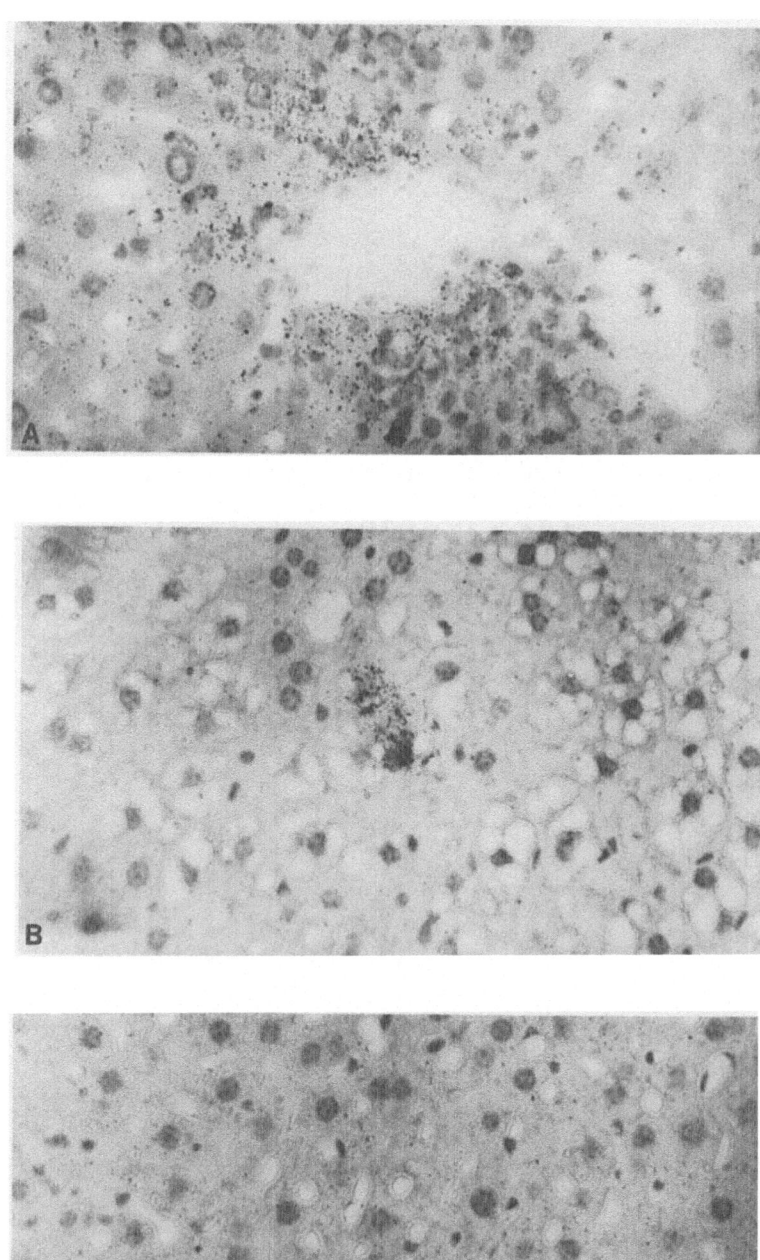

Fig. 4.   MHV-A59 RNA detected by <u>in situ</u> hybridization with an
          H^3-labeled probe and autoradiographically exposed for one
          week.   H&E   x385.

          A)   Spinal cord section from a mouse 5 days after i.c.
               inoculation with 3×10^3 pfu of MHV-A59.   Viral RNA is
               detected in a few cells in the anterior columns of
               white matter.
          B)   Spinal cord of a mouse 10 months after i.c. inoculation
               with 3×10^3 pfu of MHV-A59.   Viral RNA is detected in a
               few white matter cells near the anterior horn.
          C)   Spinal cord section from a mock infected mouse process-
               ed in parallel.   No hybridization is seen.

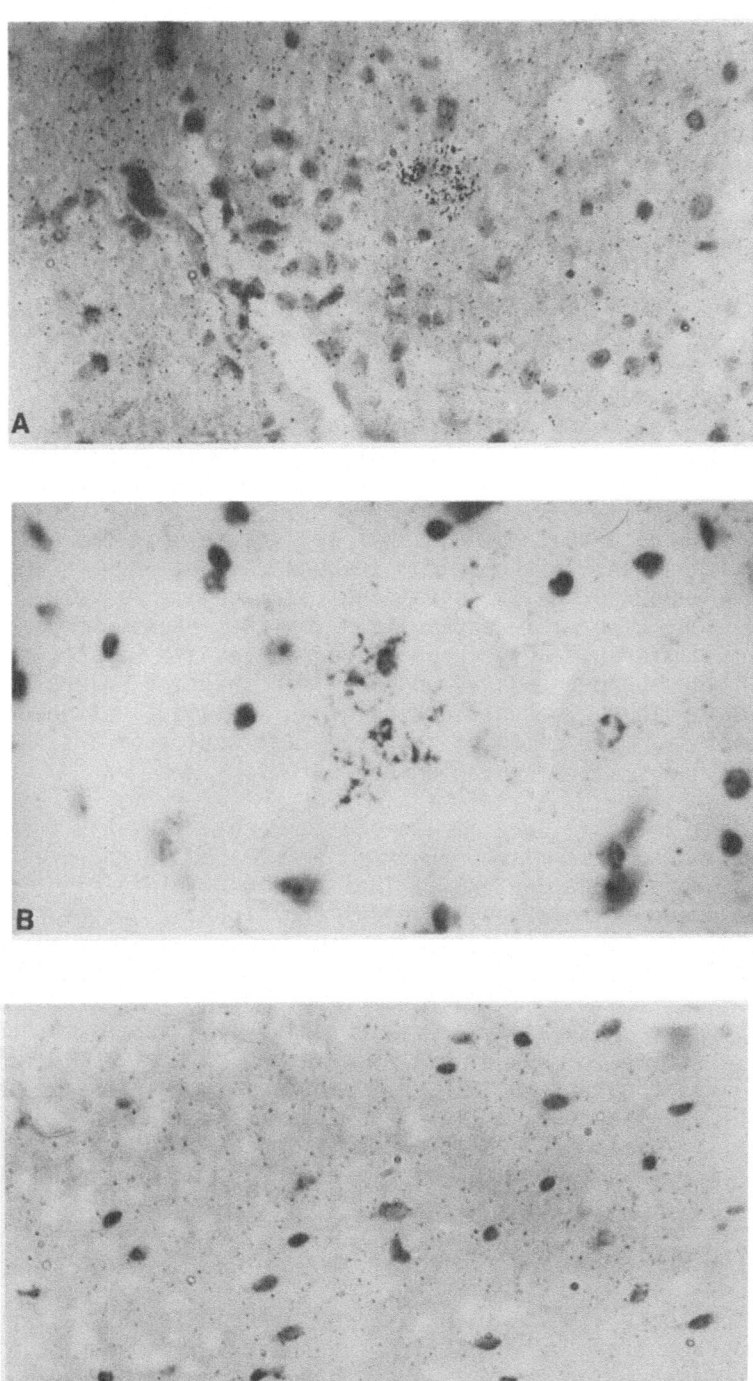

DISCUSSION

Viral persistence is a possible explanation for a broad array of chronic diseases in animals and humans. Two examples of chronic diseases attributed to coronavirus persistence are MHV-3 chronic vasculitis and MHV-JHM chronic demyelinating disease. The two diseases differ in pathogenic mechanism and apparently in target cell. Nevertheless, viral persistence has been shown in both. MHV-3 was recovered from chronically infected mice[8] and infectious JHM could be recovered from chronically infected mice[9] and rats.[10]

In MHV-A59 infected mice that develop chronic demyelination, there is persistence of virus-specific nucleic acid. Whether or not persistence of a low level of virus as evidenced by viral nucleic acid sequences is the mechanism of chronic demyelination is not yet clear. In another model system, Theiler virus infection of mice, viral persistence[11] as well as an immune-mediated mechanism[12] has been shown to be involved in chronic demyelination.

We show here that MHV-A59 RNA persists in both the CNS and the liver while chronic pathological changes develop only in the CNS. Since the number of cells containing viral genome is very low in both tissues, a possible explanation for this phenomenon can be an essential difference between oligodendrocytes and hepatocytes. A single oligodendrocyte is responsible for covering several axons with myelin. Thus, the destruction of an individual oligodendrocyte is potentially more damaging than the destruction of a single hepato-cyte, which has little pathological effect.

It has thus far been impossible to recover MHV-A59 from chronically infected mice. This may be related to the small number of cells containing viral RNA. The in situ hybridization technique has been shown to be a very powerful tool for the detection of small amounts of viral nucleic acid,[13] as our study reienforces. It is still unclear whether a small amount of infectious virus is present.

The number of grains seen in chronically infected tissue cells is similar to the number of grains detected in acutely infected cells. This suggests that there is not a large difference in the amount of viral RNA per cell in the tissues from acutely or chronically infected animals, and that there is not a significant block in the amount of total viral transcription during persistent infection.

ACKNOWLEDGEMENTS

The authors wish to thank Suzanne Amrhein for assistance with the preparation of the manuscript and Audrey Gilden for printing the photographs. This work was supported by grants RG-1421-A-1 and RG-894-C3 from the National Multiple Sclerosis Society and

grants AI 17418 and NS 11037. E. Lavi was the recipient of a
Penn-Israel Wexler Fellowship award and was supported in part by
the Kroc Foundation.

REFERENCES

1. E. Lavi, D. H. Gilden, Z. Wroblewska, L. B. Rorke, S. R. Weiss,
    Experimental demyelination produced by the A59 strain of
    mouse hepatitis virus, (abs), Neurology, (Suppl. 2), 33:106
    (1983).
2. I. W. McLean, P. K. Nolsan, Periodate lysin paraformaldehyde
    fixative: A new fixative for immunoelectron microscopy,
    J. Histochem. Cytochem., 22:1077-1083 (1974).
3. M. Brahic, A. T. Haase, Detection of viral sequences in low
    reiteration frequency by in situ hybridization, Proc. Nat.
    Acad. Sci., 75:6125-6129 (1978).
4. S. R. Weiss and J. L. Leibowitz, Characterization of murine
    coronavirus RNA by hybridization with virus-specific cDNA
    probes, J. Gen. Virol., 64:127-133 (1983).
5. N. M. Gough, E. A. Webb, S. Corey and J. M. Adams, Molecular
    cloning of seven mouse immunoglobulin K chain messenger
    ribonucleic acids, Biochemistry, 19:2702-2710 (1980).
6. M. Grunstein and D. S. Hogness, Colony hybridization: A
    method for the isolation of cloned DNAs that contain a
    specific gene, Proc. Nat. Acad. Sci., 72:3961-3965 (1975).
7. P. W. J. Rigby, M. Dieckmann, C. Rhodes, P. Berg, Labeling
    deoxyribonucleic acid to high specific activity in vitro
    by nick translation with DNA polymerase I., J. Mol. Biol.,
    113:237-251 (1977).
8. J. L. Virelizier, A. D. Dayan, A. C. Allison, Neuropathological
    effects of persistent infection of mice by mouse hepatitis
    virus, Infect. Immun., 12:1127-1140 (1975).
9. R. L. Knobler, P. W. Lampert, M. B. A. Oldstone, Virus per-
    sistence and recurring demyelination produced by a tempera-
    ture-sensitive mutant of MHV-4, Nature, 298:279-280 (1982).
10. H. Wege, M. Coga, H. Wege, V. ter Meulen, JHM infections in
    rats as a model for acute and subacute demyelinating disease,
    in: "Biochemistry and Biology of Coronaviruses," V. ter
    Meulen, S. Siddell, H. Wege, eds., Plenum Press, New York,
    327-340 (1981).
11. M. Brahic, W. G. Stroop, J. R. Baringer, Theiler virus persists
    in glial cells during demyelinating disease, Cell, 26:123-
    128 (1981).
12. H. D. Lipton, M. C. Dal Canto, Theiler's virus induced demyelina-
    tion: Prevention by immunosupression, Science, 192:62-64
    (1976).
13. A. T. Haase, P. Ventura, K. P. Johnson, E. Norrby, C. J. Gibbs,
    Jr., Measles virus in infection of the central nervous system,
    J. Inf. Dis., 144:154-160 (1981).

VIROLOGICAL AND IMMUNOLOGICAL ASPECTS OF CORONAVIRUS INDUCED

SUBACUTE DEMYELINATING ENCEPHALOMYELITIS IN RATS

H. Wedge, R. Watanabe and V. ter Meulen

Institute of Virology
University of Wurzburg, F.R.G.

SUMMARY

Infection of rats with the murine coronavirus JHM led to acute or subacute encephalitis. Viral and host factors greatly influenced the outcome of the infection. A number of temperature-sensitive (ts) mutants was obtained which differed widely in their capacity to induce lesions of the central nervous system (CNS) in rats. Under defined conditions a subacute demyelinating encephalomyelitis (SDE) with pronounced clinical signs was observed 14-160 days post infection (p.i.). A number of rats, which showed a remission of SDE later developed a relapse of the disease accompanied by neurological symptoms. Neuropathological examination of such animals revealed lesions of active demyelination and extended remyelinated areas. The presence of viral antigen or infectious virus in the CNS of these rats demonstrated that they were persistently infected. Further investigations indicated that this virus infection triggers a cell mediated immune response against basic myelin protein which may contribute to the development of subacute to chronic encephalomyelitides.

INTRODUCTION

Several important diseases of the human central nervous system (CNS) are associated with inflammatory demyelinating lesions. An impairment of cell functions by a virus infection, an immunopathological reaction or a combination of both are possible mechanisms which lead to myelin destruction (9,10,21). Among the experimental animal models, which allow us to study such events, infections with murine coronaviruses are of particular interest. Most studies have been carried out with the murine coronavirus JHM, a neurotropic

strain which can induce demyelination in the CNS of mice and rats
(1,7,20). In mice, acute disease and clinically silent demyelinating
lesions have been described which were associated with a persistent
infection (3,4,5,6,18). In rats similar CNS lesions can be observed
after JHM infection, but in these animals, these changes, particularly demyelination, can lead to clinically recognizable diseases which
develop after long incubation times. As has been previously described the infection of rats with wild type JHM virus was followed by
different courses of encephalomyelitis (13,14,17). Clinical disease
was observed either after a short incubation time of 3 to 11 days
(acute encephalomyelitis [AE]) or developed several weeks to months
p.i. (subacute demyelinating encephalomyelitis [SDE]). AE represented a rapidly progressing fatal disease course with marked paralysis. Necrotic lesions were found in all parts of the CNS, with
involvement of neurons and glial cells. The clinical signs of SDE
started with slight hindleg paresis and ataxic gait. Lesions of
primary demyelination with relative sparing of axons were restricted
to selected areas of the white matter, and in contrast to AE glial
cells were preferentially infected. The outcome of SDE was not always fatal, and areas of extended remyelination were detectable
after recovery. A high rate of SDE was readily obtained by infection
of rats with certain ts mutants (19). These preliminary studies in
rats indicate that viral and host factors play an important pathogenic role in the development of the different CNS diseases. In the
following communication we summarize our recent findings on these
parameters.

RESULTS

Influence of host-age and viral properties on the type of CNS disease

Infection of 21-25 day old rats by wild type JHM virus was
followed by both AE and SDE with variable frequencies. Randomly
selected clones of tissue culture adapted JHM virus (by plaque
passages) caused predominantly AE (Table 1) and not SDE regardless
of the dose inoculated. To select virus mutants with altered neurovirulence a collection of ts-mutants was produced by growth in the
presence of fluoruracil. These mutants differed widely in their biological properties including neurovirulence (19). Most of these
mutants were of low neurovirulence if inoculated into 21-25 days old
rats. However, if rats less than 3 weeks old were inoculated with
certain mutants a high rate of SDE developed after an incubation time
of several weeks to months. Table 2 gives an example of an age
dependent development of SDE following infection with ts43. In rats,
which showed clinical symptoms, viral antigens were detectable by
immune histology and infectious virus could be reisolated. These
reisolates were still temperature sensitive, even after months of
persistence as shown in Table 3.

TABLE 1   CORONAVIRUS JHM INFECTION IN RATS

VIRUS INOCULATED	AGE OF ANIMALS AT INFECTION	
	SUCKLING	WEANLING
	(< 20 DAYS)	(> 20 DAYS)
WILD TYPE VIRUS PASSAGED IN MICE	AE*	AE AND SDE**
PLAQUE PURIFIED VIRUS (CELL ADAPTED)	AE	AE
TS-MUTANTS	DEPENDING ON MUTANT AND AGE OF RATS AE AND/OR SDE	SDE

```
 *  AE  = ACUTE ENCEPHALOMYELITIS
**  SDE = SUBACUTE DEMYELINATING ENCEPHALOMYELITIS
```

TABLE 2   COMPARISON OF NEUROVIRULENCE OF JHM wt and JHM ts 43

AGE AT TIME OF INFECTION (± 1 DAY)	VIRUS*	DISEASED TOTAL	INCUBATION TIME (DAYS)	RECOVERY FROM DISEASE	TYPE OF DISEASE
4	wt **	7/10	3-5	None	AE
	ts 43	26/26	10-17	4/26	AE > SDE
10	wt	8/10	3-6	None	AE
	ts 43	23/43	14-158	11/23	SDE
15	wt	7/12	4-11	None	AE
	ts 43	1/12	92	-	SDE

```
 * 4x10³ PFU/RAT were inoculated into outbred rats, strain CHBB/Thom.
** JHM wild type virus cloned by plaque passages in Sac(-) cells
```

TABLE 3   TEMPERATURE SENSITIVITY OF REISOLATED VIRUS FROM
RATS INFECTED WITH ts43*

DESIGNATION OF ISOLATE	ONSET OF CLINICAL DISEASE DAYS p.i.	TEMPERATURE SENSITIVITY[**] OF REISOLATED VIRUS
ts43-1	45	1.3×10^{-4}
ts43-2	48	1.5×10^{-4}
ts43-3	50	6.7×10^{-3}
ts43-4	50	5.0×10^{-4}
ts43-5	65	5.0×10^{-3}
ts43-6	76	2.0×10^{-2}
ts43-7	90	4.0×10^{-3}

* 4×10^3 PFU WERE INOCULATED INTO RATS AT AN AGE OF 9-11 DAYS
**   EFFICIENCY OF PLAQUING (EOP) = PFU AT $39.5^{\circ}C$: PFU AT $34^{\circ}C$.
EOP OF ts43 USED FOR INOCULATION = 1.3×10^{-5}

Relapse of SDE

The course of the CNS disease after infection with ts-mutants
was highly variable. Many rats with clinical symptoms of SDE showed a
partial or complete remission. Among 43 rats with complete remission
9 rats developed a second attack of SDE 2-18 weeks after recovery
from the first attack (Table 4). These rats revealed hindleg paresis
and severe ataxic gait 14-33 days after virus inoculation. These
symptoms gradually disappeared, but returned with the second attack.
The neuropathological changes clearly indicated a chronic disease
process as documented in Fig. 1. In all animals fresh demyelinating
lesions with infiltrations of mononuclear cells were detectable in
pons, thalamus or spinal cord, and remyelination of axons by Schwann
cells (PNS-type) or oligodendroglia (CNS-type) was also observed.
The spinal cord section shown in Fig. 1 examplifies active demyelination (Fig. 1a and c), remyelination of the CNS-type (Fig. 1d) and
remyelination by Schwann cells (Fig. 1b, e). All rats investigated
revealed viral antigens in glia cells in and near to the demyelinating plaques and infectious virus could be isolated from brain tissue
or spinal cord.

TABLE 4   CORONAVIRUS JHM INDUCED RELAPSING OF SDE

CASE NO.	MUTANT INOCU- LATED*	RAT STRAIN	ONSET OF SYMPTOMS DAYS P.I.	DURATION OF SYMPTOMS DAYS	RELAPSE OF SDE DAYS P.I.
1	ts6	Thomae	14	9	70
2	ts6	Thomae	14	15	47
3	ts6	Lewis	14	8	41
4	ts42	Thomae	19	18	56
5	ts43	Thomae	21	23	71
6	ts43	Lewis	22	15	50
7	ts43	Lewis	33	22	95
8	ts43	Lewis	33	12	138
9	ts43	Thomae	20	25	173

* Rats were inoculated at an age of 10-15 days with 4×10^3 PFU of virus (i.c.)

Cell-mediated immune reactions against myelin basic protein

The observation of a chronic relapsing disease course after JHM infection of Lewis rats with lymphocyte infiltrations has certain similarities with experimental allergic encephalomyelitis (EAE). This disease results from sensation of animals with mixtures of basic myelin protein (BMP) or CNS-tissue extracts in combination with complete Freund's adjuvants (CFA). It is known that this massive immunisation leads to sensitisation of lymphocytes which are mainly responsible for the course of disease. Animals which recover from EAE are no longer susceptible to repeated sensations with CFA and BMP.

Fig. 1   Relapse of SDE 138 days p.i.

a)   Fresh demyelination in the anterior and lateral area of
     white matter (upper half) and remyelinating area in the
     dorsal column (arrow heads) of the spinal cord. The rat
     was perfused with buffered glutaraldehyde-paraformal-
     dehyde solution. Hematoxilin-eosin and luxol-fast blue
     stain, x76.

b)   Higher magnification (x312) of remyelinating area.
     Increased number of Schwann cells and darker staining
     (thin arrows) compared to CNS type myelin (thick arrow)
     indicated PNS-type remyelination.

c)   Naked axons (arrow heads) and macrophage infiltration
     (arrow) in fresh demyelination. 1 /um section from same
     area as a) embedded in epon and stained with toluidin
     blue, x662.

d)   Remyelination of the CNS type in same spinal cord. Note
     very thin myelin sheaths around many axons. Stained
     with toluidine blue, x800.

e)   Electron microscopy from same level as a) showing
     remyelination of the PNS type. Basement membrane and
     cytoplasm of Schwann cell around axon, x32000.

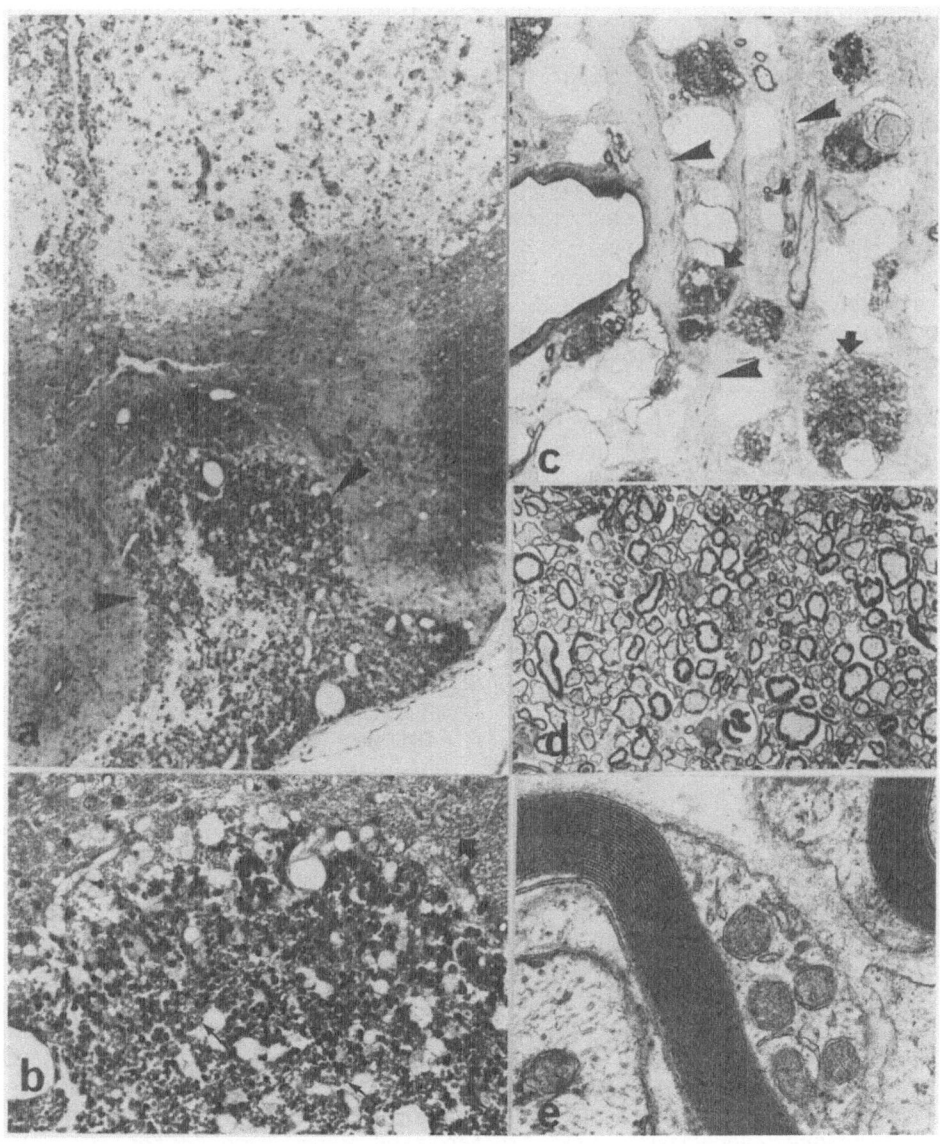

TABLE 5   SUSCEPTIBILITY TO EAE IN RATS RECOVERING FROM SDE

GROUP OF ANIMALS	INCUBATION TIME FOR EAE (DAYS)	CLINICAL SCORE AVERAGE
I CONTROL	11.7 + 1.2	4.7
II RECOVERED FROM SDE	12.8 + 2.2	1.6
III ACTIVELY SUPPRESSED (BMP/IFA)	11	0.5

The following experiments were performed to determine whether an immunopathological reaction could play a pathogenic role as shown for EAE during the course of SDE. Firstly, rats which recovered from SDE were challenged with BMP plus CFA. As shown in Table 5 normal rats developed a clinical EAE within 12 days, whereas SDE rats revealed a reduced susceptibility to BMP. A further control consisted of rats, which were repeatedly pretreated with BMP and incomplete Freund's adjuvants, a procedure which is known to result in suppression of susceptibility to induction of EAE. Rats from this group rarely developed EAE upon sensitation.

Secondly, we measured the stimulation of lymphocytes derived from SDE animals with BMP and JHM virus antigen (purified, inactivated virus). Lymphocytes were collected from spleen, thymus and peripheral blood and cultured with or without antigens (Table 6). The stimulation index was determined by incorporation of 3-H-thymidine. As can be seen in Table 6, lymphocytes from diseased rats were not only stimulated by virus antigen but also by BMP. Similar stimulation values were observed for lymphocytes derived from rats with EAE. No stimulation was found if histone, a protein with similar physicochemical properties as BMP, was used as antigen.

Thirdly, we transferred these BMP restimulated cells into healthy rats by intravenous inoculation. These lymphocytes induced slight clinical symptoms and perivascular cell infiltrations in the recipients within 5-10 days (Table 7). These perivascular infiltrations were located mainly in the dorsal area of the white matter of the spinal cord, the pons, the cerebellar white matter and thalamus. No extended demyelination was found near to the perivascular cuffs. These lesions are unlikely to be the result of transferred virus. No virus was detectable by immunohistology in transferred rats. Intravenous infection with high doses of JHM-virus or virus-lymphocyte mixtures did not lead to any CNS changes in recipients. Furthermore, no virus could be isolated from lymphocytes of rats with SDE. These experiments suggest that during JHM virus infection in Lewis rats a cellular immune response against neuroantigens develops which can influence the course of disease.

TABLE 6   STIMULATION OF LYMPHOCYTE CULTURES BY ANTIGENS*

GROUP OF RATS	ANTIGEN ADDED TO CULTURE MEDIUM		
(strain Lewis)	BASIC MYELIN PROTEIN	JHM VIRUS	HISTONE
SDE	x 4.3 + 2.7	x 6.6 + 4.8	x 1.0 + 0.1
Uninfected Controls	x 0.9 + 0.2	x 1.0 + 0.1	x 0.8

*Figures indicate the stimulation index measured by incorporation
of 3-H-thymidine relative to cultures without antigen. Lymphoid
cells from spleen, thymus and peripheral blood were cultured for
72 hours in microplates as described by Richert et al. (1979).
Before incubation, 1 µg/well of the required antigen was added.
After 48 hours, 1 µCi/well 3-H-thymidine was added and the
incorporated radioactivity was measured 24 hours later.

TABLE 7 ADOPTIVE TRANSFER OF LYMPH CELLS RESTIMULATED BY BMP*

SOURCE OF TRANSFERRED CELLS		EAE-LIKE LESIONS IN RECIPIENTS	
DONOR RATS (Lewis)	ANTIGEN	CLINICAL	HISTOLOGICAL
SDE	BMP	6/26	13/26
SDE	None	0/5	0/5
Control	BMP	0/8	0/8

*Lymphocytes from spleen, thymus and peripheral blood were cultured
for 3 days with or without antigen (Richert et al., 1979). 1x10^8
viable lymph cells were then inoculated intravenously into Lewis-
rats. Recipient rats without clinical symptoms were dissected about
10 days after transfer for histology.

COMMENTS

    The CNS disease processes observed in rats in the course of JHM
infections provide a model to study the pathogenic mechanisms which
are responsible for the different CNS changes. In particular, the
observation of lymphocyte stimulation by basic myelin protein in SDE
rats represents an interesting finding since generally brain damage
involving the release of myelin does not evoke an autoimmune response. Moreover, experimental studies have proven that EAE can only
be induced if brain antigen in combination with Freund's complete
adjuvants is given. Obviously, in SDE rats the viral infection of the

central nervous system substitutes for the Freund's complete adjuvants effect which is followed by a specific lymphocyte response against myelin basic protein.

It has been shown in JHM infections of mice and rats that the virus replicated preferentially in oligodendroglia cells (5,13). Replication in these cells may either lead to cell destruction resulting in an acute disease or to a persistent infection of glial cells. This infection could then result in an interference with cell functions followed by myelin breakdown. Cellular dysfunctions associated with persistent viral infections have been recently demonstrated in studies of neuronal cells ·in culture. It has been shown that interference with special neural cell functions such as a production of acetylcholine, acetyltransferase or acetylcholine esterase occurs in persistent virus infections with lymphocytic choriomeningitis, measles or rabies and do not always effect cell morphology, growth rate or protein synthesis (8,11,12,15). In the case of measles virus persistence in a neural cell line the presence of antiviral antibodies could overcome a specific virus-induced cellular defect (2). In C6 rat glioma cells, measles virus persistence interferes with β-adrenergic receptor stimulated cAMP synthesis. This function was restored when viral proteins were removed from the cell membrane by the action of antiviral antibodies. It is possible that immune responses could limit the damage caused by JHM virus infection of rats until a disease with clinical signs develops after a long incubation period. On the other hand the occurrence of lymphoid cells which are sensitized against basic myelin protein during the course of JHM-infection in rats suggests that viral replication in oligodendroglia cells triggers an autoimmune reaction. It is possible that either JHM virus structural proteins which are formed in CNS cells cross-react with myelin or the infection leads to changes of the oligodendroglia membrane. This may then result in the development of immunogenic structures which are also recognized on uninfected glia cells. Furthermore, infected oligodendroglia cells could release myelin material which is itself immunogenic.

At the present time none of these different mechanisms have been proven but the rat model allows us to analyze these suggested different pathogenic mechanisms. Moreover, further experiments may provide valuable information which could be of help in the study of human demyelinating disease processes associated with viral infections.

Acknowledgements. We thank Margarete Sturm, Renate Abt and Hanna Wege for excellent technical assistance and Helga Kriesinger for typing the manuscript. The work was supported by Deutsche Forschungsgemeinschaft and Humboldt-Stiftung.

REFERENCES

1) Bailey, O.T., Pappenheimer, A.M., Cheever, F.S. and Daniels,
    J.B. (1949). A murine virus (JHM) causing disseminated encepha-
    lomyelitis with extensive destruction of myelin. II. Pathology.
    Journal of Experimental Medicine 90, 195-212.

2) Barrett, P.N. and Koschel, K. (1983). Effect of antibody-induced
    modulation of measles (SSPE) virus membrane proteins on β-adre-
    nergic receptor-mediated adenylate cyclase activity. Virology
    127, in press.

3) Haspel, M.V., Lampert, P.W. and Oldstone, M.B.A. (1978). Tempe-
    rature-sensitive mutants of mouse hepatitis virus produce a high
    incidence of demyelination. Proceedings of the National Academy
    of Sciences USA 75, 4033-4036.

4) Herndon, R.M., Griffin, D.E., McCormick, U. and Weiner, L.P.,
    (1975). Mouse hepatitis virus-induced recurrent demyelination.
    Archives of Neurology 32, 32-35.

5) Knobler, R.L., Dubois-Dalcq, M., Haspel, M.V., Claysmith, A.P.,
    Lampert, P.W. and Oldstone, M.B.A. (1981). Selective localizat-
    ion of wild type and mutant mouse hepatitis virus (JHM strain)
    antigens in CNS tissue by fluorescence, light and electron mi-
    croscopy. Journal of Neuroimmunology 1, 81-92.

6) Knobler, R.L., Tunison, L.A., Lampert, P.W. and Oldstone, M.B.A.
    (1982). Selected mutants of mouse hepatitis virus type 4 (JHM
    strain) induce different CNS diseases. American Journal of Pa-
    thology 109, 157-168.

7) Lampert, P.W., Sims, J.K. and Kniazeff, A.J. (1973). Mechanism
    of demyelination in JHM virus encephalomyelitis. Electron micro-
    scopic studies. Acta Neuropathologica (Berlin) 24, 76-85.

8) Lunden, R., Vahlne, A. and Lycke, E. (1980). Measles virus in-
    fection of mouse neuroblastoma (C1300) cells. Proceedings of the
    Society of Experimental Biology and Medicine 165, 55-62.

9) McFarlin, D.E. and McFarland, H.F. (1982). Multiple Sclerosis.
    New England Journal of Medicine 307, 1246-1251.

10) ter Meulen, V., Kreth, H.W., Carter, M.J. (1982). Immunological
    aspects of slow virus infections of the nervous system. Clinics
    in Immunology and Allergy 2, 425-455.

11) Miller, C.A., Erlech, S. and Raine, C.S. (1981). Persistent measles virus infection of a clonal line of neuroblastoma: effect on neural differentiation. Life Sciences 29, 2473-2480.

12) Münzel, P. and Koschel, K. (1981). Rabies virus decreases agonist binding to opiate receptors of mouse neuroblastoma-rat glioma hybrid cells 108-CC-15. Biochemical and Biophysical Research Communications 101, 1241-1252.

13) Nagashima, K., Wege, H., Meyermann, R. and ter Meulen, V. (1978). Coronavirus induced subacute demyelinating encephalo myelitis in rats. A morphological analysis. Acta Neuropathologica 44, 63-70.

14) Nagashima, K., Wege, H., Meyermann, R. and ter Meulen, V. (1979). Demyelinating encephalomyelitis induced by a long-term coronavirus infection in rats. Acta Neuropathologica 45, 205-213.

15) Oldstone, M.B.A., Welsh, R.M. and Joseph, B.S. (1975). Pathogenic mechanisms of tissue injury in persistent viral infections. Annals of the New York Academy of Sciences 256, 65-72.

16) Richert, J.R., Driscoll, B.F., Kies, M.W. and Alvord, E.C. (1979). Adoptive transfer of experimental allergic encephalomyelitis: incubation of rat spleen cells with specific antigen. Journal of Immunology 122, 494-496.

17) Sörensen, O., Percy, D. and Dales, S. (1980). In vivo and in vitro models of demyelinating diseases. III. JHM virus infection of rats. Archives of Neurology 37, 478-484.

18) Stohlman, S.A. and Weiner, L.P. (1981). Chronic central nervous system demyelination in mice after JHMV virus infection. Neurology 31, 38-44.

19) Wege, H., Koga, M., Watanabe, R., Nagashima, K. and ter Meulen, V. (1983). Neurovirulence of murine coronavirus JHM temperature sensitive mutants in rats. Infection and Immunity 39, 1316-1324.

20) Weiner, L.P., Johnson, R.T. and Herndon, R.M. (1973). Pathogenesis of demyelination induced by a mouse hepatitis virus (JHM virus). Archives of Neurology, 28, 293-303.

21) Wisniewski, H. (1977). Immunopathology of demyelination in autoimmune diseases and virus infections. British Medical Bulletin 33, 54-59.

A ONE YEAR STUDY OF CORONAVIRUS SD INFECTION IN MICE

L.D. Jankovsky, J.S. Burks, P. Licari, B.L. Devald, and
M.C. Kemp

Center for Neurological Diseases/Rocky Mountain Multiple Sclerosis Center, Veterans Administration Medical Center, University of Colorado School of Medicine, Denver, Colorado, U.S.A.

INTRODUCTION

Coronavirus SD was isolated in mouse brain following intracerebral inoculation of autopsy brain material from a multiple sclerosis patient (1). This isolate is serologically related to the human coronavirus OC-43 and the murine coronavirus A59. It is antigenically distant from JHM, the prototype demyelinating strain of mouse hepatitis virus (2). As previously reported, intracerebral (IC) inoculation of SD into mice induces prominent demyelinating lesions in the spinal cord during the first 30 days post inoculation (PI) (3). This paper describes the pathogenesis of SD infection of mice through PI day 365.

Clinical Course of the Disease

Three hundred and eighty eight 3 to 4 week old, C57Bl/6J, specific pathogen free mice were inoculated IC with 10^4 plaque forming units of plaque purified SD produced in DBT cells (3). An additional 137 control animals received uninfected DBT cell extract in a similar manner. Evidence of central nervous system (CNS) involvement, including extreme hyperexcitability and/or hind limb paresis, was first observed between 4 and 9 days PI in 21.6% (84/388) of the infected mice. All mice were clinically normal at 30 days PI except for growth retardation in a few mice which had previous neurological signs.

271

Morbidity and impending mortality influenced selection of animals sacrificed for histopathology and virus studies in the initial study. Therefore, a second group of mice (80 infected, 10 control) were inoculated and evaluated to day 365 PI. Of these animals, 25% (20/80) exhibited neurologic signs in the first 8 days PI. Seven clinically ill mice died. Of the 13 remaining mice with neurological signs, 10 recovered by day 10 PI and 3 continued to exhibit signs. The 3 mice with neurologic signs were sacrificed on day 12. Five of the 10 recovered mice either died or experienced recurrent neurologic signs between day 52 and 146 PI. Six mice which had not demonstrated clinical signs early, developed neurological signs between day 109 and 290 PI. The remainding 35 mice had no neurologic signs at any time before being sacrificed at various points throughout the study.

Virus Studies

Infectious virus, by plaque assay, was recoverable up to PI day 6 from brain and spinal cord (3). Virus could be detected occasionally by cocultivation between PI days 7 and 12. Infectious virus was not detectable after day 12 PI by any method. Viral antigen was consistently demonstrated in CNS lesions by indirect immunofluorescence through day 10 and by autoradiography techniques (4) through day 30 PI.

Histopathology

Fixation and preparation of tissues for light and electron microscopy have previously been described (3). In the initial study 95% of the infected mice examined had histologic evidence of CNS involvement occurring during the first 30 days PI. In the first week an acute meningoencephalitis was noted. During the second, third and fourth weeks, well circumscribed demyelinated lesions of the spinal cord were the prominent histopathologic feature. Initially, the demyelinated lesions were small, subpial and devoid of inflammatory cells other than macrophages. Large demyelinated lesions extending over several vertebral segments were observed on PI day 12 (Fig. 1). Perivascular demyelination was associated with prominent lymphoid cuffs (lymphocytes, plasma cells and macrophages). Demyelination was not observed by light microscopy beyond PI day 30. However, by electron microscopy, myelin breakdown was observed in the spinal cord of two animals 90 days PI. Remyelinating activity was detected by day 12 PI and was prominent by day 20 PI. Thinly myelinated axons, with oligodendroglial cell cytoplasm interposed between myelin lamellae and axonal membranes, were numerous at the periphery of spinal cord lesions (Fig. 2).

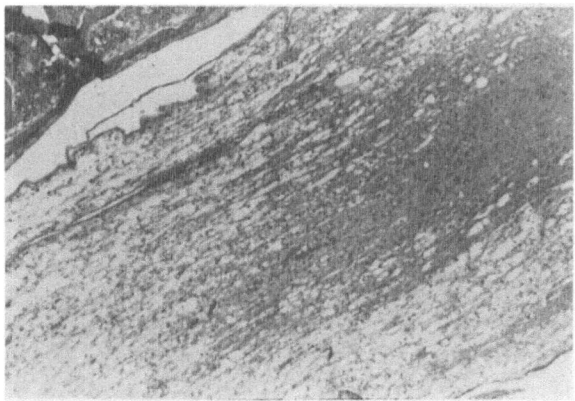

Figure 1: Diffuse Demyelination. In this longitudinal section of
mouse spinal cord on day 12 PI, diffuse demyelination extends over
several vertebral segments (light micrograph 40X).

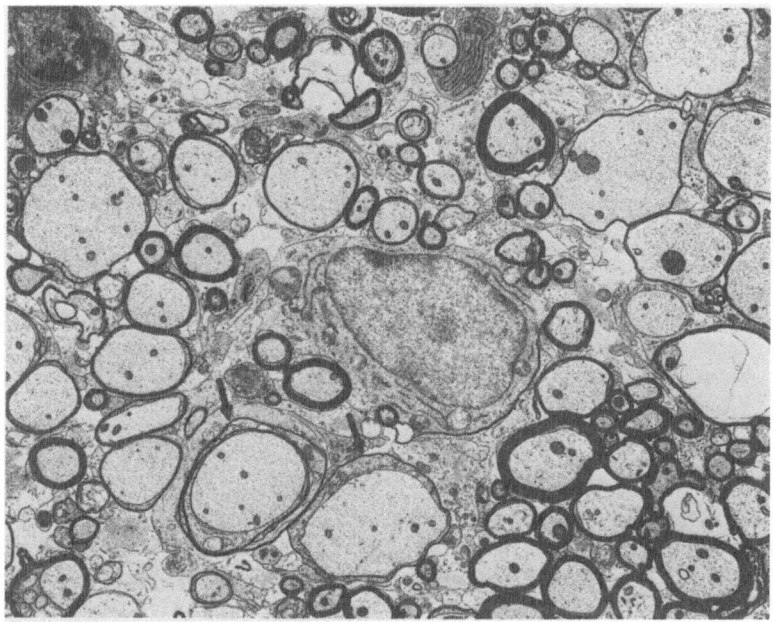

Figure 2: Remyelination. Several thinly myelinated axons surround
an oligodendroglial cell in the center of this cross section of
mouse spinal cord on day 20 PI. Dark staining oligodendroglial cytoplasm (arrows) is interposed between axonal membranes and myelin
lamellae (electron micrograph, 5600X).

Hydrocephalus was the major neuropathologic feature of SD infection beyond PI day 30 (Fig. 3). Temporal cortices of hydrocephalic mice exhibited a loss of neurons and an abundance of reactive atrocytes. Aqueductal stenosis was not observed in any animal. Of the 35 mice which had no neurologic signs throughout the course of this study, 8 (23%) were found to be hydrocephalic when examined histologically between days 164 and 335 PI. Of the 6 mice which had no neurologic signs early in the study but developed neurologic signs between day 109 and day 290 PI, all had hydrocephalus. Of the 5 mice which had early signs but remained clinically normal after day 10 PI, 2 (40%) had hydrocephalus. Of the 5 mice which had early signs and recovered and later developed a recurrence of neurological signs or were found dead in their cages, only one was examined and it had hydrocephalus.

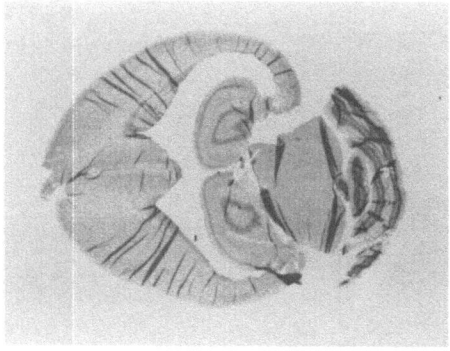

Figure 3: Hydrocephalus. In this horizontal section of mouse brain 109 days PI, temporal cortices are extremely thin and lateral ventrical are markedly dilated (light micrograph, 6.5X).

Immunoglobulin G was first detected in brain and spinal cord lesions by autoradiography (3) on PI day 6 and remained detectable in lesions for the first 30 days PI. The presence of IgG has not been evaluated beyond day 30 PI.

Comment

Virus induced demyelination may result directly from viral mediated cellular dysfunction/destruction or indirectly through an immunopathologic process (5). The mechanism of SD induced demyelination is unclear. An immunopathologic process is less likely since treatment with cyclophosphamide does not inhibit demyelination (6). Although infectious virus could only be recovered for the first six days PI, viral antigen persisted and corresponded with the period of active demyelination in the first 30 days PI. Therefore, viral antigenic expression correlated with demyelination, but production of infectious virus did not.

Hydrocephalus was prominent after 30 days PI in all mice with clinical signs and 23% of mice which never developed clinical signs. Virus induced hydrocephalus has been reported following obstruction of the aqueduct of Sylvius (7), as a compensatory change secondary to destructive lesions in the cerebral hemispheres and as a function of insufficient reabsorption of the cerebrospinal fluid. Residual destructive changes in temporal cortices and the absence of aqueductal stenosis suggests SD induced hydrocephalus is of a compensatory nature. Late clinical signs associated with hydrocephalus may indicate continuing or intermittent tissue destruction.

Are the mechanisms of demyelination in this SD infection in mice similar or different from demyelination seen in multiple sclerosis? Similarities include: 1) A biphasic disease occurs in some SD infected animals, and a relapsing/remitting course is seen in most MS patients; 2) Axons are spared in a fulminant demyelinating process in both; 3) Lesions are commonly located along surfaces or perivascular areas in both; 4) Prominent lymphocytic perivascular inflammation is noted at certain stages in both; 5) IgG is present in the demyelinating lesions in both and 6) Remyelination occurs at the periphery of the demyelinated lesions in both.

Significant differences between SD infection in mice and MS include: 1) Obvious clinical signs are absent in SD infection in mice during the period of active demyelination between PI days 10 and 30; 2) There is a paucity of demyelinating lesions after PI day 30 in SD infected mice; 3) MS is not known to be associated with an encephalitis preceeding demyelination as is observed in SD infection, and 4) some SD infected mice develop marked hydrocephalus.

The relationship between coronavirus SD and multiple sclerosis is uncertain and will remain uncertain until MS brain tissue and control tissue are evaluated for the presence or absence of SD viral genome.

REFERENCES:

1. Burks, J.S., B.L. DeVald, L.D. Jankovsky, J.C. Gerdes, 1980. Two Coronaviruses Isolated from Central Nervous System Tissue of Two Multiple Sclerosis Patients. Science. 209:933-934.
2. Gerdes, J.C., I. Klein, B.L. DeVald, J.S. Burks, 1981. Coronavirus Isolates SK and SD from Multiple Sclerosis Patients Are Serologically Related to Murine Coronavirus A59 and JHM and Human Coronavirus OC-43, but not to Human Coronavirus 229E. J. Virol. 38:231-238.
3. Mendelman, P.M., L.D. Jankovsky, R.S. Murray, P. Licari, B.

DeVald, J.C. Gerdes, J.S. Burks, 1983. Pathogenesis of Coronavirus SD in Mice I. Prominent Demyelination in the Absence
of Infectious Virus Production. Arch. of Neurol.

4.   J.C. Gerdes, I. McNally, L. Hileman, J.S. Burks, 1982. Autoradiographic Detection of IgG and Viral Antigens. J. Immunol.
Meth. 54:191-202.

5.   Weiner, L.P., S.A. Stohlman, 1978. Viral Models of Demyelination. Neurology 28:111-114.

6.   J.S. Burks, L. Jankovsky, I.T. McNally, M.C. Kemp. 1983. Im-
munosuppression with Cyclophosphamide Does Not Prevent
Demyelination or Result in Uncontrolled Viral Replication in
Coronavirus SD Infected Mice. 1983. See these proceedings.

7.   Johnson, R.T., K.P. Johnson, C. Jill Edmonds, 1967. Virus
Induced Hydrocephalus: Development of Aqueductal Stenosis
After Mumps Infection. Science. 157:1066-1067

This study was supported by grants from the Veterans
Administration and the Kroc Foundation. We thank Karon Keys for
her patience and typing in preparation of this manuscript.

IMMUNOSUPPRESSION WITH CYCLOPHOSPHAMIDE DOES NOT PREVENT DEMYELINATION OR RESULT IN UNCONTROLLED VIRAL REPLICATION IN CORONAVIRUS SD INFECTED MICE

J.S. Burks, L. Jankovsky, P.A. Licari,
I.T. McNally and M.C. Kemp

Center for Neurological Diseases/Rocky Mountain Multiple
Sclerosis Center, University of Colorado School of
Medicine, Veterans Administration Medical Center
Denver, Colorado, U.S.A.

Coronavirus SD following intracerebral inoculation has been shown to precipitate demyelination in the brains and spinal cords of weanling mice (1). Demyelination occurs at a time when virus cannot be isolated and some areas of demyelination are associated with a perivascular inflammatory response. Also, IgG is present in demyelinated areas. Since demyelination may be immunologically mediated, this study evaluates the effect of immunosuppression with cyclophosphamide (CY) on demyelination and viral replication.

Coronavirus SD was inoculated intracerebrally into 3 – 4 week old C57Bl/6J mice at 10^4pfu/.03ml. Half of the mice were immuno-suppressed with CY (200mg/kg) at day 1, 5, 9, 13, and 17 post-inoculation (PI). Mice were sacrificed at days 5, 12, and 20 PI.

With the non-immunosuppressed mice, 27% exhibited neuro-logical signs on days 4 through 7, with 100% recovery by day 8. Of the immunosuppressed mice, 90% exhibited no clinical signs on days 4 through 12 with a mortality rate of 27%.

The mice treated with CY had no serum antibody to coronavirus SD by an EIA assay, while the non-treated mice had a mean titer of 1:2560 on days 12 and 20 PI. Spleens and thymuses of CY treated animals were markedly reduced in size. Histologically, thymic cortices were hypocellular and splenic white pulp was depleted.

Virus concentrations in brain, determined by a plaque assay, reached a maximum of 10^4 pfu/ml and 10^5 pfu/ml in CY treated and untreated mice, respectively, at day 5 PI. By day 12 PI, virus

277

could not be isolated from mice in either group. The mechanism(s) by which SD was eliminated from the mice by day 12 PI in the CY treated mice is unknown. Viral antigen was detected by auto-radiography in the brain and spinal cord at days 12 and 20 PI in both groups. Bound IgG, which was abundant in demyelinated areas of non-immunosuppressed mice, was absent in CY treated mice.

Coronavirus SD induced demyelination was not prevented by CY treatment. Small focal subpial and large deep perivascular demyelinating lesions were produced in both groups. Although macrophage infiltration remained, perivascular lymphocyte accumulations were not present in the CY treated mice (Fig. 1).

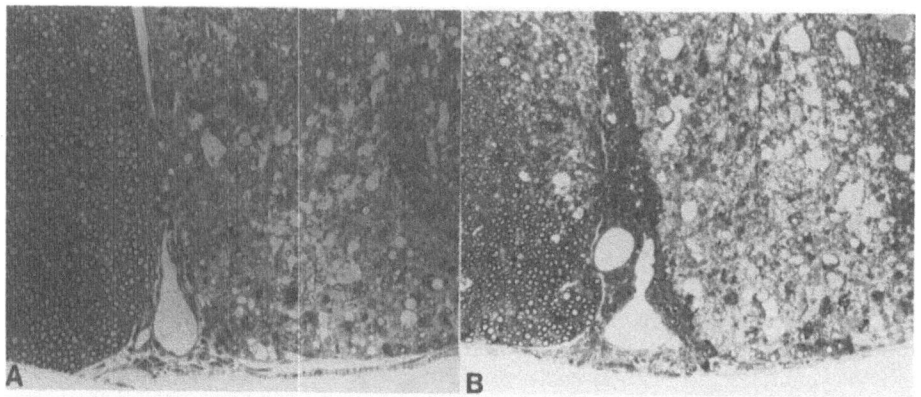

Fig. 1: Demyelinated lesions in the spinal cord of SD infected mice were similar in size and location in CY treated (A) and untreated mice (B). However, CY treatment prevented the peri-vascular accumulation of lymphocytes and plasma cells commonly seen in demyelinating lesions; 640 X.

REFERENCES

1.   Mendleman, P.M., L.D. Jankovsky, R.S. Murray, P. Licari, B.L. DeVald, J.C. Gerdes & J.S. Burks, 1983. Pathogenesis of Coronavirus SD in Mice. I Prominent Demyelination in the Absence of Infectious Virus Production. Arch. Neurol. In Press.
2.   Gerdes, J.C., I. McNally, L. Hileman, J.S. Burks, 1982. Autoradiographic Detection of IgG and Viral Antigens. J. Immunol. Meth. 54:191-202.

This work was supported by the Kroc Foundation and the Veterans Administration.

IN VIVO AND IN VITRO MODELS OF DEMYELINATING DISEASES - VIII: GENETIC, IMMUNOLOGIC AND CELLULAR INFLUENCES ON JHM VIRUS INFECTION OF RATS

O. Sorensen, S. Beushausen, S. Puchalski, S. Cheley, R. Anderson, M. Coulter-Mackie and S. Dales

Department of Microbiology and Immunology
University of Western Ontarie
London, Ontario, Canada, N6A 5C1

Introduction

A number of mouse hepatitis viruses, including MHV-A59, MHV-3, and JHM, have been used as in vivo models of neurotropic viral infections (Hirano et al., 1980; Knobler et al., 1981; Lampert et al., 1973; Le Prevost et al., 1975). The majority of experiments with these agents have involved mice as the host, a system which may be complicated by the viscerotropism of some of these coronaviruses. Previous work in our laboratory (Sorensen et al., 1980, 1982) and by others (Nagashima et al., 1978, 1979; Hirano et al., 1980) demonstrated that rats injected intracerebrally (IC) with JHM virus (JHMV) offer a challenging model for studies of neurotropic agents interacting with the central nervous system (CNS). The presence of anti-coronavirus antibodies in a high proportion of the human population (MacNaughton, 1982) give these models added relevance in regard to enquiries into the viral etiology of human diseases of the central nervous system (CNS), among them multiple sclerosis.

Age-related Genetic Resistance of Rats to CNS Disease

Our studies revealed that rat strains can be classified as either "sensitive" or "resistant" to an IC inoculation of JHMV (Sorensen et al., 1980, 1982). In our experience, the inbred Wistar Furth (WF) strain (obtained from Microbiological Associates, Bethesda, Maryland and Harlan Sprague Dawley, Walkersville, Maryland) is more sensitive at 5 to 21 days of age than the Wistar Lewis (WL) rat (obtained from Charles River Canada Inc., St.-Constant, Quebec). The WL strain used in these experiments was highly susceptible to experimental allergic encephalomyetitis (unpublished data). In a comparable study Nagashima et

279

al., (1979) were able to infect weanling Chbb.THOM rats with JHMV
suggesting that these and WF rats may be equally sensitive.
Eventually, at >21 days of age, the WF strain becomes completely
resistant. With WF rats inoculated at 2 days of age the mortality
rate is over 90% and remains quite high at 5 days of age and
beyond (Table 1, Sorensen et al., 1980, 1982). In contrast, when
WL rats are inoculated at 2 days of age their mortality rate is
only about 50%. By 5 days only about 10% of WL rats are killed by
the injection and by 10 days the mortality rate declines further
(Table 1). The increased resistance is, however, accompanied by a
shift in neurologic disease, from an acute encephalomyelitis,
involving primarily the grey matter of the cerebrum, to a
demyelinating disease characterized by lesions confined to the
myelinated tracts of the rhombencephalon and spinal cord.

Table 1 - AGE AND STRAIN DEPENDENT SUSCEPTIBILITY OF INBRED RATS
            TO PARALYSIS AND DEATH FOLLOWING INTRACEREBRAL
                      INOCULATION WITH JHMV

Strain	Age at Inoculation (days)	Number Paralyzed/no. dead at post-inoculation days[a]				No. Inoculated
		1-7	8-14	15-21	>21	
WL	10	0	0	1/1	0	12
	15	0	0	0	0	17
	21	0	0	0	0	14
	30	0	0	0	0	15
WF	10	0	6/8	9/9	5/5	33
	15	0	0	3/3	2/2	14
	21	0	0	1/1	0	8
	30	0	0	0	0	18
WF (immuno-suppressed)	5				6/6[b]	9

a - Rats which died or were killed in extremis.
b - 2 rats recovered from paralysis and are not included in this
    column

The heritable control of the development of resistance to the disease was analyzed in the F_1 and F_2 generations of (WF x WL) and among the (F_1 x WF) and F_1 x WL) backcrosses. In all cases the animals were challenged IC with JHMV at 10 days of age. The results of these breeding experiments are summerized in Figure 1. Along with the experimental data are the predicted (p) values calculated from a genetic model which assumes that (a) a single gene controls the resistance trait and (b) in the WF strain the

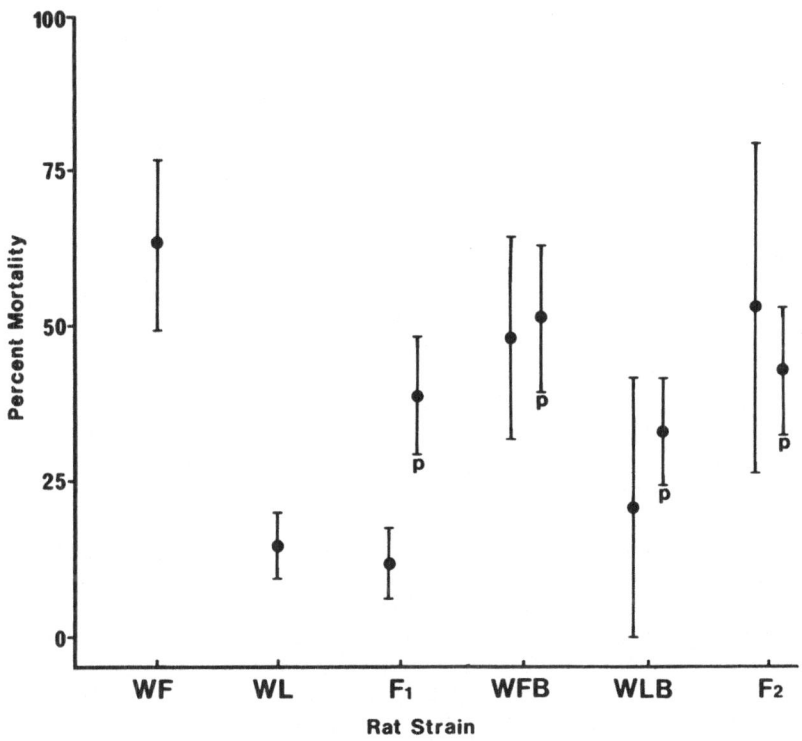

Fig. 1 - The average percent mortalities (with standard errors) of 10 day old WF or WL rats and various cross matings of these strains following intracerebral inoculation with JHMV. Bars desginated "p" indicate values predicted on the assumption that a single gene controls the acquisition of resistance and WF rats were homozygous recessive (rr) and the WL strain was heterozygous (RR,Rr,rr).

WF - Wistar Furth   WL - Wistar Lewis
F_1 - WF x WL F_2 - F_1 x F_1
WFB - F_1 x WF (Wistar Furth Backcross)
WLB - F_1 x WL (Wistar Lewis Backcross)

gene behaves as a homozygous recessive (rr) while in WL rats it is present in the heterozygous form i.e. RR, Rr, or rr. Generally, the observed values fit reasonably well with those predicted by this model. Only the F_1 generation appeared to be more resistant than predicted (Fig. 1). Although the reason for departure from the predicted value is unknown it is conceivable that among the relatively few WL rats which were bred to produce the F_1 generation, those of the RR genotype predominated. The model, furthermore, presumes an equal representation of homozygous and heterozygous genotypes, an assumption which may not reflect accurately the genetic makeup of the general population or of those individual WL rats selected to produce the F_1 hybrids. These findings suggest that, in the rat, susceptibility to CNS disease provoked by JHMV is under genetic control.

Humoral and Intracerebral Antibody Responses.
     A survey of serum JHMV-neutralizing antibody titers indicated that, upon a single IC or intraperitoneal (IP) injection of JHMV or MHV-3, the neutralizing antibody in the serum was not significantly different from that present in uninoculated controls (Sorensen et al., 1982). The low titers, usually <1:10, of endogenous antibodies were most probably the consequence of an endemic infection with SDA or Parker's rat coronavirus, agents possessing some serologic cross-reactivity with members of the mouse hepatitis group (Robb and Bond, 1979). A single injection might be expected to function as a booster to an endogenous coronavirus response. However, inoculation of small amounts of antigen, only 10^4-10^5 pfu/animal and absence of replication outside the CNS may explain the lack of a secondary-type increase in serum antibody titers. Furthermore, the injections were made at about the age when an initial exposure to the endemic agents would be expected to occur.

     To determine whether virus introduced IC could elicit localized production of antibody, the cerebrospinal fluids (CSF) of control and infected rats were analyzed for the presence of anti-JHMV IgG. All CSF samples were checked for the presence of erythrocytes and those CSF's contaminated with blood were discarded. The data from radioimmune assays (RIA), summarized in Table 2, revealed that when symptoms of the acute or chronic virus-induced disease were evident, an accompanying 300-600 fold increase in anti-JHMV IgG CSF:serum ratio occurred, implying local production within the CNS (Schliep and Felgenhauer, 1978; Fleming et al., 1983). Among injected rats without clinical or histological indications of disease, including all animals examined after IC inoculation with MHV-3 and some inoculated IC with JHMV, increases in CSF anti-JHMV IgG concentrations were small (Table 2) when compared with control rats inoculated IP with JHMV. Thus, CSF antibody appeared to be formed only in those animals in which JHMV-induced disease occurs, presumably

contingentupon, and associated with, viral replication in the CNS.
Nevertheless, localized production of I_gG in the CNS was unable to
protect rats from either the acute or chronic neurologic disease
     The RIA method employed here detected all subclasses of IgG
reactive against all JHMV antigens. Thus, those antibodies
relevant to neutralization probably comprised only a fraction of
the total IgG detected. The levels reported here for CSF IgG are
comparable to those reported for other viral infections of the CNS
(Schliep and Felgenhauer, 1978; Martin et al., 1982). By

Table 2 - Anti-JHMV I_gG Concentrations in Cerbrospinal
Fluid (CSF) and Serum of Rats after Virus Inoculation

Virus and Inoculation Route	Mean Concentration of Anti-JHMV IgG (ug/ml)		Ratio $\frac{CSF}{Serum}$ X 100
	Serum	CSF	
Controls JHMV 1P No Disease[1] (21 dpi)	1370.0 ± 383.8[2]	0.019 ± 0.016	0.003 ± 0.002
MHV_3 IC No Disease (7-21 dpi)	2225.7 ± 940.6	0.30 ± 0.20	0.032 ± 0.028
JHMV IC No Disease (7-40 dpi)	2384.3 ± 766.0	1.60 ± 0.70	0.071 ± 0.017
JHMV IC Acute Disease (<15 dpi)	3018.0 ± 1235.1	50.5 ± 24.2	1.97 ± 0.89
JHMV IC Chronic Disease (>21 dpi)	1408.3 ± 588.7	6.1 ± 1.7	1.11 ± 0.35

1- No disease judged by lack of clinical and histological
   indications
2- Standard error of the mean.

contrast, serum antibody levels were much lower than those
prevailing during the infection of sheep CNS by the neurotropic
Visna virus (Martin et al., 1982).

The latency of JHMV in the CNS of some asymptomatic rats has
been demonstrated following abrogation of the immune response by
immunosuppression with cyclophosphamide (Sorensen et al., 1982).
Thus, when 9 WF rats were immunosuppressed 28 days after IC
inoculation with JHMV, 8/9 animals developed clinical signs of
disease and infectious virus could be isolated (Sorensen et al.,
1982). Immunosuppression, however, was unable to negate the
genetically controlled age-related resistance of WL rats, when
placed on the immunosuppressive regimen either 7 days prior to or
at the time of virus injection at 17 days of age. These
observations are consistent with those on mice, which reveal that
cell-mediated immunity is of paramount importance in the
development of resistance to infections by mouse hepatitis viruses
(Sorensen et al., 1982).

Histopathology
Our previous work, based on electron microscopic examination,
suggested that in the more prolonged demyelinating disease, viral
infection was confined to the glia (Sorensen et al., 1980).
However, analysis of viral antigen distribution by indirect
immunofluorescent microscopy has demonstrated that cells with the
morphology of neurons, contain viral antigen (Fig. 2b).
Similarily, Knobler et al., (1980) showed that the neuron was an
essential target cell for JHMV infection of SJL mice, a strain
shown to have an age-dependent resistance to IC JHMV inoculation.
The neuron may also be the initial target or a repository for JHMV
during the CNS disease process in rats.

Antigen-containing cells were usually not present in areas
with lesions, identified in hematoxylin and eosin (H & E) stained
sections (Fig. 2a,3a). Immunofluorescent microscopy revealed that
cells with viral antigen were distributed in tissue of relatively
normal appearance (Fig. 2a) or adjacent to a lesion (Fig. 3b).
Electron microscopic surveys, described previously (Sorensen et
al., 1980), were likewise unsuccessful in demonstrating virus
particles within lesion areas identified in 1 µm toluidine blue
stained sections, but were successful in locating coronavirus
particles in cells of adjacent apparently normal tissue.

The current observations imply that JHMV can persist and
replicate within neurons and perhaps oligodendrocytes of the CNS
without causing rapid death of the cell or eliciting an immune
reaction leading to tissue necrosis and possible suppression of
the infection. The absence of antigen-positive cells within areas
of necrosis implies that virus infection may occur at a time
preceeding the development of lesions. It is also conceivable
that the demyelination evident in the chronic disease is the

consequence of oligodendrocyte killing by the host's immunologic
response rather than cellular dysfunction and death provoked
directly by the virus.

Detection of Virus-Related RNA
        Detection of antigen-positive cells in the CNS enabled us to
pinpoint cells expressing viral protein(s) but provided no data
concerning cells which may be latently infected without antigen
expression. To examine latency, CNS tissues were surveyed
employing a cDNA probe against the murine coronaviruses. The
probe was prepared against the smallest mRNA (RNA-A) of MHV-A59
because this molecular species possesses a high degree of homology
with JHMV mRNA A. This mRNA species is homologous with the 3' end
of all 7 mRNA species found in murine coronavirus infected cells
(Cheley et al., 1981a). The isolated and purified mRNA was copied
by reverse transcription into cDNA with ^{32}P-dCTP as described

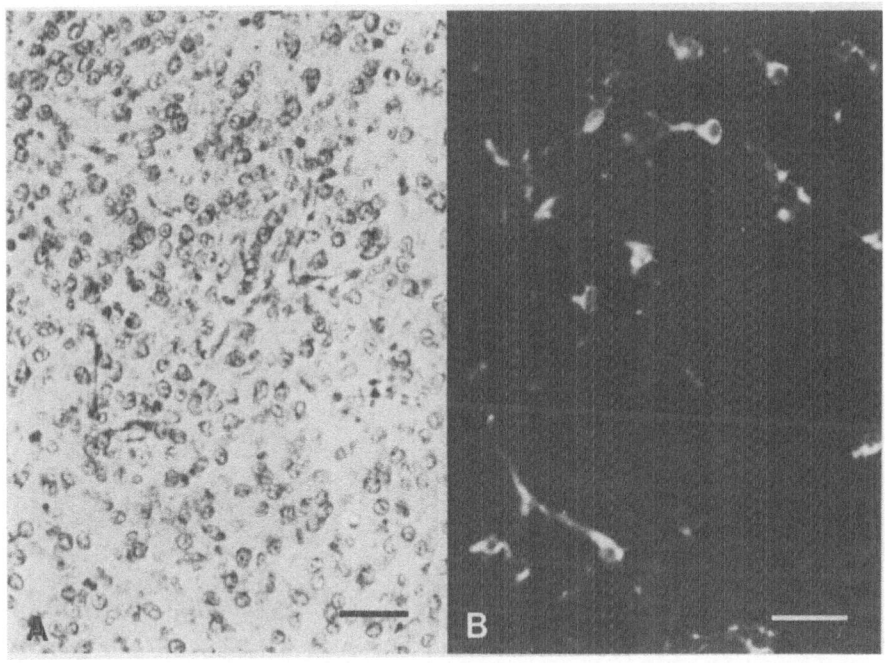

Fig. 2 - A sagittal section through the cerebrum of a 6 day old
rat 4 days after IC inoculation with JHMV. H & E staining (a)
reveals an apparently normal area of grey matter. However,
indirect immunofluorescence staining for JHMV antigens (b) reveals
a number of cells, probably neurons, containing viral antigens.
Bar - 25 μm.

previously by Cheley$_8$et al., (1981b). The product had a specific
activity of about 10^8 cpm/µg DNA and was deemed to be adequate for
detecting subpicogram quantities of RNA by the dot-blotting
procedure.

Animals killed for conducting dot-blot hybridizations on CNS
tissues were anesthetized, then dissected to expose and remove the
CNS. Selected regions of tissue from half the CNS were cut into
samples and snapfrozen. Included were the telencephalon,
diencephalon and mesencephalon, cerebellum, pons and
myelencephalon, cervical spinal cord, lumbar spinal cord, and
whenever possible, the optic nerves. The contralateral half of
the CNS was fixed and prepared for histological and
immunofluorescent microscopy. RNA extracts from the CNS were

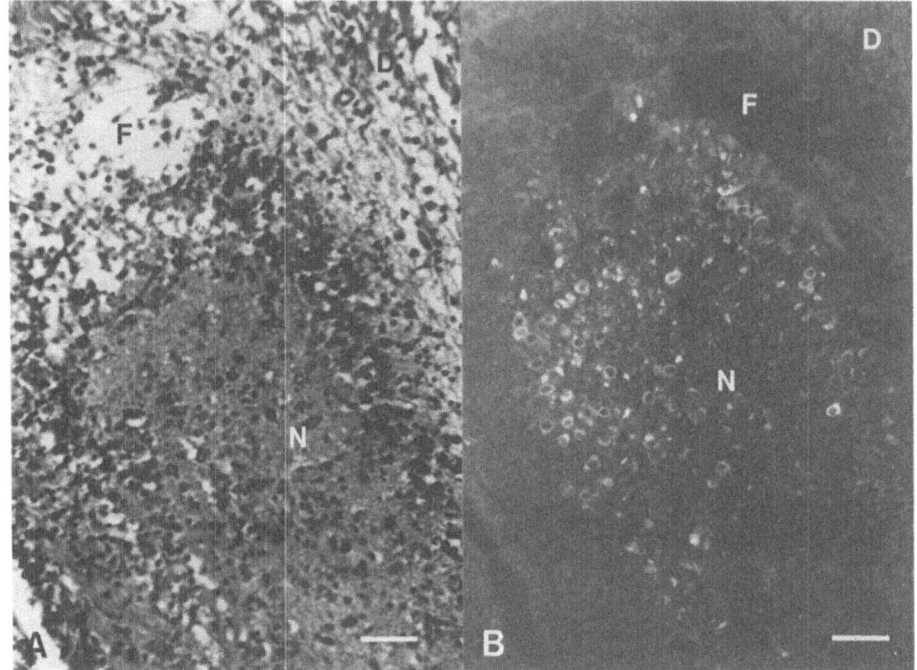

Figure 3

Fig. 3 - A sagittal section showing the hippocampus of a 6 day old
rat 4 days after ic inoculation with JHMV. H & E staining (a)
reveals a focus of necrosis (F) as well as considerable demyelination (D) while unaffected tissue is seen at N. Indirect immunofluorescent staining for JHMV antigens of an adjacent section (b)
reveals presence of a large numer of infected cells in the apparently normal tissue. Note also that the necrotic (F) and demy-
linated (D) areas are devoid of cells containing JHMV antigens.
Bar - 25 µm.

obtained by a modification of the method previously reported
(Cheley et al., 1981a). Briefly, frozen tissues were defrosted in
7.6M guanidine-HCl, 0.1M potassium acetate, pH 7.5, to give a
final concentration of 100 mg or less tissue/ml. The tissue was
disrupted by forcing it several times through a 21g needle at
-20°C. The homogenate was then mixed with 0.6 volumes of 95%
ethanol, allowed to stand overnight at -20°C, then centrifuged at
5800xg for 20 min. The resultant pellet was dissolved in 1.5 ml
20 mM EDTA, pH 7.0, and extracted with 4.5 ml chloroform/butanol
(4:1 v/v). The solvent phase was re-extracted twice more and the
3 aqueous extracts were pooled, made 3M with respect to sodium
acetate, pH 6.0, and allowed to stand overnight at -20°C. The
suspension was centrifuged at 1,800xg for 1 hour and the RNA
pellet was washed with 95% ethanol and dried at -20°C. The dry
RNA pellet was then dissolved in 150 µl water, 100 µl formalin and
250 µl of 20 x SSC (300 mM sodium chloride, 30 mM sodium acetate,
pH 7.6), heated at 50°C for 15 min and stored at -70°C. For RNA-
cDNA hybridization, samples were applied undiluted or at dilutions
of 0.5, 0.25, or 0.1 to cellulose acetate then hybridized under
stringent conditions.

    In general, RNA samples from uninoculated control rats failed
to specifically bind the ^{32}P-cDNA. Each extract applied at the
cited dilutions was examined for the intensity and size of the dot
produced by autoradiography. The data were deemed valid only when
an appropriate dose response was obtained, judged by gradation in
the size and intensity of dots. The wet weight of tissue in the
original sample extracted for RNA in these analyses ranged from
about 5 mgm of spinal cord or optic nerves to 50 mgm of
telencephalon.

    Previous examinations of CNS from diseased rats (Sorensen et
al., 1980, 1982) revealed that histopathological lesions
frequently had a bilateral distribution although usually not at
identical positions in the CNS. Thus, we believe that the
histopathology on one hemisphere of the CNS and the detection of
viral RNA from the contralateral side provided a valid comparison
of these two parameters of the infectious process. The selected
examples of dot-blotting data, shown in Figure 4, illustrate the
results achieved from uninoculated rats, animals with acute
encephalomyelitis, or those in which a chronic, prolonged,
demyelinating disease prevailed. Although the data are not shown
in this figure, extracts of spinal cord from the animal with acute
encephalomyelitis were also positive. It appears that during
acute encephalomyelitis JHMV RNA can be detected throughout the
CNS, perhaps with the exception of the cerebellum. By contrast,
during chronic demyelinating disease viral RNA is present
predominantly in the posterior portions of the brain and in the
spinal cord (Fig. 4). With respect to the concordance between the
presence of viral RNA (determined by dot-blots) and
histopathology, ascertained on the opposite side of the brain,

Figure 5 illustrates that correlation could not always be
demonstrated. In the selected example of an animal with acute
encephalomyelitis there was no agreement between the presence of
JHMV RNA and the histopathology observed in the telencephalon,
cerebellum or spinal cord. In another rat, with chronic
demyelinating disease, no correlation could be demonstrated in the
diencephalon or mesencephalon. It should, however, be emphasized
that the lack of concordance might be due to the limitation on the
number of sections selected for histopathological evaluation.

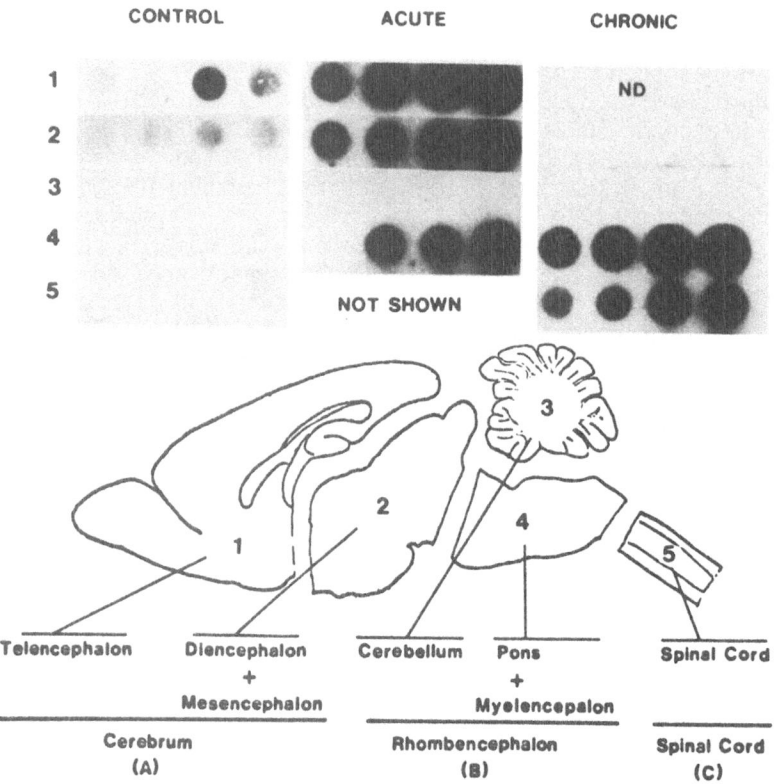

Fig. 4 - Autoradiograms of dot-blot cDNA hybridizations with
extracts of the 5 tissues from rat brain identified in the
diagram. Representative blots are presented from an uninoculated
control animal, a rat suffering an acute encephalomyelitis and an
animal with a chronic demyelinating disease. The 4 dots represent
1/10, 1/5, 1/2 and undiluted samples of each extract. The spinal
cord of the animal with acute encephalomyelitis (not shown) was
also JHMV RNA positive.
ND - not determined.

More likely, it is due to an absence of viral antigens in necrotic
lesions and the presence of viral proteins in cells located within
tissues with a histologically normal appearance, as documented by
immunofluorescent microscopy. It was, therefore, not surprising
to encounter acutely or chronically affected animals, like those
exemplified in Figure 5, in which regions such as the
diencephalon, mesencephalon, and the cerebella were negative for
JHMV RNA but positive in histopathological analysis. Conversely,
in areas with a histologically normal appearance, such as the
telencephalon of the acutely affected rat, viral RNA was found.
Similarily, the presence of JHMV RNA in the histologically normal
cervical spinal cord of a rat with acute encephalomyelitis implies
that virus infection may precede the development of lesions.

Our previous work revealed that there are profound time-
related changes in the distribution of grey and white matter
lesions in the CNS due to JHMV infection (Sorensen et al., 1980).
The current survey, using JHMV specific cDNA in the dot-blotting

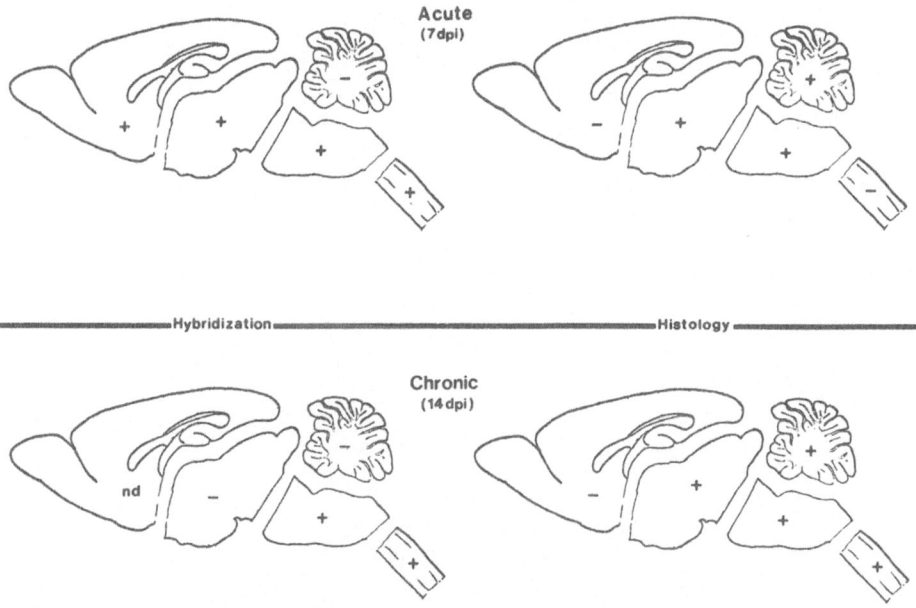

Fig. 5 - A comparison of results from cDNA hybridizations on
tissue extracts prepared from half the rat brain with histological
examination of the contralateral hemisphere. In hybridization "+"
indicates a positive series of dot-blots. In the histology a "+"
indicates the presence of lesion(s), identified in of H & E
stained sections.
ND - not determined.

hybridization analysis revealed that 7 to 17 days post-inoculation the CNS of animals succumbing to JHMV infection contained virus specific RNA in regions where neuropathology was not evident (Fig. 6) also suggesting that the infection precedes lesion formation.

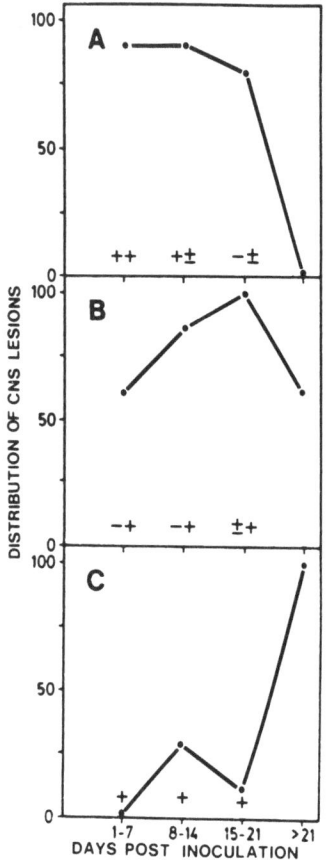

Fig. 6 - Concordance between presence (+) or absence (-) of JHMV RNA and the distribution of histological lesions (the percent of the animals examined with lesion(s) in a particular region of the CNS) plotted as a function of the number of days after IC inoculation.
Panel A - Cerebrum (telencephalon, diencephalon and mesencephalon)
Panel B - Rhombencephalon (Cerebellum, Pons and Myelencephalon)
Panel C - Spinal cord.

JHMV and MHV-3 Infection of Dissociated CNS Cultures

Despite considerable progress with regard to the factors important to coronavirus-induced disease in rats (Bailey et al., 1949; Nagashima et al., 1978, 1979; Hirano et al., 1980; Sorensen et al., 1980, 1982), little is known about the initial cell-virus interactions that occur following IC inoculation, nor how these events might regulate the resulting neurologic disease. Electron microscopic studies of JHMV infected CNS tissues have demonstrated the presence of virus particles in oligodendrocytes and neurons during chronic demyelinating disease (Nagashima et al., 1978; Sorensen et al., 1980) and in astrocytes during acute encephalomyelitis in rats (Nagashima et al., 1978). The nature of the initial tropism of JHMV for particular cells in the CNS, however, remains to be elucidated. To examine these early cell-

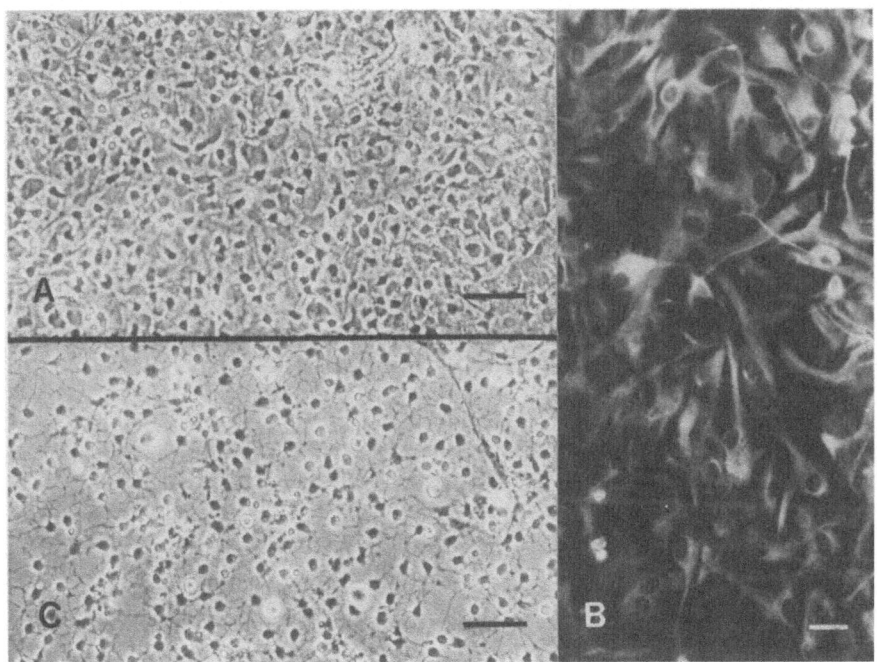

Figure 7

Fig. 7 - The appearance of a 10 day old primary dissociated CNS culture prepared from neomatal rats. A stratified mixed culture (a) consisting of a lower layer of adherent astrocytes and less adherent cells forming a superficial layer. Adherent astrocyte layer (b) stained, by the indirect method, with anti-GFAP anti-bodies. A shaken culture (c) established by plating less asherent cells removed from the mixed culture. Note the presence of fluorescing intracellular intermediate filamentous structures. Bar - 25 μm virus interactions under controlled and defined conditions, dissociated primary CNS cultures were prepared from the cerebral corticies of neonatal rats by a modified procedure of McCarthy and de Vellis (1978), using a mechanical dissociation of tissue by serial passages through pipettes of decreasing bore diameter. The cell suspensions, containing astrocytes, oligodendrocytes and neurons, were seeded onto plastic tissue culture dishes and incubated at 37°C.

Such mixed cultures (Fig. 7a) when examined microscopically were observed to contain a layer of adherent cells identified as astrocytes, by presence of glial fibrillary acidic protein (GFAP)in them as revealed by immunofluorescent microscopy (Fig. 7b), and a superficial layer of less adherent cells presumed, on morphological criteria, to be neurons and oligodendrocytes (Bhatt et al., 1980). The less adherent superficial cells could be removed by shaking (McCarthy and de Vellis 1981) so as to produce two types of cultures, one of the adherent cells, enriched in astrocytes (Fig. 7b) and the other consisting of cells from the superficial layer, enriched in oligodendrocytes and neurons but devoid of astrocytes (Fig. 7c).

Since IC inoculation of very young rats with JHMV elicits neurological disease but a similar inoculation with MHV-3, even into the newborns, fails to do so (Hirano et al., 1980; Sorenson et al., 1981, 1982), it was surprizing to discover that in the mixed cultures MHV-3 could replicate at 32.5°C to high titers (Table 3, Fig. 8) and cause cytopathic effects (CPE) among the adherent astrocytic layer. This CPE was characterized by the formation of syncytia similar to those described for L cells and cells of neural origin (Lucas et al., 1977). MHV-3 replication was arrested when infected cultures were shifted to 39.5°C but resumed upon shift-down to 32.5°C (Fig. 9). A similar temperature restriction of coronavirus infection has been reported for cells of neural and other origin (Lucas et al., 1978). In contrast to MHV_3, JHMV replicated only briefly in mixed cultures yielding low titers and failing to cause any apparent CPE (Table 3, Fig. 9). JHMV replicated for more extended periods in only 2/12 cultures still to low titers and without apparent CPE. Variability in the duration from the time of birth, when the cultures were established, until infection was initiated did not influence the infectious process of mixed cultures, despite the continued in vitro maturation processes shown to occur among astrocytes, oligodendroyctes and neurons (Abney et al., 1981).

To determine which cell layer was associated with the replication of which agent the shaken and mixed cultures were inoculated separately with MHV-3 or JHMV. The data, summarized in Table 3, revealed that MHV-3 was unable to replicate efficiently in the shaken cultures consisting primarily of neurons and oligodendrocytes, whereas JHMV replicated equally well in the shaken and mixed cultures. By comparison MHV-3 was replicated for

Table 3 - IN-VITRO REPLICATION OF CORONAVIRUSES IN TOTAL OR
SELECTED RAT CORTICAL CELL CULTURES

Days after inoculation	Mixed Cultures		Shaken Cultures	
	MHV_3 *	JHMV *	MHV_3 *	JHMV *
1	1,000-10,000	100-1,000	10-100	100-1,000
2	10,000	100	0-10	100
4	10,000-100,000	0-100	0	0-10
8	10,000-1,000,000	0	0	0

M.O.I.-0.1 pfu/cell
* pfu/ml of supernatant

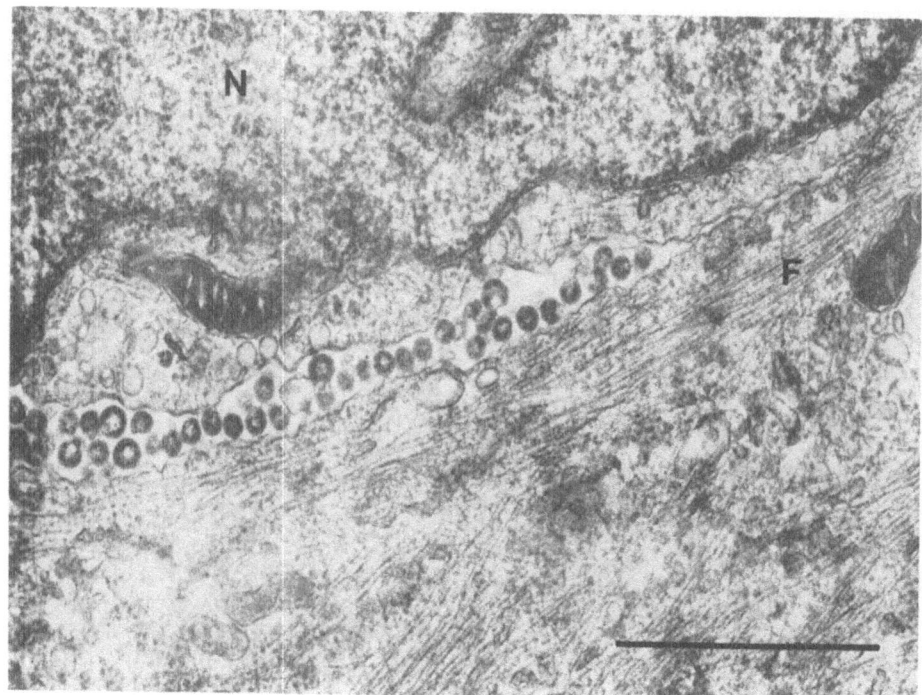

Fig. 8 - A representative electron micrograph of an adherent
astrocyte from the lower layer of a mixed culture sampled 28 days
after infection with MHV-3. Note numerous coronavirus particles
within a cytoplasmic vesicle in the vicinity of a nucleus (N) and
organized bundles of cytoplasmic intermediate filaments (F).
Bar - 1.0 μm.

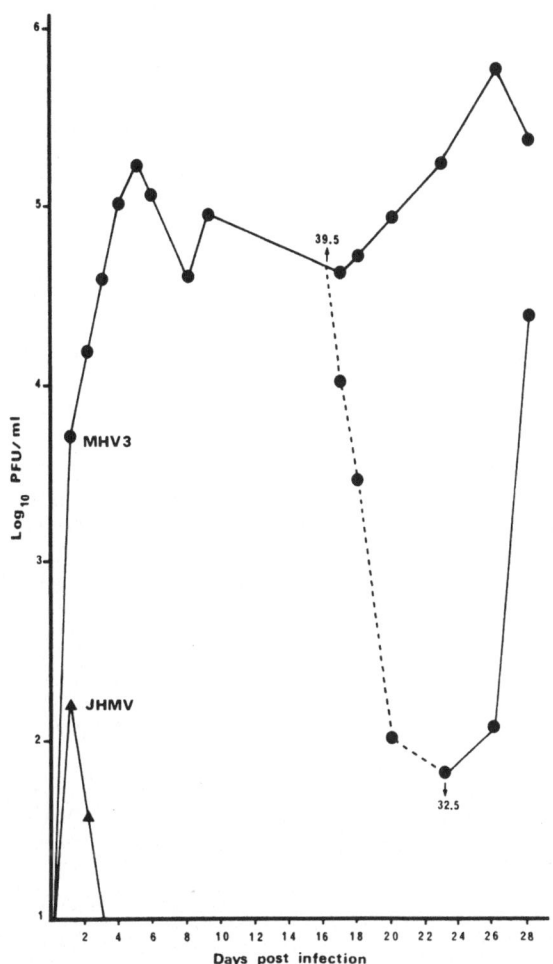

Fig. 9 - Replication of JHMV (▲) and MHV-3 (●) in mixed cultures
at the permissive (32.5°C) and restrictive (39.5°C) temperatures.
Arrows indicate temperature shifts (↑ up, ↓ down). The M.O.I. in
each experiment was about 0.1 pfu/cell.

prolonged periods,   >21 days, and to high titers (∽10^5 pfu/ml)
in the adherent astrocytic cultures. Thus, an efficient and
persistent MHV-3 replication appears to be confined to the
primarily astrocytes while JHMV replication, limited in quantity
and duration, appears to be associated with cells transferrable to
the shaken cultures, presumed to be enriched in neurons and
oligodendrocytes.

Conclusions and Prospective

Data obtained to date show that JHMV-induced neurologic disease in rats represents an interesting model for CNS diseases and might have human relevance. In future analysis of this model it will be essential to (a) obtain explanations for the ability of JHMV but not MHV-3 to cause disease in rats despite the ability of both viruses to replicate in rat cells of neural origin; (b) establish the identity of the primary target cell(s) in the CNS for JHMV; and (c) elucidate the mechanisms for viral persistence and the maintenance of prolonged latency. Host factors are also important and must be investigated further, including the genetically controlled influence on age-related acquisition of resistance to this disease and the manner in which humoral and/or cell-mediated immunity affects the disease process, particularly that connected with the formation of demyelinating lesions.

REFERENCES

Abney, E.R., Bartlett, P.P., and Raff, M.C. 1981. Astrocytes, ependymal cells, and oligodendrocytes develop on schedule in dissociated cell cultures of embryonic rat brain Developmental Biol. 83:301-310.

Bailey, T.O., Pappenheimer, A.M., Cheever, F.S., and Daniels, J.B. 1949. A murine virus (JHM) causing disseminated encephalomyelitis with extensive destruction of myelin. II. Pathology. J. Exp. Med. 90:195-231.

Brahic, M., and Haase, A.T. 1978. Detection of viral sequences of low reiteration frequency by in situ hybridization Proc. Natl. Acad. Sci. U.S.A. 55:6125-6129.

Cheley, S., Anderson, R., Cupples, M.J., Chan, E.C.M.L., and Morris, V.L. 1981a. Intracellular murine hepatitis virus-specific RNA's contain common sequences. Virology 112:596-604.

Cheley, S., Morris, V.L., Cupples, M.J., and Anderson, R. 1981b. RNA and polypeptides homology among murine coronaviruses. Virology 115:310-321.

Fleming, J.O., Ting, J.Y.P., Stohlman, S.A., and Weiner, L.P. 1983. Improvements in obtaining and characterizing mouse cerebrospinal fluid. Application to mouse hepatitis virus-induced encephalomyelitis. J. Neuroimmunol. 4:129-140.

Hirano, N., Goto, N., Ogawa, T., Ono, K., Murakawi, T., and Fujiwara, K. 1980. Hydrocephalus in suckling rats infected intracerebrally with mouse hepatitis virus, MHV-A59. Microbiol. Immunol. 24:825-834.

Knobler, R.L., Haspel, M.V., and Oldstone, M.B.A. 1981. Mouse hepatitis virus type 4 (JHM strain)-induced fatal central nervous system disease. I. Genetic control and the murine neuron as the susceptible site of disease. J. Exp. Med. 153:832-843.

Lampert, P.W., Sims, J.K., and Kiazeff, A.J., 1973. Mechanism of demyelination of JHM virus encephalomyelitis, Electron microscopic studies. Acta Neuropathol. 24:76-85.

Le Prevost, C., Virelizier, J.L., and Dupuy, J.M. 1975. Immunopathology of mouse hepatitis virus type 3. III. Clinical and virologic observations of a persistent viral infection. J. Immunol. 115:640-643.

Lucas, A., Coulter, M., Anderson, R., Dales, S., and Flintoff, W. 1978. In vivo and in vitro models of demyelinating diseases. II. Persistence and host-regulated themosensitivity in cells of neural derivation infected with mouse hepatitis and measles viruses. Virology 88:325-337.

Lucas, A., Flintoff, W., Anderson, R., Percy, D., Coulter, M., and Dales, S. 1977. In vivo and in vitro models of demyelinating diseases: Tropism of the JHM strain of murine hepatitis virus for cells of glial origin. Cell 12:553-560.

MacNaughton, M.R. 1982. Occurrence and frequency of coronavirus infections in humans as determined by enzyme-linked immunosorbent assay. Infect. Immun 38:419-423.

Martin, J.R., Goudswaard, J., Palsson, P.A., Georgsson, G., Petursson, G., Klein, J., and Nathanson, N. 1982. Cerebrospinal fluid immunoglobulins in sheep with Visna, a slow virus infection of the central nervous system. J. Neuroimmunol. 3:139-148.

McCarthy, K.D., and de Vellis, J. 1978. Alpha-adrenergic receptor modulation of beta-adrenergic, adenosine and protaglandin E_1 increased adenosine 3':5'-cyclic monophosphate levels in primary cultures of glia. J. Cyclic Nuc. Res. 4:15-26.

Nagashima, K., Wege, H., Meyermann, R., and ter Meulen, V. 1978. Coronavirus induced subacute demyelinating encephalomyelitis in rats: a morphological analysis. Acta Neuropathol. 44:63-70.

Nagashima, K., Wege, H., Meyermann, R., and ter Meulen, V. 1979. Demyelinating encephalomyelitis induced by long-term coronavirus infection in rats, A preliminary report. Acta Neuropathol. 45:205-213.

Robb, J.A., and Bond, C.W. 1979. Coronaviridae. Comp. Virol. 14:193-247.

Schliep, G., and Felgenhauer, K. 1978. Serum-CSF protein gradients, the blood-CSF barrier and the local immune response. J. Neurol. 218:77-96.

Sorensen, O., Dugre, R., Percy, D., and Dales, S. 1982. In vivo and in vitro models of demyelinating disease: Endogenous factors influencing demyelinating disease caused by mouse hepatitis virus in rats and mice. Infect. Immun. 37:1248-1260.

Sorensen, O., Percy, D., and Dales, S. 1980. In vivo and in vitro models of demyelinating disease. III. JHM virus infection of rats. Arch. Neurol. 37:478-484.

Stroop, W.G., Baringer, J.R., and Brahic, M. 1981. Detection of Theiler's virus RNA in mouse central nervous system by in situ hybridization. Lab. Invest. 45:504-509.

RESTRICTED REPLICATION OF A TEMPERATURE SENSITIVE MUTANT OF MHV–

A59 IN MOUSE BRAIN ASTROCYTES

Mario van Berlo, Guus Wolswijk, Jero Calafat*, Marian Horzinek
and Ben van der Zeijst

Institute of Virology, State University Utrecht, The
Netherlands and *The Netherlands Cancer Institute, Antoni van
Leeuwenhoekhuis, The Netherlands

Temperature-sensitive (ts) mutants of mouse hepatitis virus
(MHV-A59) are drastically attenuated in their pathogenic
properties: intracerebral inoculation of mice with mutants results
in more prolonged infection of the central nervous system without
clinical signs (Koolen et al., 1983, Virology 125, 393-402). This
was surprising in the case of mutant ts-342 which was "leaky" and
grew well in tissue culture cells at 37oC. We have studied the
replication of mutant ts-342 in primary cultures of mouse brain

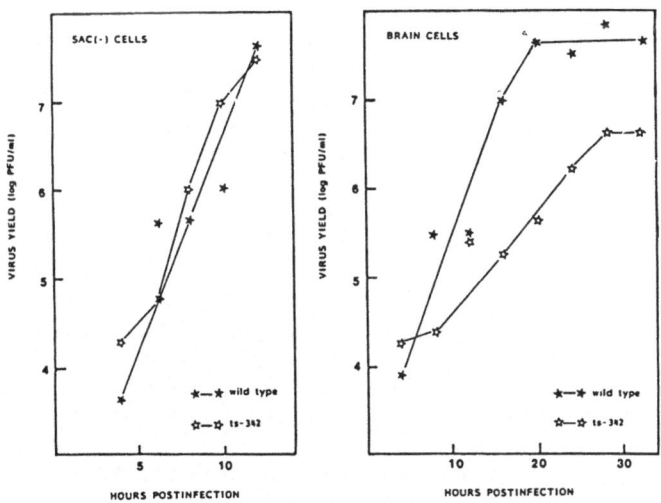

Fig.1. Growth kinetics of MHV-A59 and its mutant ts-342 in Sac(-)
cells (A) or in mouse brain cells (B). The cells were
infected with 50 PFU/cell.

cells,   derived   from   approximately   14–day–old   Balb/c   mouse
embryos. Cultures   became confluent after seven days.   The   cells
were   identified   as   astrocytes   since   they   contained   glial
fibrillary acidic protein (GFAP).

Virus   growth in Sac(–) cells was similar for wild type   MHV–
A59   and   ts–342. In mouse brain cells, however, production of
infectious   ts–342   virions was only about 5% of wild type virus
(Fig.1).   Using   immunofluorescence   no   difference   was   noticed
between wild type and ts–342 virus–infected cells.

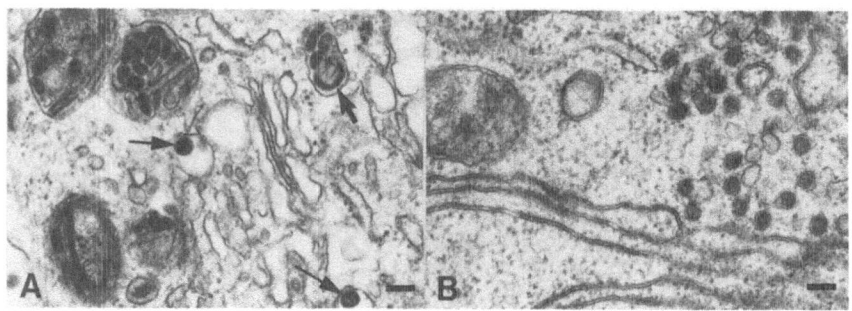

Fig.   2.   Electron   micrographs of mouse brain astrocytes infected
            with   MHV–A59 (A) and its mutant ts–342 (B).   26 h   post
            infection. Bar = 100 nm

Electron   microscopy   (Fig.2) showed that in wild type   virus–
infected cells virus particles were abundant and matured in smooth
membrane cisterns closely associated with the Golgi system (A;bud–
ding site at thick arrow; free virus at thin arrows). Tubular
structures   about   30 nm in diameter were also present in these
cisterns.   (B):In   mutant–infected cells no virus particles as in
(A)   were   seen but sometimes spherical particles of about   70   nm
were present in the cytoplasmic matrix,   consisting of two concen–
tric double membranes. The core was electron–lucent and no nucleo–
capsid   strands as in (A) were seen.   Stacked profiles of double
membranes similar to those surrounding the particles were present.

Infected   cells   were   labeled   with ^{35}S–methionine   and ^{3}H–
glucosamine. In Sac(–) cells (labeled from 7 to 9 h p.i.) no
difference   in   intracellular virus–specific proteins was found
between wild type virus and ts–342. Also mouse brain cells
infected with wild type virus contained the normal set of viral
proteins (labeling from 16 to 22 h p.i.). However,   ts–342
infected   brain   cells   contained no E2 and pp 24/E1 and only a
reduced amount of gp 26.5/E1 and gp 25.5/E1 (data not shown).

The   restricted replication of ts–342 in mouse brain cells is
probably due to a second site mutation, which affects the host
range by causing a reduced level of glycoproteins in astrocytes.

REPLICATION OF MURINE CORONAVIRUSES IN SOMATIC CELL HYBRIDS FORMED
BETWEEN A MOUSE FIBROBLAST CELL LINE AND EITHER A RAT SCHWANNOMA
LINE OR A RAT GLIOMA LINE

Wayne F. Flintoff

Department of Microbiology and Immunology
University of Western Ontario
London, Ontario, CANADA N6A 5C1

INTRODUCTION

The murine hepatitis viruses can readily establish persistent
infections both in vivo and in vitro. In vivo, persistent
infections, dependent upon the virus strain, and the age and
genetic background of the host, can occur resulting in chronic
hepatitis or chronic demyelination of the central nervous system
(1). In vitro, these agents can establish persistent infections
in both neural and non-neural cell lines (2,3,4) without the
requirements for viral modifications or environmental
manipulations such as the presence of viral antibody or
interferon.

Our previous results have indicated that when infection of
various cell lines with either the MHV_3 or JHM strain of the
murine coronaviruses resulted in persistence, virus replication
was almost invariably thermosensitive and this was due to unknown
factors under host control, since the progeny virions themselves
were not temperature-sensitive (2,3). In addition, one cell line,
the rat RN2 Schwannoma, had the unique ability to discriminate
between the MHV_3 and JHM strains (2). JHM was replicated
persistently in this line, whereas, MHV_3 replication was aborted.
Another rat cell line, the C6 glioma, did not support the
replication of either agent (3). At present, it is unclear as to
the mechanism of persistence or restriction demonstrated by these
cell lines. These observations coupled with others (4,5) strongly
imply that the host cell has a profound influence in regulating
the replication of these agents.

As a further approach to analyzing the host functions involved in viral persistence and restriction, somatic cell hybrids have been formed between mouse L2 cells, a cell line totally permissive for both MHV_3 and JHM replication, and either the RN2 or the C6 cells. The results described in this report, indicate that the L cell functions appear to be dominant over the RN2 and C6 ones, since both viral agents replicated lytically in the somatic cell hybrids.

MATERIALS AND METHODS

Cells and Virus. The sources and routine propagation of the L2 and RN2-2 cell lines, and the MHV_3 and JHM strains of mouse hepatitis virus were as previously described (2,3) except that alpha medium (6) was used in place of Eagle's minimal essential medium. The C6 thymidine kinase minus (C6TK⁻) cells were obtained from Dr. B.P. Schimmer, Banting and Best Institute, Toronto, Ontario, Canada.

Virus propagation was monitored by a plaque assay on L2 cell monolayers as previously described (2). Yields are expressed as PFU/ml (plaque forming units/ml).

Selection of genetically marked L2 cells. L2 cells were treated for 3 hours in the presence of 0.2 µg/ml   N-methyl-N'-nitro-N-nitrosoguanidine at 34⁰, washed, and resuspended in fresh medium. Survival was usually about 50%. The cells were allowed to grow 6 days to allow for expression of putative mutations before selections were carried out. The basic procedure for mutant selections is described elsewhere (7). Cells, at 5 x 10^5/100 mm tissue culture dish, were exposed to 0.2 µg/ml 6-thioguanine (TG) (Sigma Chemical Co.) for 8 days at 34⁰ with replacement of drug and medium every 2 days. Colonies surviving at a frequency of 4 x 10^{-6} were picked, cloned by limit dilution, and tested for resistance. One clone, L2 TG , was resistant to at least 50 µg/ml TG, a concentration 10^3 higher than was cytotoxic for the wild-type cells, and contained   0.1% of the wild-type hypoxanthine phosphoribosyl transferase activity as determined by the assay described by Chasin and Urlaub (8).

The L2 TG^R7 cells were exposed to 3 mM ouabain (Oua) to select for Oua resistant cells (9). Colonies surviving at a frequency of 10^{-5} were isolated, cloned, and shown to be resistant to at least 3 mM Oua. Wild-type cells were unable to grow at concentrations above 0.5 mM. One doubly marked clone, L2 TG^R Oua^R7-1, and designated L2 TG^R Oua^R was used in the hybridization experiments.

Neither resistance to TG, nor Oua, nor the presence of both of these markers affected the ability of the cells to support the replication of either the MHV_3 or JHM strains of mouse hepatitis virus.

Cell-cell hybridizations. Somatic cell hybrids were formed between the L2 TG^R Oua^R and RN2-2 cells, and the L2 TG^R Oua^R and C6Tk⁻ cells by exposure to polyethylene glycol (PEG) 6000 (British Drug House) for 1 min using the procedure described by Pontecorva (10). Cells were plated in complete medium for 1 day to allow recovery from the fusion process prior to the addition of HAT (1) + Oua selection medium (7 x 10^{-5}M hypoxanthine, 2 x 10^{-8}M methotrexate, 4 x 10^{-5}M thymidine, 2 x 10^{-3}M Oua) for the L2 TG^R Oua^R x RN2-2 cells, or HAT (2) medium (7 x 10^{-5}M hypoxanthine, 10^{-6}M methotrexate, 4 x 10^{-5}M thymidine) for the L2 TG^R Oua^R x C6TK⁻ cells. In the latter hybridization, the Oua resistant marker was not used in the selection scheme. Hybridization frequencies are shown in Table 1. After 8 to 10 days incubation at 34⁰, surviving colonies were picked, expanded, maintained in normal medium, and used for study. Subclones of some of these isolates were obtained by limit dilution. There were no differences in the response of these subclones and the original isolates to virus infection.

Karyotypic analyses. Exponentially growing cells were incubated with 0.25 µg/ml colcemid (Grand Island Biological Co. for 1.5 hrs at 34⁰. The cells were washed with hypotonic and fixing solutions and chromosome spreads prepared (11). To distinguish between mouse and rat chromosomes the formamide-Giemsa staining procedure of Marshall (12) was used. With this technique a majority of mouse chromosomes contain centromeric regions which stain intensely, whereas, the centromeric regions of the rat chromosomes do not. From 5 to 10 chromosome spreads were examined for each cell line. In addition standard trypsin-banding techniques were also employed (11).

Lactate Dehydrogenase Assay. The preparation of cell extracts and the assay for lactate dehydrogenase was essentially as described by Weiss and Ephrussi (13) using Gelman Sephraphore III cellulose acetate strips. In vitro hybridizations were carried out in 1M NaCl and 70 mM Na phosphate pH 8.0 as described by Markert (14).

RESULTS

Properties of hybrid cells. Using the genetically marked cell lines, cell-cell hybrids were formed between either the mouse L cells and rat RN2 cells or the L cells and rat C6 cells. Although the frequency of hybrid formation was greater than the survival of either the mouse or rat parental cell lines under

Table 1 Hybridzation Frequencies

Cross	PEG		Experiment
L2 TG^R Oua^R x L2 TG^R Oua^R a,b	+	6 x 10^{-7}	2.5 x 10^{-6}
RN2-2 x RN2-2^a	+	1 x 10^{-7}	--
C6TK$^-$ x C6TK$^-$	+	--	2.5 x 10^{-6}
RN2-2 x L2 TG^R Oua^R a	-	6 x 10^{-6}	--
RN2-2 x L2 TG^R Oua^R a	+	4 x 10^{-5}	--
C6TK$^-$ x L2 TG^R Oua^R b	-	--	2.5 x 10^{-5}
C6TK$^-$ x L2 TG^R Oua^R b	+	--	1.7 x 10^{-3}

[a]Determined by growth in HAT (1) + Oua selection medium.

[b]Determined by growth in HAT (2) selection medium.

these selective conditions (Table 1), it was conceivable that parental cells might have survived the selection scheme. Thus, it was important to distinguish between authentic cell hybrids and parental survivors. Hybrid cells formed between these mouse and rat cells could be readily distinguished from the parental cells on the basis of their chromosome content and on the production of species-specific gene products.

As shown in Table 2, the mouse-rat hybrid cells had average chromosome numbers that were greater than those of either the rat or mouse parental cells used to form them.

To demonstrate that the chromosome content of the hybrid cells consisted of both mouse and rat chromosomes, a centromeric-staining procedure for mouse chromosomes using formamide-Giemsa was employed (12). As shown in Figure 1, the mouse chromosomes can be readily distinguished from the rat chromosomes because of the intense centromeric staining of the former. It is also evident form this Figure that in the two L2 TG^R Oua^R x RN2-2 cell hybrids shown, both mouse and rat chromosomes were present. Using this procedure and standard trypsin-Giemsa chromsome banding techniques, it was possible to identify both mouse and rat chromosomes in the hybrid cells. The chromosome compositions of

Table 2   Chromosome Content of Hybrids

Cell Line	Chromosome Number[a]	Mouse Chromosomes[b]	Rat Chromosomes[b]
Parental L2 TG^R Oua^R	42 + 3		
RN2-2	42 + 1		
C6TK$^-$	35 + 5		
Hybrids (A) L2 TG^R Oua^R x RN2-2			
Hybrid 1	82 + 5	38 + 5	43 + 4
2	80 + 8	34 + 3	46 + 4
3	72 +7	40 + 3	32 + 3
4	70 + 6	33 + 4	37 + 5
5	75 + 5	35 + 3	38 + 2
6	60 + 2	22 + 3	37 + 3
7	69 + 7	30 + 4	40 + 4
8	76 + 4	36 + 5	37 + 5
(B) L2 TG^R Oua^R x C6TK$^-$			
Hybrid 21	55 + 5	27 + 7	28 + 8
22	65 + 8	27 + 7	38 + 5
23	71 + 4		
24	69 + 7		
25	70 + 6		
26	73 + 2	36 + 2	38 + 4

[a]Average chromosome number based on 5 to 10 chromosome spreads with standard deviation indicated.
[b]Determined by standard trypsin-Giemsa banding and the centrometric staining procedure of Marshall (12).

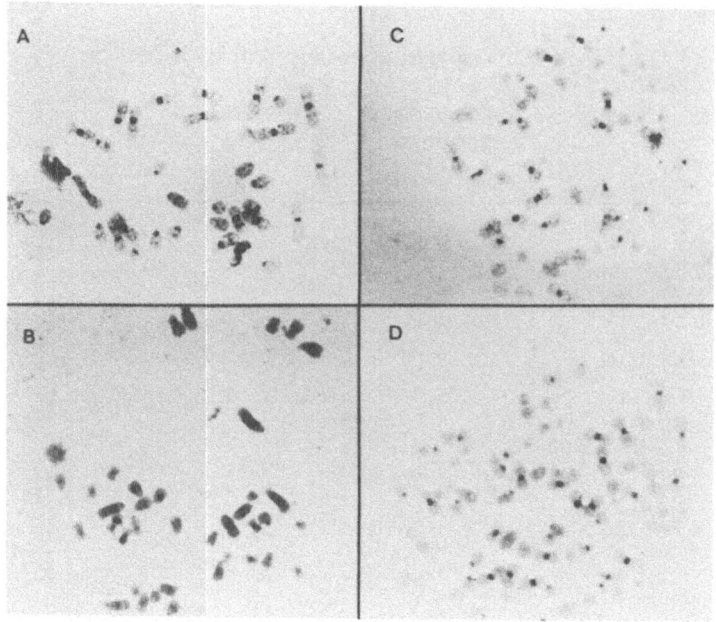

Figure 1

Figure 1.   Chromosomes of selected cell lines.   Chromosomes were
            prepared and treated with trypsin and formamide and
            stained with Giemsa as described in Materials and
            Methods.   Chromosomes from (A) L2 TG^R Oua^R, (B) RN2-2,
            (C) HYBRID 6, and (D) HYBRID 2 cells.

the hybrids are summarized in Table 1.   For the most part for both
types of hybrids, a majority of the parental rat chromosomes was
present with some variability in the parental murine chromosomes.

    The authenticity of the hybrid cells was also demonstrated by
the presence of both murine and rat lactate dehydrogenase
isozymes.   As shown in Figure 2 the rat RN2-2 cells produced a
lactate dehydrogenase enzyme that migrated more cathodally than
similar enzyme from mouse L2 TG^R Oua^R cells.   When a mixture of
rat and mouse lactate dehydrogenase was dissociated and
reassembled in vitro, four major bands and a faint fifth band of
enzymatic activity were obtained (Figure 2, lane D).   Such a
pattern was absent in a mixture of parental extracts (Figure 2,
lane C).   When extracts of hybrid cells were assayed for lactate

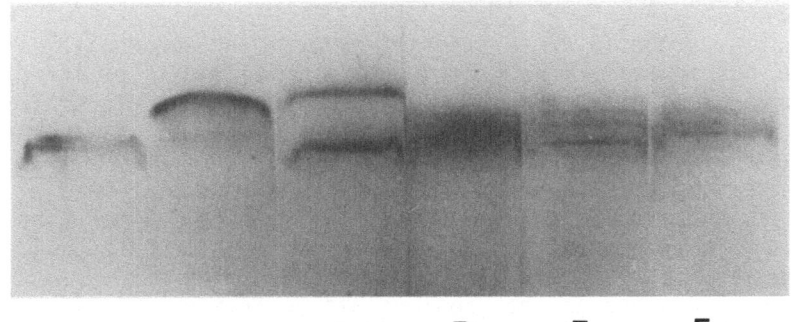

Figure 2.   Lactate dehydrogenase isozymes in hybrid cells.
            Lactate dehydrogenase was assayed as described in
            Materials and Methods. Lactate dehydrogenase from (A)
            L2 TG^{R}Oua^R extract. (B) RN2-2 extract; (C) a 1:1
            mixture of L2 TG^{R}Oua^R and RN2-2 extracts; (D) a 1:1
            mixture of L2 TG^{R}Oua^R and RN2-2 extracts assembled in
            vitro; (E) HYBRID 6 extract; and (F) HYBRID 2 extract.

dehydrogenase activity (Figure 2, lanes E,F) an isozyme pattern
similar to that of the in vitro assembled isozymes was obtained.
These results are consistent with the presence and association of
both mouse and rat forms of lactate dehydrogenase in the hybrid
cells. Similar results were obtained for the L2 TG^R Oua^R x C6 TK$^-$
cells.

Replication of JHM and MHV$_3$ in hybrids between mouse
fibroblasts and rat Schwannoma cells. Previous results indicated
that mouse L2 cells supported the replication of both the JHM and
MHV$_3$ virus strains in a lytic fashion which involved extensive
cell destruction through syncytial formation. When RN2 cells were

used as host, JHM replicated persistently with restricted
cytopathology in a temperature sensitive manner. MHV_3 replication
was totally restricted in the RN2 cells (2,3). The availability
of somatic cell hybrids between these 2 cell lines permitted an
examination of which host cell type dominantly affected the virus
replication process.

Confluent monolayer cultures of several independently
selected hybrid cells were infected at a multiplicity of infection
(moi) of 0.05 with either JHM or MHV_3, maintained at either 32^0 or
39^0, and virus production determined after 24 hours. As shown in
Table 3, the hybrid cells could replicate both JHM and MHV_3 at
both temperatures. The virus yields for the most part were
similar to those obtained with the L2 TG^R Oua^R cell line as host
and considerably higher than those obtained with the RN2 cell.
Accompanying these high levels of virus production was an
extensive cytopathic effect (cpe) resulting from syncytial
formation. By 24 hours at 39^0, essentially all the cells in the
monolayer were involved and total destruction and cell lifting had
occurred. A similar cpe was observed at 32^0, however, total
destruction was delayed until 30 to 36 hours post-infection.
These effects were apparent with the L2 TG^R Oua^R, and hybrid lines
1, 2, 3, 4, 5, 7, and 8. Hybrid 6 showed some differences. This
hybrid, which produced lower yields of virus than the other hybrid
lines at 24 hours (Table 3), showed very little, if any, cpe, at
both temperatures with JHM virus. If a cpe was present it was
restricted to less than 10% of the cells in the population.
Similar results were also obtained with MHV_3 infections, although
the cpe was somewhat more extensive, perhaps involving 20 to 30%
of the cells in the population. The cpe observed with either
virus in this line appeared to be restricted since longer
incubation periods up to 7 days did not result in a more extensive
cpe even though 30-80% of the cells scored as infectious centers.
The extent of the cpe was also not affected by increasing the moi
to 5 even though the number of cells scoring as infectious centers
was 80%. Initially hybrid 6 cells could produce either JHM or MHV_3
virus at 39^0. However, after about 1 week in culture these
infected cells lost the ability to shed virus at 39^0 even though
they continued to produce virus in a cyclical manner at 32^0. At
this time, if cells shedding virus at 32^0 were shifted to 39^0
there was a cessation of virus production. The properties of
cyclical release of virus and restricted virus replication at the
elevated temperature is reminiscent of the JHM infection of RN2
cells in which from 0.1 to 10% of the cells are infected (2,3).
In the case with hybrid 6 cells, however, both JHM and MHV_3 were
replicated and the number of infected cells was from 50 to 80%.
Ten subclones of the hybrid 6 cells behaved similarly when
challenged with virus.

Table 3 Replication of JHM and MHV_3 in Parental
and Hybrid Cell Lines

| | Virus Yield (pfu/ml) | | | |
| | JHM | | MHV_3 | |
CELL LINE	32^0	39.5^0	32^0	39.5^0
L2 TG^{R}Oua^R	4×10^5	2×10^5	5×10^5	4×10^5
RN2-2	4.5×10^2	5	50	5
HYBRID 1	5×10^5	4×10^5	1×10^5	1.5×10^5
2	3×10^5	2×10^5	5×10^5	3×10^5
3	2×10^5	1.5×10^5	1.8×10^5	1.1×10^5
4	5×10^5	3×10^5	5×10^5	3×10^5
5	2×10^5	3×10^5	5×10^5	7×10^4
6	6.5×10^3	2.9×10^3	7.5×10^4	3.3×10^4
7	2×10^5	2×10^5	5×10^5	3.6×10^5
8	4×10^5	3×10^5	3×10^5	1×10^5

[a]Confluent monolayers of the various cell lines were infected at a moi of 0.05 with either JHM or MHV_3 at either 32^0 or 39^0. After 1 hr to allow for virus adsorption, the infected cells were washed 2 times with phosphate buffered saline, fed fresh medium, and incubated at the appropriate temperature. Virus released into the medium was assayed at 24 hrs post-infection by the plaque assay at 32^0 on L2 monolayer as described in Materials and Methods.

Replication of JHM and MHV_3 in hybrids between mouse fibroblasts and rat glioma cells. Previously results indicated that the rat C6 glioma cell line was restrictive to the replication of both the JHM and MHV_3 strains (3). The availability of somatic cell hybrids between the L and C6 TK$^-$ cells permitted an examination of which host functions were dominant.

Confluent monolayers of several independently selected hybrid cells were infected at an moi of 0.05 with either virus strain at 32^0, and virus production monitored after 30 hours. The hybrids could replicate both JHM and MHV_3 (Table 4). The virus yields from the hybrid cells were similar to those from the parental mouse cells (L2 TG^R Oua^R). Accompanying this virus production in all the lines tested with both viruses was extensive syncytial formation involving about 80-100% of the cells in the culture.

DISCUSSION

The results described in this report indicate that the permissive or lytic state of coronavirus infection, characteristic of the mouse L fibroblast cell was a genetically dominant trait over the persistent or restrictive host states of the rat RN2 Schwannoma or rat C6 glioma cells. This conclusion is based on the observation that when somatic cell hybrids, formed between either the L and RN2 cells or the L and C6 cells, were infected with either JHM or MHV_3, virus yields and cytopathic effects were

TABLE 4   Virus Production From Mouse Fibroblast X Rat Glioma Cells

Cell Line	JHM	MHV_3
L2 TG^R Oua^R	5×10^5	5×10^5
C6TK$^-$	5	5
Hybrid 21	5×10^5	3×10^5
22	2×10^5	5×10^5
23	3×10^5	7×10^5
24	4×10^5	1×10^5
25	5×10^5	3×10^5
26	2×10^5	2×10^5

[a]Confluent monolayers of the various cell lines were infected at a moi of 0.05 with either JHM or MHV_3 at 32^0. After 1 hr to allow for virus adsorption, the infected cells were washed 2 times with phosphate buffered saline, fed fresh medium, and incubated at 32^0. Virus released into the medium was assayed at 30 hrs post-infection by the plaque assay at 32^0 on L2 monolayers as described in Materials and Methods.

similar to those of the L2 parental cell line. Such features are
not characteristic of the infections of RN2 or C6 cells (2,3).
However, one hybrid, hybrid 6, formed between RN2 and L2 TG^R Oua^R
cells, and its subclones differed from the others of its type in
their response to virus infection. These cells could initially
replicate both virus strains at 32° and 39° without extensive
syncytial formation. After about one week in culture such cells
lost the ability to produce virus at 39° but continued to produce
virus at 32°. The reason for the difference between this hybrid
and the others is at present unclear. It may be related in some
way to the chromosome content of this hybrid cell since its
chromosome number is lower than that of the others (Table 2).

     Since chromosome loss does occur in cell-cell hybrids (15) it
is conceivable, however, that one of the rat chromosomes codes for
a dominantly acting factor which is responsible for virus
resistance or persistence. This chromosome may be among those
that are frequently lost in the hybrids. This would thus lead to
the viral susceptibility of the hybrids. Preliminary karyotyping
results have indicated that the mouse-rat hybrids appear to
contain a majority of the parental rat chromosomes. The
individual hybrids do not appear to have consistently lost the
same rat chromosomes. However, more extensive studies will be
required to address this possibility. Once established these
hybrids appear to be phenotypically stable since several of the
lines have been kept in continuous culture for up to 8 months and
periodically screened for susceptibility to lytic virus infection.
Todate, all lines after prolonged culture behaved similarly in
their responses to infection as they did shortly after isolation.
The result that the totally permissive state (ie. the L cell) is
dominant over the restrictive/persistent state (ie. the RN2 cell)
or the totally restrictive state (i.e. the C6 cell) is not unlike
other host-virus systems where it has been demonstrated that
permissive host functions are dominant over nonpermissive ones
(16,17,18). At present, it is unclear as to the nature and role
that the L2 functions play in overcoming the RN2-2 controlled
persistent, thermosensitive replication of JHM, and the
restriction of MHV$_3$ and the C6 restriction of both viruses.
Knowledge of these L cell functions might prove useful in an
understanding of both coronavirus persistence and restriction. It
is of interest to note that although MHV$_3$ replication is
restricted in RN2 cells, if it is permitted to initiate
replication as it does in hybrid 6 then after about 1 week in
culture a persistent infection not unlike that of the JHM
infection of RN2-2 cells can be obtained.

Since there are available several different cell lines that can
become persistently infected with the JHM and MHV$_3$ virus strains
(3) it will be of interest to determine whether these cell lines

behave in a manner similar to the RN2 cells when somatic cell hybrids are formed with the mouse L2 cells. Such studies are currently in progress.

ACKNOWLEDGEMENTS

The author wishes to thank M. Weber, C. Nagainis, and F. Williams for technical assistance, and Dr. S. Dales for use of the light microscope.

REFERENCES

1. H. Wege, St. Siddell, and V. ter Meulen. The biology and pathogenesis of coronaviruses, Curr. top. Microbiol. Immunol. 99:165(1982).

2. A. Lucas, W. Flintoff, R. Anderson, D. Percy, M. Coulter, and S. Dales. In vivo and in vitro models of demyelinating diseases: Tropism of the JHM strain of murine hepatitis virus for cells of glial origin, Cell 12:553 (1977).

3. A. Lucas, M. Coulter, R. Anderson, S. Dales, and W. Flintoff. In vivo and in vitro models of demyelinating diseases: II Persistence and host-regulated thermosensitivity in cells of neural derivation infected with mouse hepatitis and measles viruses, Virol. 88:325 (1978).

4. S.A. Stohlman, and L.P. Weiner. Stability of neurotropic mouse hepatitis virus (JHM strain) during chronic infection of neuroblastoma cells, Arch. Virol. 57:53 (1978).

5. K.V. Holmes, and J.N. Behnke. Evolution of a coronavirus during persistent infection in vitro, Adv. Exptl. Med. Biol. 142:287 (1982).

6. C.P. Stanners, G.L. Elicieri, and H. Green. Two types of ribosomes in mouse-hamster hybrid cells, Nature (New Biol.) 230:52 (1971).

7. W.F. Flintoff, S.V. Davidson, and L. Siminovitch. Isolation and partial characterization of three methotrexate resistant phenotypes from Chinese hamster ovary cells, Somat. Cell Genet. 2:245 (1976).

8. L.A. Chasin, and G. Urlaub. Mutant alleles for hypoxanthine phosphoribosyl transferase: Codominant expression, complementation, and segregation in hybrid Chinese hamster cells, Somat. Cell Genet. 2:453 (1976).

9. R.M. Baker, D.M. Brunette, R. Mankovitz, L.H. Thompson, G.F. Whitmore, L. Siminovitch, and J.E. Till. Ouabain-resistant mutants of mouse and hamster cells in culture, Cell 1:9 (1974).

10. G. Pontecorvo. Production of mammalian somatic cell hybrids by means of polyethylene glycol treatment, Somat. Cell Genet. 1:397 (1975).

11. R.G. Worton, and C. Duff. Karyotyping, Methods Enzymol. 58:322 (1979).

12. C.J. Marshall. A method for analysis of chromosomes in hybrid cells employing sequential G-banding and mouse specific C-banding, Exptl. Cell. Res. 91:464 (1975).
13. M.C. Weiss, and B. Ephrussi. Studies of interspecific (rat x mouse) somatic hybrids. II. Lactate dehydrogenase and B-glucuronidase, Genetics 54:111 (1966).
14. C.L. Markert. Lactate dehydrogenase isozymes: dissociation and recombination of subunits. Science 140:1329 (1963).
15. U. Francke, and B. Francke. Requirement of the human chromosome 11 long arm for replication of Herpes simplex virus type 1 in nonpermissive Chinese hamster x human diploid fibroblast hybrids, Somat. Cell Genet. 7:171 (1981).
16. D.A. Miller, O.J. Miller, V.G. Dev, S. Hasmi, R. Tantravahi, L. Medrano, and H. Gree. Human chromosome 19 carries a poliovirus receptor gene, Cell 1:167 (1974).
17. J.J. Graver, P.L. Pearson, P.J. Pearson, and A.J. V.d. Eb. Control of SV40 replication by a single chromosome in monkey-hamster cell hybrids, Somat. Cell Genet. 6:443 (1980).
18. R.S. Lemons, W.G. Nash, S.J. O'Brien, R.E. Benuiste, and C.J. Sherr. A gene (Bevi) on human chromosome 6 is an integration site for baboon type C DNA provirus in human cells, Cell 14:995 (1978).

PERSISTENT IN VITRO INFECTION WITH MOUSE HEPATITIS VIRUS 3

Lucie Lamontagne and Jean-Marie Dupuy

Armand-Frappier Institute
Immunology Research Center, University of Quebec
Laval, Quebec, Canada H7N 4Z3

SUMMARY

Mouse hepatitis virus 3 (MHV_3) infection in mice displays various types of sensitivity according to mouse strains: resistance, full susceptibility and semisusceptibility. MHV_3 infections were carried out in primary cultures of embryonic fibroblasts originating from various mouse strains and in mouse lymphoid cell lines. Persistent infection was induced in 2 out of 3 primary embryonic fibroblast cultures. A high production of virus was obtained, as tested by viral titers and cell membrane antigen detection. Cytopathic effects characterized by cell lysis were related to in vivo phenotypes. Persistent MHV_3 infection established in vitro in YAC mouse lymphoid cell line was characterized by virus production, occurence of cellular viral antigens and cell lysis. Cell cloning and antibody treatment experiments indicated that the type of viral transmission was horizontal and not vertical. These data indicate that persistent infection induced by MHV_3 in lymphoid cell lines is characterized by a viral "carrier state" where production of infectious viral particles remains in equilibrium with cell permissiveness.Biological and biochemical properties of MHV_3 variants derived from persistently infected YAC lymphoid cells were characterized. Similar heterogeneous thermosensitive properties were observed when YAC-derived cloned substrains (YAC-MHV_3) were compared to parental-derived cloned viruses, indicating that no selection of temperature-sensitive mutants was induced in persistently infected YAC cells. The capacity, however, of YAC-MHV_3 to induce a lethal acute disease when injected into susceptible mice was lost very rapidly and seemed to be regulated by host factors.

INTRODUCTION

Mouse hepatitis virus 3 (MHV_3) infection in mice leads to various types of evolution according to strain, age and immune status of animals[1,2]. Three types of viral sensitivity were observed: resistance, full susceptibility and semisusceptibility. The latter is characterized by a chronic disease with occurrence of paralyses and viral persistency since MHV_3 can be recovered during the first 3 months postinfection in most animals from brain, liver, spleen and lymph nodes[3]. Genetic analysis indicated that acute and chronic diseases are under the influence of at least 2 major genes, or gene complexes, which are different for both diseases[4]. In addition, it was observed that resistance to the development of paralyses in semisusceptible F_1 hybrids was governed by genes of the H-2 complex[4]. During the chronic phase of the disease, a progressive immunodeficiency occurs, which is related to marked involvement of the lymphoid system, presence of MHV_3 in lymphoid cells[5] and capacity of the virus to replicate in lymphocytes[6], all factors leading to lympholysis and inhibition of antigen-driven lymphocyte proliferation[5]. Natural resistance also plays an important role in MHV_3 sensitivity since in vivo susceptibility was correlated in vitro with the capacity of MHV_3 to replicate or not in hepatocytes[7,8]. Persistent viral infections induced in vitro with coronaviruses (MHV_3 and JHM strains) have mainly been established in continuous cell lines of neural origin[9,10] and in mouse myeloblasts or rat hepatoma cells[9]. Mechanisms involved in such persistent infections are still unknown.

In order to study the mechanism involved in MHV_3 persistency, we have established persistent in vitro infections in lymphocyte cell lines as well as in embryonic fibroblast cells originating from various mouse strains with different genetic sensitivity to MHV_3.

RESULTS AND DISCUSSION

MHV_3 persistent infection in embryonic fibroblast cells

MHV_3 infection was carried out in primary cultures of embryonic fibroblasts originating from various mouse strains (resistant: A/J, susceptible: C57Bl/6 and semisusceptible (C57Bl/6 x A/J)F_1). Embryonic fibroblast cells were obtained from 15 to 18 day-old mouse embryos. Virus-induced cytopathic effects and membrane antigens as well as virus replication and interferon synthesis were studied. Persistent infection was induced in 2 out of 3 primary embryonic fibroblast cultures.

In infected primary cell cultures (Fig. 1), high virus titers were observed in A/J and in (C57Bl/6 x A/J)F_1 cells. In C57Bl/6 cells, virus titers were high at days 2 to 4 postinfection, but decreased regularly thereafter to become negative by day 10. MHV_3-induced cytopathic effects (CPE) exhibited striking differences according to mouse strains. No CPE were seen in fibroblast cultures derived from the resistant A/J

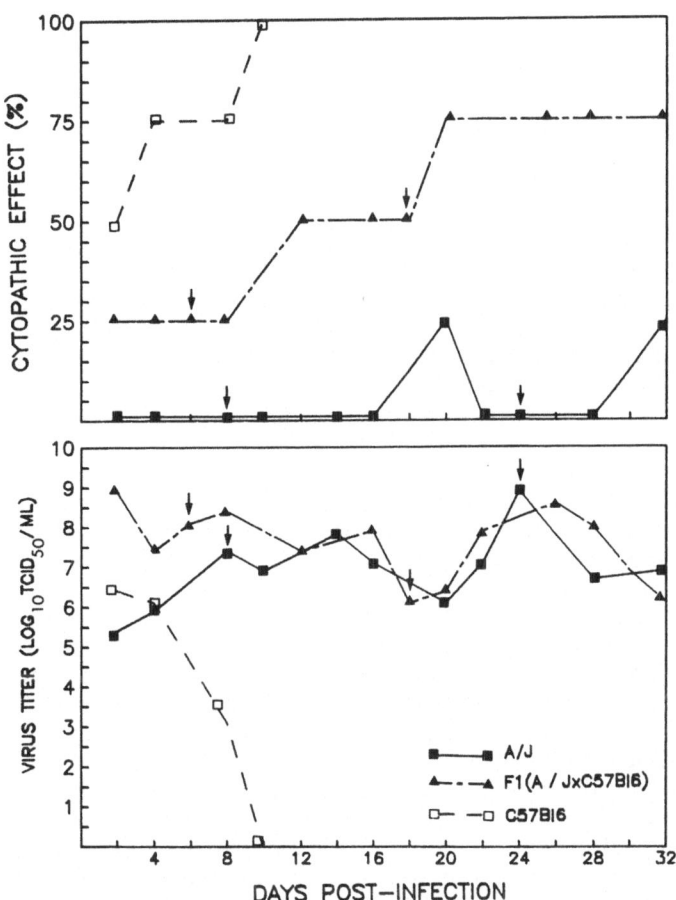

Figure 1.   MHV$_3$ infection in primary cell cultures of embryonic fibroblasts originating from A/J, B$_6$ and B$_6$AF$_1$ mouse strains.

strain, whereas cells from susceptible C57Bl/6 mice expressed a high percentage of CPE by day 2 postinfection and were entirely lysed by day 10. Fibroblast cultures derived from (C57Bl/6 x A/J)F$_1$ hybrids displayed an intermediate behaviour as CPE, already present by day 2 postinfection, regularly increased thereafter without reaching, however, total cell lysis. Search for interferon production was carried out at 5 day intervals in supernatants from MHV$_3$ infected embryonic fibroblast cell cultures. No interferon was detected during viral persistency. Results indicate that genetically determined sensitivity of mice to MHV$_3$ infection can be exhibited in embryonic fibroblasts with regard to establishment of persistent infections and resistance to virus-induced cell lysis.

MHV$_3$ persistent infection in YAC cells

In an attempt to investigate a causal relationship between virus persistency and lymphocytes, in vitro studies of MHV$_3$ replication in lymphocyte cell lines were undertaken. YAC cells (YAC-1 substrain) are derived from a Moloney virus induced T-cell lymphoma of A/Sn origin and have been propagated as a suspension line in culture for several years. Cells were grown in suspension culture in RPMI 1640 (Flow Laboratories, McLean) medium containing 10% of fetal calf serum, penicillin (100 U./ml) and streptomycin (100 mg/ml). Subcultures were performed by dilution with fresh culture medium when cell density reached 5×10^5 cell/ml. The doubling time of lymphoid cells was 18 h.

Persistent infections were established in YAC cells (Fig. 2) and were maintained up to 100 days in some experiments. They were stopped at that time for convenience. In every culture, the number of viable cells was regularly counted and virus persistency was determined by both virus production and detection of cellular viral antigens using the indirect immunofluorescence test. A marked difference in cell number was observed when infected and uninfected YAC cells were compared. In addition, a cell "crisis", characterized by a drastic decrease in cell number, occurred in infected cell populations at passages 7 and 15 (Fig. 2). Infectious virus was produced by persistently infected YAC cell cultures. Titers varied with time and no significant difference was seen between free-virus and cell associated virus titers. Indirect immunofluorescence examination performed on infected and control cells displayed different patterns of fluorescence according to time of infection. Large fluorescent syncytia were frequently seen during the first 2 passages postinfection, whereas small fluorescent cells, without fusion   were observed thereafter.

Persistent MHV$_3$ infection was characterized by several factors, e.g.: virus production, occurence of cellular viral antigens and cell lysis. Although some variations were observed, a general relationship was seen between the 3 factors during cell cultures. High virus titres were associated with a decrease of fluorescent cell number and of cell lysis. Conversly, low virus titers were associated with high numbers of fluorescent

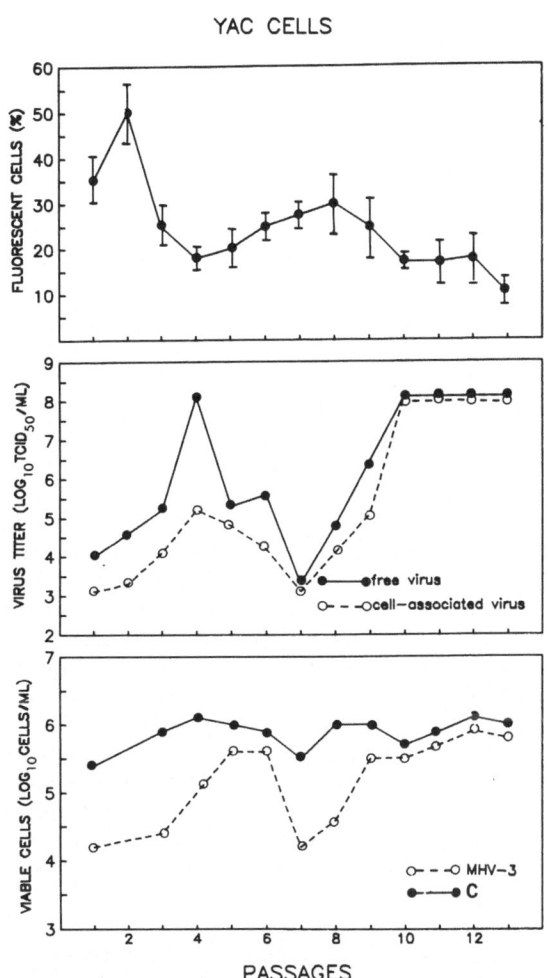

Figure 2.   MHV$_3$ persistent infection induced in YAC cells.

cells and increased lysis. Such a relationship suggests sequential events where virus production would be followed by accumulation of viral antigen and cell death. This relationship was particularly remarkable when "crisis" occurred. Such "crisis" were manifested by a sharp increase of cell lysis and of fluorescent cells and, concomitantly, by a marked decrease of virus titers. Similar cell "crisis" have already been demonstrated in mouse L cells persistently infected with VSV[11,12] in human lymphoblastoid cells infected with parvoviruses[13] or with HSV[14].

Mode of viral transmission in MHV$_3$ persistently infected YAC cells

In order to study the mode of viral transmission, two experiments were performed: cell cloning of infected and uninfected YAC cells, and treatment of cells undergoing a persistent infection with high concentrations of specific anti-MHV$_3$ antibody.

Cell cloning of persistently infected and uninfected YAC cells was performed using the limit dilution method. Cloning efficiency was estimated as the ratio between numbers of growing and expected clones. Cloning efficiency of infected (I) versus uninfected control (C) cells, resulted in a I/C ratio. Results obtained in 2 experiments of cell cloning showed that I/C ratios were 0.77 and 0.72. Virus did not persist in any of the cell clones as evidenced by absence of virus production, of immunofluorescent cells, and of resistance to superinfection. In order to evaluate the role of extracellular transmission of infection in virus persistency in YAC cells, anti-MHV$_3$ Ab was added during 4 successive passages at a final concentration of 1:25. Free or cell-associated virus was not recovered after the first passage and the number of fluorescent cells progressively decreased. No evidence of viral infection was detected in subsequent passages after extensive washings followed by culture in antibody-free medium. Results obtained with anti-MHV$_3$ Ab treatment are in favor of a horizontal transmission as the route of viral persistency in YAC cell cultures. This was further evidenced by the absence of viral informations detected in cell clones, indicating that clone producing cells either underwent abortive infection without effect on clone growth, or have never been infected. These data indicate, therefore, that persistent infection induced by MHV$_3$ in lymphoid cell lines is characterized by a viral "carrier state" where production of infectious viral particles remains in equilibrium with cell permissivity.

Properties of MHV$_3$ isolated from persistently infected YAC cells

Several viral factors have been involved in the establishment and maintenance of persistent infections, such as defective interfering particles, occurrence of thermosensitive mutants, antigenic drift or interaction between selection of viral mutants and interferon system.

In order to study the viral properties, virus cloning was performed on virus progeny derived from persistently infected YAC and L2 cells.

Parental virus and MHV$_3$ from persistently infected YAC cells (YAC-MHV$_3$) were used as starting materials for the preparation of viral clones. Virus cloning was performed on L2 cells using the limit dilution assay at 48 hrs.

Thermosensitivity of cloned virus. Determination of thermosensitivity was carried out in L2 cells in microtitration plates, infected with cloned viruses (0.01 m.o.i.) and maintained in culture at 33°C, 37°C or 39.5°C for various times. Each titration was done in triplicate. A virus yield ratio was calculated according to the difference in virus titers obtained when cells were cultured at 2 different temperatures for 18 or 24 hours. Viral populations derived from L2 or YAC cells cultured at 33°C, 37°C and 39.5°C exhibited a heterogeneous pattern of thermosensitivity. Mean titers of cloned virus substrains derived from YAC cells cultured at the 3 different temperatures were similar to those obtained with cloned viruses isolated from L2 cells and cultured at the same temperature. For each cloned virus, a yield ratio was calculated according to the difference of virus titers observed for 2 temperatures tested. As shown in Table 1, a similar heterogeneity in yield ratios was observed when YAC-derived cloned substrains were compared to L2 derived cloned viruses. It is

Table 1.   Replication at different temperatures of viral clones isolated from MHV$_3$ infected L2 and YAC cells

Yield (log 10)	33°C - 37°C				37°C - 39.5°C			
	YAC-MHV$_3$ No. clones (%)		L2-MHV$_3$ No. clones (%)		YAC-MHV$_3$ No. clones (%)		L2-MHV$_3$ No. clones (%)	
-1	3	(7.5)	0	(0)	1	(3)	0	1
0	1	(2.5)	2	(13.3)	2	(6)	2	(18)
1	10	(25)	1	(6.7)	9	(28)	5	(45)
2	7	(17.5)	3	(20)	9	(28)	3	(27)
3	6	(15)	3	(20)	8	(25)	1	(9)
4	7	(17.5)	5	(33.3)	3	(9)	0	(0)
5	5	(12.5)	1	(6.7)	0	(0)	0	(0)
6	1	(2.5)	0	(0)	0	(0)	0	(0)
7	0	(0)	0	(0)	0	(0)	0	(0)
Total No. of clones tested	40		15		32		11	

1. Yield ratio was calculated according to the difference in virus titers obtained when cells were cultured at various temperatures for 18 hours (37°C -39.5°C) or 24 hours (33°C -37°C).

interesting to note that parental MHV$_3$ exhibited heterogeneous viral populations with respect to thermosensitivity. Viral heterogeneity was maintained in persistently infected YAC cell cultures and no selection of ts mutants appeared to be induced. Similar negative results were observed with neuroblastoma cells persistently infected with JHM virus where no ts mutants could be detected[9]. In addition, Lucas et al. have demonstrated that the rapid inhibition of MHV$_3$ and JHM viral synthesis resulting from a high temperature shift was not associated with the appearence of ts mutants but was related to host factors[10].

Defective-interfering (DI) particles and interferon. Sekellick and Marcus have proposed that initiation and maintenance of persistent infections in cell cultures, competent for the interferon system, may be related to the development of DI particles or virus mutants with an increased capacity of cells to induce interferon[15].

A volume of 0.1 ml of 10-fold dilutions of virus suspension was injected intraperitoneally (i.p.) into each of 3 adult C$_{57}$Bl/6 mice per dilution. The number of dead animals per group was recorded. For in vitro interference assay, different concentrations (10^2 to 10^4 TCID$_{50}$) of parental virus were mixed with 10^4 TCID$_{50}$ of a virus suspension obtained from persistently infected cell cultures (35 days postinfection). Interferon assay was carried out according to a published method[16] after destruction of viral infectivity by heat or irradiation. Neither interferon nor DI particles were detected in MHV$_3$ persistently infected YAC cell cultures. Similar negative results were obtained in persistent infections induced in vitro with other coronaviruses either in animal[10] or in human cell lines[17].

In vivo pathogenicity. Virus evolved from persistently infected cell cultures can differ from parental virus by virulence markers such as in vivo pathogenicity. The capacity of YAC cell-derived MHV$_3$ substrain to induce an acute disease upon injection into susceptible mice was tested. YAC cells were inoculated with 1 m.o.i. of parental MHV$_3$. In vitro virus titers as well as in vivo pathogenicity were determined in culture supernatants at various times postinfection. It was observed that eight days after infection, YAC cell culture supernatants had lost their property to induce an acute disease when injected into susceptible C$_{57}$Bl/6 mice. Subsequent in vivo experiments revealed that virus could be recovered, at low titers, during several months postinfection from peritoneal macrophages, liver and brain in animals infected in vivo with non-pathogenic (NP) virus.

In vivo pathogenicity of uncloned and cloned MHV$_3$ derived from YAC or L2 cells, was determined after subsequent passages carried out either in vitro on L2 cells or in vivo in susceptible mice. As shown in Table 2, YAC-MHV$_3$ which was devoid of in vivo pathogenicity property even

Table 2:   In vivo pathogenicity of YAC cell-derived MHV$_3$ after in vitro or in vivo passages.

Origin of cell-derived MHV$_3$ (No. of clones)	No. of passages (days)		In vivo pathogenicity[1]	
	In vitro	In vivo	No.survival/No. tested (%)	
			Newborns	Adults
YAC-MHV$_3$, uncloned	-	-	5/7 (71)	19/19 (100)
YAC-MHV$_3$, cloned (21)	2 (2)	-	11/135 (8)	21/21 (100)
YAC-MHV$_3$, cloned, (4)	4 (4)	-	ND[2]	5/15 (33)
YAC-MHV$_3$, uncloned	-	1 (4)	ND	1/3 (33)
L2-MHV$_3$, uncloned	-	-	ND	0/15 (0)
L2-MHV$_3$, cloned (14)	2 (2)	-	ND	0/42 (0)

1.   0.1 ml of culture supernatant was injected i.p. in C57Bl/6 mice. In all experiments, virus titers as determined in vitro ranged from 10^5 to 10^7/ml.

2.   ND: not done.

upon injection in newborns regained its ability to induce an acute disease after in vivo or in vitro passages. After 2 passages in L2 cells, YAC-MHV$_3$ became pathogenic for newborns but not for C$_{57}$Bl/6 adult mice, whereas pathogenicity was reached in the latter after 4 passages. Although NP-MHV$_3$ injection into susceptible mice led to the persistence of a virus which recovered its pathogenicity 4 days postinfection, it was surprising that infected animals did not succumb.

    In order to study the responsibility of persistency in the loss of in vivo pathogenicity, virus progeny derived from persistently infected embryonic cell cultures was tested. Viruses isolated from embryonic fibroblasts retained their in vivo pathogenic property even after 32 days of viral persistency. The loss of pathogenicity was related, therefore, not to the state of viral persistency itself, but rather to the origin of replicating cells as this was observed in lymphoid cells and not in fibroblasts. In addition, the rapid reversion to pathogenicity undergone by MHV$_3$ passaged into susceptible mice, suggests that viral pathogenicity may be regulated by the host.

CONCLUSION

Our work indicates that embryonic fibroblast cells originating from various mouse strains support MHV$_3$ replication which leads to in vitro persistency. In addition, a genetically determined sensitivity to MHV$_3$ infection in fibroblasts is expressed according to virus-induced cell lysis. Persistent infection induced by MHV$_3$ in lymphoid cell lines is characterized by a viral "carrier state" where production of infectious viral particles remains in equilibrium with cell permissivity. The ability of MHV$_3$ to induce in vitro persistent infections in lymphoid cell lines suggests that a similar mechanism may be involved in vivo. Carrier-type transmission of infection would also result, during the chronic phase of the disease, in atrophy of lymphoid organs leading to progressive development of immunodepression[5]. Conversely, high anti-MHV$_3$ antibody titers should block transmission of infection and cure the animals. During the chronic disease, a second and higher rise of anti-MHV$_3$ Ab levels occurs during the third month of infection. Although MHV$_3$ can easily be recovered from organs of infected mice during the first trimester of infection, after that time all usual methods of virus recovery failed[5]. Our results suggest that MHV$_3$ replication in lymphoid cell lines leads to induction or selection of variants which maintain in vitro pathogenicity but display reduced in vivo pathogenic effects. In addition, such variants are responsible for the development, in susceptible mice, of a subclinical infection. Persistent MHV$_3$ infection in lymphoid cell lines and in embryonic fibroblast cells represent an interesting model for studying virus-host cell interactions as well as cellular mechanisms involved in the resistance to virus-induced cell lysis and in the loss of pathogenicity. The in vivo significance, however, of the latter phenomenon has to be established and its existence in normal lymphocytes would be an observation of major importance.

REFERENCES

1.   Le Prevost, C., E. Levy-Leblond, J.L. Virelizier, and J.M. Dupuy. Immunopathology of mouse hepatitis virus type 3 infection. I. Role of humoral and cell mediated immunity in resistance mechanism. J. Immunol. 114: 221 (1975).

2.   Dupuy, J.M., E. Levy-Leblond, and C. Le Prevost. Immunopathology of mouse hepatitis virus type 3 infection. II. Effect of immuno-suppression in resistant mice. J. Immunol. 114: 226 (1975).

3.   Le Prevost, C., J.L. Virelizier, and J.M. Dupuy. Immunopathology of mouse hepatitis virus type 3 infection. III. Clinical and virologic observation of a persistent viral infection. J. Immunol. 115: 640 (1975).

4.   Levy-Leblond, E., D. Oth, and J.M. Dupuy. Genetic study of mouse sensitivity to MHV$_3$ infection: influence of the H-2 complex. J. Immunol. 122: 1359 (1979).

5.   Leray, D., C. Dupuy, and J.M. Dupuy. Immunopathology of mouse hepatitis virus type 3 injection. IV. MHV$_3$ induced immunosuppression. Clin. Immunol. Immunopathol. 23: 1457 (1982).

6.   Krzystyniak, K., and J.M. Dupuy. Early interaction between mouse hepatitis virus 3 and cells. J. Gen. Virol. 57: 53 (1981).

7.   Arnheiter, H., T. Baechi, and O. Haller. Adult mouse hepatocytes in primary monolayer culture express genetic resistance to mouse hepatitis virus type 3. J. Immunol. 129: 1275 (1982).

8.   Taguchi, F., S. Kawamura, and K. Fujiwara. Replication of mouse hepatitis viruses with high and low virulence in cultured hepatocytes. Infect. Immun. 39: 955 (1983).

9.   Lucas, A., M. Coulter, R. Anderson, S. Dales, and W. Flintoff. In vivo and in vitro models of demyelinating diseases. II. Persistence and host-regulated thermosensitivity in cells of neural derivation infected with mouse hepatitis and measles viruses. Virology 88: 325 (1978).

10.   Stohlman, S.A., and L.P. Weiner. Stability of neurotropic mouse hepatitis virus (JHM strain) during chronic infection of neuroblastoma cells. Arch. Virol. 57: 53 (1978).

11.   Ramseur, J.M., and R.M. Friedman. Prolonged infection of L cells with vesicular stomatitis virus. Defective interfering forms and temperature-sensitive mutants as factors in the infection. Virology 85: 253 (1978).

12.   Youngner, J.S., E.J. Dubovi, D.O. Quagliana, M. Kelly, and O.T. Preble. Role of temperature-sensitive mutants in persistent infections initiated with vesicular stomatitis virus. J. Virol. 19: 90 (1976).

13.   Bass, L.R., and F.M. Hetrick. Persistent infection of a human lymphocyte cell line (Molt-4) with the Kilham rat virus. J. Infect. Dis. 137: 210 (1978).

14.   Cummings, P.J., R.J. Lakomy, and C.R. Renaldo, Jr. Characterization of herpes simplex virus persistence in a human T lymphoblastoid cell line. Infect. Immun. 34: 817 (1981).

15.   Sekellick, M.J., and P.I. Marcus. Persistent infection. II. Interferon-inducing temperature sensitive mutants as mediators of cell-sparing: possible role in persistent infection by vesicular stomatitis virus. Virology 95: 36 (1979).

16.   Dahl, H., and M. Degré.   A microassay for mouse and human interferon. Acta. Path. Microb. Scand. Sec. B. 80: 863 (1972).

17.   Chaloner-Larson, G., and M. Johnson-Lussenburg. Establishment and maintenance of a persistent infection in L 132 cells by human coronavirus strain 229E. Arch. Virol. 69: 117 (1981).

CHARACTERIZATION OF MHV–A59 PERSISTENTLY INFECTED CELLS

Reinald Repp, Teruko Tamura, Hans-Dieter Klenk
and Heiner Niemann

Institut fuer Virologie, Fachbereich Humanmedizin der
Justus–Liebig–Universitaet Giessen, Frankfurter Str. 107
D 6300 Giessen, FRG

The aim of our work is to characterize MHV–A59 persistently infected cloned 17C11 cell lines on a molecular level. These cell lines were obtained by three consecutive infections of 17C11 cells (2 PFU/cell) and cloned three times by limited dilution in the presence of conditioned medium which contained 30 percent ultrafiltrated supernatant from 17C11 cells.

The obtained cell lines showed fusion area to a different extent and a reduced growth rate. None of them produced plaquing virus except the uncloned lines at an early passage number. At this stage small plaque mutants could be isolated. After cloning no intracellular particles could be detected by electron microscopy.

Dot blot hybridization with reverse transcribed viral cDNA showed the presence of virus specific RNAs. No hybridization was obtained with the DNA fraction.

All cell lines were resistant to MHV–A59 reinfection. Only the cloned lines were also resistant to infection with VSV.

   The   presence of virus specific proteins was shown   by
immunofluorescence using a mouse antiserum highly enriched for
anti El antibodies or monoclonal anti El. Unlike during lytic
infections the detected antigens were located in small clusters
outside the golgi area. (see Fig.1). From the sizes and location
these positively stained organelles might constitute lysosomes.

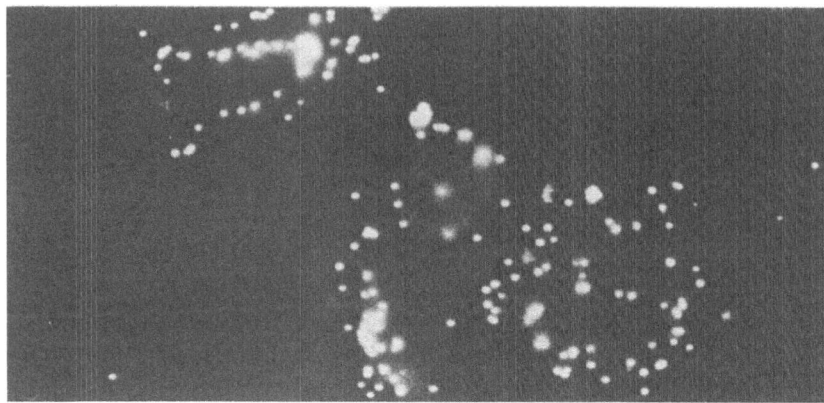

Fig.1. Intracellular clusters of viral antigens in persistently
       infected cloned cells (3iC2). Cells were incubated with
       mouse anti El and stained with FITC goat anti mouse. In a
       similar experiment a rabbit anti golgi serum kindly
       provided by Brian Burke, EMBL Heidelberg, FRG was added in
       a second step.

Table 1 shows a summary of the results:

TABLE I

CHARACTERIZATION OF THE CELL LINES

	Persistently infected cells uncloned	3iC1 cloned	3iC2 cloned	3iC3 cloned
Cell passage time (days)	7	7	7	7
Cell dilution at passsage	1:10	1:10	1:3	1:3
Need of conditioned medium	–	only during cloning	+	+
Cell fusion area	(+)	+	+++	++
Number of lytic crises (=CPE after passage)	2	–	–	–
Virus specific RNA	+	+	+	+
Virus specific DNA (tested in hybridization with reverse transcribed viral cDNA)	–	–	–	–
Expression of viral antigens (immunofluorescence)	+	+	++	++
Production of small plaque mutants	+ (at passage 12 earlier passages were not tested)	–	–	–
Intracellular virus particles	not tested	–	–	–
Resistance to MHV–A59 reinfection	+	+	+	+
Resistance to infection with VSV	–	–	+	+

FINE SPECIFICITY AND GENETIC RESTRICTION
OF T CELL CLONES SPECIFIC
FOR MOUSE HEPATITIS VIRUS, STRAIN JHM

Jerold G. Woodward, John O. Fleming, Glenn K. Matsushima,
Jeffrey A. Frelinger, and Stephen A. Stohlman

University of Southern California, School of Medicine
2025 Zonal Avenue, Los Angeles, CA 90033

INTRODUCTION

Mouse hepatitis viruses are members of the coronavirus group of animal viruses. Although named for their propensity to induce acute hepatitis in animals stressed by a variety of conditions, it has become clear that as a group they possess the ability to cause a diverse group of diseases in their natural host (Wege, et al, 1982). One strain of MHV, named JHM virus (JHMV), was isolated from mice found to have demyelinated lesions of the central nervous system (Bailey, et al, 1949). More recently it has been found that JHMV is not only capable of causing acute encephalomyelitis with demyelination but also chronic demyelination probably due to the establishment of a latent infection of oligodendroglia, the cells of myelin within the central nervous system (Herndon, et al, 1975; Stohlman and Weiner, 1981).

In our attempts to understand the role of the host in the establishment and maintance of latent JHMV infection and chronic demyelination we first examined a panel of inbred mice and found that only one, SJL, of the 13 strains tested was resistant to JHMV infection (Stohlman and Frelinger, 1978). Backcross analysis using two H-2 identical strains, SJL and B10.S, indicated that two genes were required for resistance. One of these genes is dominant, designated Rhv-1, and one is recessive, designated Rhv-2. This analysis using two strains of mice identical at the major histocompatibility complex is compelling evidence that H-2 linked genes are not involved in conferring resistance to JHMV. Inspite of the lack of H-2 linkage, resistance to fatal disease in SJL mice is abolished by X-irradiation, suggesting that the cell-mediated immune system plays a crucial role in protection (Stohlman, unpublished data).

331

In susceptible mice, which in opposition to SJL, become latently infected following survival from the acute encephalomyelitis, we have also found suggestive evidence that cell-mediated immunity plays a crucial role in protection from acute disease. First, we have found, as have others (M. Happel, personal communication), that anti-viral antibody is incapable of protecting mice from acute JHMV encephalomyelitis. Second, we found that mice immunized by intraperitoneal injection with JHMV were refractory to intracranial infection with JHMV by 4 days post immunization. Additional evidence has accumulated that antibody is capable of interacting with the viral proteins on the surface of infected cells resulting in the cessation of production of infectious virus (Stohlman and Weiner, 1978). Virus persists in these cells even after the removal of the anti-viral antibody, suggesting that antibody is not effective in protection and in fact it may be a very detrimental host response leading to the establishment of latently infected cells in the CNS.

In order to better characterize the mechanisms of host resistance to JHMV infection we have produced T cell clones reactive to JHMV antigens. In this paper, we describe the detailed analysis of four T cell clones in terms of antigen specificity, genetic restriction and capacity to function in the delayed type hypersensitivity response to JHMV antigen.

MATERIALS AND METHODS

Mice: The C57BL/6 (B6) mice immunized to obtain the T cell clones were obtained from Jackson Laboratories, Bar Harbor, MA, at 6 weeks of age and used immediately. All other mice used in this study were bred and housed in the Immunogenetics mouse colony, University of Southern California, School of Medicine.

Virus: The plaque purified small plaque variant of the neurotropic JHM strain of MHV was used throughout. The isolation and propagation of this virus, designated JHMV-DS, have been previously described (Stohlman, et al, 1982). The immunogen for these studies was prepared by infecting 5 x 150 cm tissue culture plates of DBT cells with JHMV-DS at an MOI of approximately 0.1. At complete viral induced fusion (14-16 hrs post infection) the cell sheets were first washed 2x with sterile PBS and then the cells were removed from the plates by scraping. The cells from each plate were placed in 5 ml of PBS, sonicated, and the resulting suspension clarified by centrifugation at 500 x g for 10 min. The clarified sonicate was stored at -70°C. Uninfected monolayers of DBT cells processed in a like manner served as control antigen. Infected cell lysates were prepared from two additional viruses, MHV-A59 and MHV-2. The lysates were prepared as described above except that the MOI used was 1.0. The lysates were prepared from MHV-A59 cells at 8 hrs post infection and from MHV-2 infected cells at 24 hrs post infection.

Purified JHMV was prepared as previously described (Lai and Stohlman, 1978). Briefly, supernatant fluids from infected cultures were clarified by centrifugation at 10,000 x g for 30 min. The virus was pelleted through 20% sucrose by centrifugation for 2.5 hrs at 27,000 RPM in an Beckman SW28 rotor, resuspended, and banded by centrifugation on a 20-42% sucrose gradient at 40,000 RPM for 2 hrs.

Isolation of T cell clones: B6 mice were immunized in the hind footpads with JHMV antigen in Freund's complete adjuvant and 8 days later, their draining popliteal lymph nodes (DLN) were removed and teased into a single cell suspension. In early experiments, the proliferative capacity of these cells was determined by culturing 1×10^5 DLN cells in microtiter plate wells along with varying concentrations of JHMV or control antigen. Cell proliferation was determined by adding 1 uCi of ^{3}H-thymidine, specific activity 2 Ci per mM (New England Nuclear, Boston, Mass.), to each well 24 hrs prior to harvest. Cells were collected onto glass fiber filters, rinsed, dried and counted in a liquid scintillation counter. The medium used for all experiments was RPMI 1640 supplemented with 100 units/ml pencillin, 50 ug/ml streptomycin, mM glutamine, 5×10^{-5} M 2-mercaptoethanol and 10% fetal calf serum.

DLN cells destined for cloning were cultured in 24 well Linbro plates at a density of 3×10^6 DLN cells/well along with a dilution of JHMV antigen that gave optimum proliferation in the microplate assay, usually 1:100. After 4 days, blast cells were harvested, washed, and re-seeded in 24 well plates at a density of 1×10^5 cells/well containing 2 $\times 10^6$ irradiated (2000rads) syngenic spleen cells, and the optimum dilution of JHMV antigen.

After 4 additional days the T cells from this secondary stimulation were cloned at limiting dilution in 96 well plates in media containing 4×10^5 cells/well irradiated syngenic spleen cells, 5% semi-purified mouse Con A supernatant as a source of interleukin-2, and JHMV antigen. After 4 days at 37°C, each well received 50 ul of fresh medium containing the above additives. Colonies became visible after 8 days and were harvested after 10 days with a pasteur pipet. Cell clones were expanded in media containing the same additives and frozen in liquid nitrogen awaiting characterization. Clones 4B10 and 4G4 were derived from a cloning plate that received 1 cell/well and had 13 wells with positive growth, or a cloning efficiency of 13.5%. Clones 3B10 and 3C4 were derived from a plate that received 0.5 cells/well and had a 6 wells with positive growth or a cloning efficiency of 12.5%. All clones were recloned under the same conditions and colonies were taken from plates that had less than 33% positive wells.

In Vitro Proliferation Assay of T cell clones: T cell clones were seeded into 96 well microplates at a density of 2×10^4 T cells/well and cultured in the presence or absence of irradiated spleen cells (4×10^5/well) from various mouse strains and JHMV, MHV-2, MHV-A59 or control antigen. Cultures were pulsed on day 2 with 1 uCi of ^{3}H-thymidine and harvested on day 3 as described above.

Delayed type Hypersensitivity Response: Normal unimmunized mice from various strains were injected in both hind footpads with 2×10^5 T cell clones and either control antigen (left foot) or JHMV antigen (right foot) in a total volume of 20 ul. Footpad thickness was measured with calipers 24, 48 or 96 hours after injection. The data is expressed as the mean difference in footpad thickness (right - left) for groups of at least 4 mice $\pm$ standard error of the mean.

Inhibition of Proliferation by Monoclonal Antibodies: The proliferative response to JHMV was carried out as described above except that the wells received an additional 0.05 ml of medium containing the monoclonal antibody supernatants. The derivation and characterization of the JHMV-specific monoclonal antibodies has been previously described (Fleming, et al, 1983). Each monoclonal antibody was used at a final dilution of 1/32. The cultures were pulsed with ^{3}H-thymidine on day 2 and harvested on day 3 as described above.

RESULTS

Isolation of JHMV-Specific T Cell Clones: In order to determine the optimum conditions for the cloning of JHMV specific T cells, a series of preliminary experiments were conducted using DLN cells from JHMV immunized mice. Initially, mice were immunized in the hind footpads with JHMV antigen in Freund's complete adjuvant and their DLN cells tested for proliferation eight days later. The data in Table 1 show the response of DLN cells to a lysate of JHMV infected cells as compared to a lysate of uninfected cells (control antigen). Although there is some response over background to the control antigen, the response to JHMV antigen is almost an order of magnitude greater. In this experiment, a 1:800 dilution of antigen gave the maximal response, therefore we used this dilution for the subsequent expansion and cloning of JHMV specific T cells.

Table 1

PROLIFERATION OF DLN CELLS FROM MICE IMMUNIZED WITH JHM VIRUS[1]

Antigen Added to Culture	Dilution	Hours in Culture[2]		
		48	72	96
None	----	3,600	4,100	4,200
Control[3]	1/200	8,100	13,600	11,300
	1/800	9,200	17,200	15,800
JHM	1/200	30,000	70,300	22,400
	1/800	93,000	139,500	90,400

1. C57BL/6 mice were immunized 8 days previously with lysate of JHM virus infected cells in Freunds complete adjuvant.

2. Incorporation of ^{3}H-thymidine added 24 h prior to harvest. Results represent mean CPM of triplicate wells.

3. Control antigens represent whole cell lysate from uninfected DBT cells.

To establish the JHMV-specific T cell clones, DLN cultures were re-stimulated once with a 1:800 dilution of JHMV antigen and fresh antigen presenting cells (APC), then cloned at limiting dilution with antigen, APC, and interleukin-2, as described in Materials and Methods. Four of the fourteen clones established by this procedure were chosen for initial characterization.

The presence of Thy-1 and Ly alloantigens on the surface of all four JHMV-specific T cell clones was determined an antibody and complement mediated microcytotoxicity assay. All clones were positive for Thy-1 as well as the Ly1 marker. The clones were negative for the Ly 2,3 markers (data not shown). This phenotype is characteristic for the T helper subset of T cells whereas the $Ly1^-,2,3^+$ phenotype serves to distinguish the cytotoxic T cell subset (Swain, et al, 1981).

In vitro Genetic Restriction: One of the common characteristics of $Ly1^+$ helper T cells is that they recognize antigen only in association with I region gene products on the surface of the antigen presenting cells (APC) (Yano, et al, 1977). The Ia antigens involved in this recognition are encoded by 2 gene loci, which code for the subunits that make up the I-A and I-E molecules respectively. The Ia antigens show considerable polymorphism, and as shown in Table 2, there are 8 commonly used inbred strains of mice defining different H-2 haplotypes. We also used 3 recombinant strains, and a mouse strain derived from B6 with a mutation in the I-Aβ chain, B6CH-2^{bm12}.

Table 2

H-2 Haplotypes of Inbred Strains

Strain	K	I-A	I-E	D
		H-2 Subregion		
C57BL/6	b	b	b	b
B10.A	k	k	k	d
B10.S	s	s	s	s
B10.P	p	p	p	p
B10.Q	q	q	q	q
B10.M	f	f	f	f
B10.RIII	r	r	r	r
B10.D2	d	d	d	d
B10.A(4R)	k	k	b	b
B10.A(3R) or (5R)	b	b	k	d
B10.MBR	b	k	k	q
B6.CH-2^{bm12}	b	b*	b	b

Lower case letters indicate different alleles at the loci indicated.

*   Site of the bm12 mutation is the β chain of the I-A molecule. .

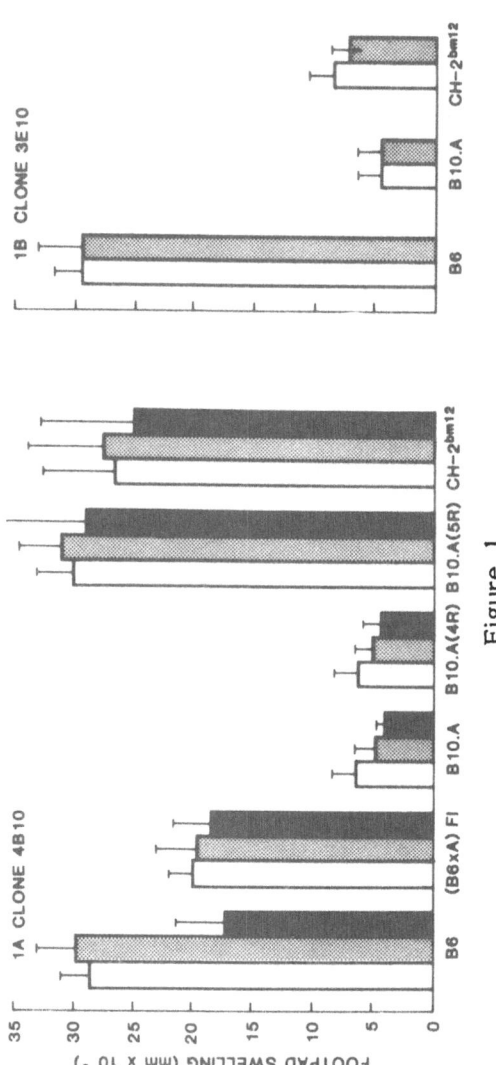

Figure 1

Delayed-Type Hypersensitivity elicited in nonimmune mice by the transfer of T cell clone 4B10 (1A) and clone 3E10 (1B) with viral antigen into the footpads of recombinant inbred strains of mice measured at 24, 48, and 96 hrs post transfer (1A) or 24 and 48 hrs (1B). Data is expressed as the mean and $\pm$ 1 std. deviation of the right foot, thickness (antigen) minus left foot thickness (control antigen) for groups of 4-6 mice.

We have utilized these inbred strains as donors of APC's to determine the Ia antigens required for the in vitro response of the 4 T cell clones. The data in Table 3 show that none of the T cell clones respond to antigen in the absense of added APC's. All clones respond quite well when B6 irradiated spleen cells as a source of APC are included along with JHMV antigen. However, none of the clones respond to JHMV antigen when presented on APC's derived from the 7 other independent haplotypes tested. These data demonstrate that the T cell clones show an absolute requirement for APC's and that they are genetically restricted to the H-2^b haplotype.

Table 3

Genetic Restriction of Antigen Presentation to
JHMV-Specific T Cell Clones

Irradiated Spleen Cells Added[2]	^{3}H-Thymidine incorporation of T cell clones cultured with and without JHMV antigen[1]							
	3E10		4B10		4G4		3C4	
	-	+	-	+	-	+	-	+
NONE	245	236	241	218	137	171	40	81
C57BL/6	421	36,543	240	82,165	347	36,520	108	21,600
B10.A	132	269	300	312	149	371	146	551
B10.S	113	165	332	1,429	97	133	47	109
B10.P	142	457	455	472	182	193	110	206
B10.Q	74	101	2,609	6,551	347	968	59	74
B10.M	49	47	256	251	174	413	58	95
B10.RIII	99	99	99	414	146	528	66	120
B10.D2	151	260	89	149	83	113	28	60
B10.A (4R)	130	696	56	309	263	557	39	156
B10.A (3R)	1,166	67,382	297	78,819	643	35,964	296	14,913
B10.MBR	89	302	14	377	93	154	55	100
B6.CH-2^{bm12}	243	233	242	32,309	434	9,815	59	107

1. T cell clones (2x10^4/well) were cultured with (+) or without (-) JHMV antigen (1:100 dilution) for 3 days. Results represent mean counts per minute of triplicate wells.

2. 2000 Rad irradiated spleen cells (4x10^5 cells/well) from the strains indicated were added at the begining of the culture period.

In order to determine whether the clones are restricted to the I-A or the I-E molecules, APC's from the recombinant inbred strains B10.A (3R) and B10.A (4R) were tested. Cells from B10.A (3R) but not B10.A (4R) were able to function as APC's in this system, indicating that the relevant I region molecule involved in presenting JHMV antigen to these T cell clones is the I-A molecule. Additional information was gained by using APC's from bm12 mice. This mutant strain differs from the wild type B6 only in a small region of the chain of the I-A molecule. As shown in Table 3, JHMV-specific T cell clone 4B10 responded well to JHMV antigen presented on bm12 APC's whereas clones 3E10 and 3C4 were totally

Table 4

Antigen Specificity of T Cell Clones

| T Cell Clone[1] | Control Cell Lysate | ^{3}H-thymidine incorporation in the presence of[2]: | | | Purified JHMV |
		JHMV	MHV-2	MHV-A59	
3E10	206	13,296	22,185	1,203	22,283
4B10	148	31,986	27,284	7,907	53,157
4G4	164	17,698	18,981	N.D.	N.D.
3C4	708	N.D.	N.D.	N.D.	14,522

1. T cell clones (2 x 10^4/well) were cultured in the presence of syngeneic (C57BL/6) irradiated spleen cells (4 x 10^5/well).

2. Cultures were pulsed on day 2 and harvested on day 3. Results represent mean CPM of triplicate wells. Antigen was diluted to 1:120 for purified JHM and 1:60 for the rest.

gp180/90. The other monoclonals specific for the viral nucleocapsid protein pp60 and the minor envelope glycoprotein gp25 had no effect on the proliferative response. These data suggest that the receptor on clone 3E10 may recognize antigenic determinants on the virion major envelope glycoprotein.

DISCUSSION

The rationale for producing JHMV-specific T cell clones is, in many ways, similar to the rationale for producing monoclonal antibodies. Because of the extremely fine specificity of binding, monoclonal antibodies are extremely useful for dissecting the functional and nonfunctional antigenic domains of individual proteins as well as for obtaining information on the role of humoral immunity in disease processes. In an analogous manner T cell clones allow the examination of the fine specificity of the antigens involved in the generation of the cell mediated immune response as well as the characterization of the individual T cell types participating in the immune response.

In our initial attempts to delve into the role of cellular immunity in the response to JHMV we have isolated fourteen independent JHMV antigen specific T cell clones and have characterized four of them. The

incapable of responding. Clone 4G4 gave a very weak response to JHMV presented on bm12 APC's. These data indicate that the bm12 mutation eliminated the sites on the I-A molecule required for antigen presentation to clones 3E10 and 3C4 but not for clone 4B10. Since the mutation in bm12 is in the β chain, these data suggest that clones 3E10 and 3C4 recognize JHMV antigen at least in part in association with the β chain whereas clone 4B10 recognizes JHMV antigen predominately in association with the α chain. Clone 4G4 may utilize a portion of the determinant affected by the bm12 mutation.

In vivo Genetic Restriction: Experiments were conducted to determine whether these JHMV-specific T cell clones could mediate a delayed type hypersensitivity (DTH) response in vivo. T cell clones in combination with either JHMV (right foot) or control antigen (left foot) were injected into the hind footpads of mice. The data in Figure 1a show that Clone 4B10 is capable of inducing a DTH response to JHMV only when the host shares the I-A subregion with B6. Thus, the same pattern of genetic restriction holds for the in vivo DTH response as is observed in the in vitro proliferative response. The data in Figure 1b show a similar result for clone 3E10. Furthermore, in agreement with the in vitro data in Table 3, clone 4B10 gives a positive DTH response in bm12 mice whereas 3E10 does not. Thus the in vitro proliferative response appears to accurately reflect the in vivo DTH response in terms of the genetic restriction of the T cell-APC interaction.

Antigen Specificity: It was important to determine whether these T cell clones were indeed specific for JHMV antigen. In preliminary experiments the T cell clones were re-titered with JHMV antigen and found to give optimal proliferation with dilutions of 1:60 to 1:100 (data not shown). The results in Table 4 show that all four clones proliferate in the presence of JHMV antigen and not with control antigen. In addition, three of these clones tested showed equivalent reponses when cultured with antigen prepared from MHV-2 infected cells. Two out of 2 clones tested also showed cross reaction with MHV-A59 antigen although considerably less than to JHMV or MHV-2. This is interesting in light of the fact that serologically, JHMV is more related to MHV-A59 than MHV-2. Finally, in order to rule out the possibility that the clones were responding to some cellular component or contaminant, JHMV was purified by sucrose gradient centrifugation and tested as an antigen. This preparation was in fact more effective at stimulating the clones and had a higher titer in dose response curves (data not shown).

The proliferative response to purified virus also indicated that the T cell clones recognize a virus structural protein and therefore monoclonal antibodies specific for these proteins were tested for their ability to inhibit proliferation. Figure 2 shows that the proliferation of three of the four clones was not inhibited by the presence of any of the anti-viral monoclonal antibodies. Clone 3E10, however, was inhibited by all three monoclonals tested which are specific for the envelope glycoprotein

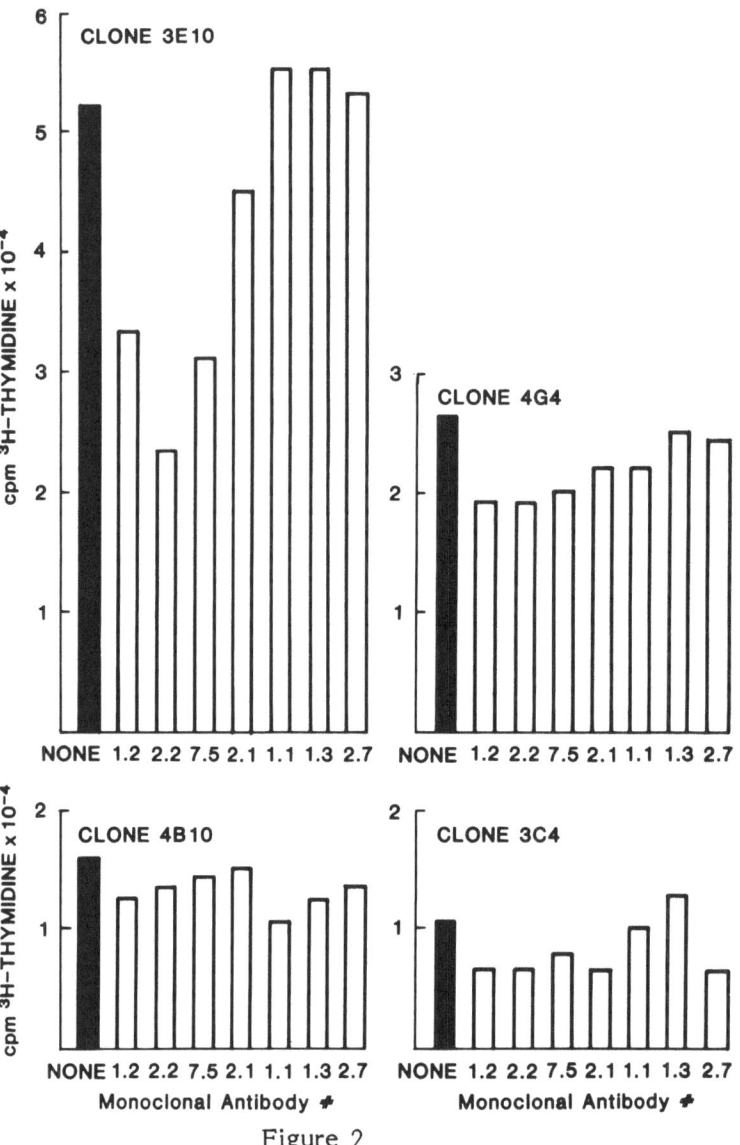

Figure 2

Inhibition of T cell clone proliferation by antigen-specific monoclonal antibody. T cell clones were cultured in the presence of antigen presenting cells, semi-purified IL-2, antigen, and monoclonal antibodies specific for viral antigens gp180 (monoclonals # 1.2, 2.2, and 2.7), pp60 (monoclonals # 2.1 and 1.1) and gp25 (monoclonals # 1.3 and 2.7). ³H-thymidine incorporation was determined at 3 days.

four clones all bear the classical "T helper cell" surface phenotype and exhibit an absolute requirement for both antigen presenting cells and the eliciting antigen. They also demonstrate a strict genetic restriction in that only APC's bearing I-A region gene products of the H-2^b haplotype function in the presentation of antigen to the T cell clones which were derived from the H-2^b C57BL/6 strain. In addition we have shown that the in vivo response is genetically restricted to the H-2^b I-A haplotype expressed on the endogenous APC's which is exactly analogous to the in vitro data presented. Finally, since the utility of the T cell clones would ultimately reside in their ability to remain functional in an in vivo setting we have shown that the four clones are capable of eliciting a delayed type hypersensitivity response.

The differential ability of the four T cell clones to recognize JHMV antigen in combination with the mutant Ia molecule expressed on the APC's derived from the B6CH-2^{dm12} mouse provides an indication that at least three of the four clones are distinct in terms of Ia receptor specificity. T cell clones 3E10 and 3C4 must have a receptor that recognizes the virus antigen in combination with a different portion of the I-A^b molecule than the 4B10 clone since the former clone cannot recognize JHMV antigen in combination with the mutant I-A^b while the latter clone does. The receptor on clone 4G4 probably represents a third distinct recognition site since it responds partially to JHMV antigen presented on bm12 APC's. This fine specificity of T cell clones to recognize determinants on the Ia molecule in conjunction with antigen was first demonstrated by Kimoto and Fathman (1980) and appears to be a general property of helper T cell clones which all show genetic restriction to the Ia molecule.

The ability of our T cell clones to induce a DTH reaction correlates well with results from other labs using various T cell-antigen combinations (Bianchi, et al, 1981; Weiss and Dennert, 1981). A large body of evidence has accumulated concerning the mechanism of this response. Antigen injected into the footpad becomes rapidly bound to Ia bearing APC's, either tissue macrophages, dendritic cells or Langerhans cells. Since the T cell clones are injected into the same site as antigen, specific Ia restricted recognition occurs resulting in proliferation and lymphokine release by the T cells. The lymphokine release results primarily in the infiltration of monocytes resulting in a demonstrable DTH type reaction.

The other facet of the signal required for a T cell proliferative response is the particular JHMV antigen recognized in combination with the Ia molecule. We have initiated three experimental avenues to examine this question. The first was to use antigens prepared from serologically distinct strains of MHV. The antigen prepared from MHV-A59 infected cells was able to stimulate some proliferation in the two clones tested. The antigen prepared from MHV-2 infected cells was recognized as efficiently as JHMV antigen, indicating that the antigenic domain recognized by the T cell clones is very conserved in MHV-2 and was less conserved in MHV-A59. The second avenue was to test the ability of gradient purified virus to be recognized by the T cell clones. All three clones tested responded to purified virus. This information indicates that the T cell clones are responding to virus structural proteins or a derivitivae of these produced by antigen processing and not to virus-specified nonstructural proteins found in the cell lysate used as an antigen.

These data therefore indicate that the proliferation induced by MHV-2 is induced by cross-reactive antigenic determinants on a virus structural protein. To examine the relative conservation of the viral proteins, a panel of monoclonal antibodies specific for the JHMV virion proteins was tested for their ability to bind to other MHV strains. These data show that the pp60 and gp25 proteins are relatively conserved, while the envelope glycoprotein gp180/90 is relatively unique. This finding led to our third approach to defining the viral antigen recognized in association with Ia. T cell proliferation assays were carried out in the presence of a number of monoclonal antibodies specific for the virus structural protein. The proliferation of three of the T cell clones was not inhibited by any of the monoclonal antibodies tested. Clone 3E10, however, was inhibited by three monoclonals (J1.2, J2.2, and J7.5) all directed against the gp180/90 envelope glycoprotein. Neither the monoclonal antibodies directed against pp60 (J2.1 and 1.1) nor those reactive with the minor envelope glycoprotein gp25 (J1.3 and 2.7) inhibited proliferation. Although the proliferative response was not completely inhibited, these data indicate that T cell clone 3E10 recognized the virion major envelope glycoprotein in association with Ia.

This work is only beginning and a large number of questions remain. We have shown that the helper T cell clones we have isolated have retained some aspects of their ability to function in vivo. The role of the various subpopulations of T cells during JHMV infection remains to be elucidated but these clones will allow a unique possibility to examine directly the role of a specific T cell population in protection from acute viral encephalomyelitis and give insight into the delicate balance between completely clearing an infection and the establishment of chronic disease. It should also be possible, either by directly inhibiting proliferation or by using immunoaffinity columns, to define the viral antigens recognized in conjunction with Ia for the stimulation of the helper T cell population.

ACKNOWLEDGEMENTS

    This work was supported by grant NS 18146 from the National Institutes of Health. J.A.F. is the recipient of an American Cancer Society Faculty Research Award. The authors wish to express their gratitude to Raymond L. Mitchell for editorial assistance.

REFERENCES

- Bailey, O.T., Pappenheimer, A.M., Cheever, F.S., and Daniels, J.B. (1949). A murine virus (JHMV) causing disseminated encephalomyelitis with extensive destruction of myelin. II. Pathology. J. Exp. Med. 90:195-212.
- Bianchi, A.T., Hooijkass, H., Benner, R., Tees, R., Nordin, A., and Schreier, M. (1981). Clones of helper T cells mediate antigen-specific, H-2 restricted DTH. Nature 290:62-63.
- Fleming, J., Stohlman, S., Harmon, R., Lai, M., Frelinger, J., and Weiner, L. (1983). Antigenic relationship of murine coronaviruses: Anaylsis using monoclonal antibodies to JHM (MHV-4) virus. Virology in press.
- Herndon, R.M., Griffin, D.E., McCormick, U., and Weiner, L.P. (1975). Mouse hepatitis virus-induced recurrent demyelination. Arch. Neurol. 32:32-35.
- Kimoto, M., and Fathman, C.G. (1980). antigen reactive T cell clones. I. Transcomplementing hybrid I-A-region gene products function effectively in antigen presentation. J. Exp. Med. 152:759-769.
- Lai, M.M.C., and Stohlman, S.A. (1978). The RNA of mouse hepatitis virus. J. Virol. 26:236-242.
- Stohlman, S.A., and Frelinger, J.A. (1978). Resistance to fatal central nervous system disease by mouse hepatitis virus strain JHM. I. Genetic Analysis. Immunogenetics. 6:277-281.
- Stohlman, S.A., and Weiner, L.P. (1978). Stability of neurotropic mouse hepatitis virus (JHM strain) during chronic infection of neuroblastoma cells. Arch. Virol. 57:53-61.
- Stohlman, S.A., and Weiner, L.P. (1981). Chronic central nervous system demyelination in mice after JHM virus infection. Neurol. 31:38-44.
- Stohlman, S.A., Brayton, P.R., Fleming, J.O., Weiner, L.P., and Lai, M.M.C. (1982). Murine coronaviruses: Isolation and characterization of two plaque morphology variants of the JHM neurotropic strain. J. Gen. Virology 63:265-275.
- Swain, S.L., Dennert, G.L., Wormsley, S., and Dutton, R.L. (1981). The Lyt phenotype of a long-term allospecific T cell line. Eur. J. Immunol. 11:175-180.
- Wege, H. Siddell, S. and ter Meulen, V. (1982). The biology and pathogenesis of coronaviruses. Curr. Tpics Microbiol. Immunol. 99:165-200.
- Weiss, S., and Dennert, G. (1981). T cell lines active in the DTH reaction. J. Immunol. 126:2031-2035.
- Yano, A., Schwartz, K.W. and Paul, W.E. (1977). Antigen presentation in the murine T lymphocyte proliferative response. I. Requriement for genetic identity at the major MHC. J. Exp. Med. 146:828-842.

THE IMMUNE RESPONSE TO MOUSE HEPATITIS VIRUS:

GENETIC VARIATION IN ANTIBODY RESPONSE AND DISEASE

Gary A. Levy[1], Robert Shaw[1], Julian L. Leibowitz[2]
and Edward Cole[1]

[1]Department of Medicine, University of Toronto,
Toronto, Ontario, Canada M4N 3M5
[2]Department of Pathology, University of California
at San Diego, La Jolla California 92093

Coronaviruses are a group of enveloped RNA viruses
which can produce a broad spectrum of diseases in their
natural hosts (1,2). These diseases include
encephalitis, hepatitis, interstitial pneumonitis,
nephritis and enteritis (3). The nature and the
severity of the resultant disease varies with the age
and the genetic background of the host, the route of
infection and the size of the virus inoculum.
Murine hepatitis virus type 3 (MHV-3) produces three
distinct patterns of disease in genetically dissimilar
inbred strains of mice. Normal adult mice of the A
strain are totally resistant to MHV-3, whereas Balb/cJ,
NZB, C57 and DBA/2 mice are all fully susceptible to
the virus and die of fulminant hepatic necrosis (4).
C3H/ebFeJ mice develop an acute hepatitis which then
progresses to chronic viral persistence with focal
hepatic inflammation and granulomatous formation (5).
It has recently been recognized that cellular elements
of the immune system are extremely important to the
host°s survival and the elimination of virus (6-8).
Cells of the monocyte/macrophage series play a vital
role in the resistance to a number of viral infections
(9). For example, the age dependent resistance to
herpes simplex virus is probably due to the inability
of the virus to replicate in the adherent cells of the
adult mice which prevents the initial multiplication
and dissemination of the virus (10). H-2 restricted

cytotoxic T-lymphocytes appear 4 days after the initial
infection and their actions peak at one week after the
primary infection (11,12). Natural killer cells have
been reported to be involved in antiviral activity
(13), interferons have been shown capable of inhibiting
herpes simplex virus multiplication in-vitro (14) and
injections of anti-interferon serum increases the
mortality (15). Observations made in murine hepatitis
infection have led to the conclusion that resistence is
dependant upon cellular immunity and specifically on
the presence of a suitable number of functionally
capable macrophages and T lymphocytes (16).

Viruses are strongly antigenic and elicit the
sequential production of IgM, IgG and IgA antibodies
during infection (17). These antibodies may inactivate
and participate in the clearance of viruses either
directly or in concert with complement and/or lymphoid
cells. The formation of antibody-virus complexes and
the resulting viral neutralization have been reported
in conjunction with a number of viral systems (18).
Antibody, by binding to the surface of a virion may
neutralize viral infectivity by several mechanisms: (1)
antibodies may bind to viral structures involved in the
adherence of the virus to a potentially susceptible
cell and thus prevent adsorption; (2) antibody may bind
to virions in a way that allows adsorption but prevents
penetration and uncoating; (3) antibody coated virions
may be taken up and degraded by macrophages which might
be otherwise permissive to the infection and (4)
antibody on the surface of the virion may activate the
complement system and or cellular elements of the
lymphoid system with resultant elimination of virus
particles.

Little attention has been directed towards the
potential role of the humoral response to MHV
infection. The studies presented here were designed
to measure the primary antibody response to MHV
infection, to determine both class and subclass
specificities of antibody response and to determine
whether the passive administration of high titered
antibodies had any effect on the course of the disease
in both semi-susceptible and fully susceptible mice.

MATERIALS AND METHODS

Cells

17 CL 1, DBT and L2 cells were grown as previously

described (17). The cells were propagated in Dulbecco°s
modified Eagles medium (DMEM) (Flow Laboratories Inc.,
Rockville, Md.) supplemented with 10% new born calf
serum (Flow Laboratories) and 25 µg/ml
chlortetracycline hydrochloride grade II (Sigma
Chemical Co., St. Louis, Mo) and buffered with 15 mM
Hepes, 3-(N-morpholine-3-propanesulfonic acid) N-tris
(hydroxymethyl)-3-methyl-2-aminoethane sulfonic acid
and 4 mM glutamine (Sigma Chemical Co.)

Virus

The origin and growth of MHV-3 has previously been
described (17). MHV-3 was obtained from the American
Tissue Type Culture Collection (Rockville, Md) and was
plaque purified twice on monolayers of DBT cells and
seed stocks prepared.
Working stocks were grown in 17CL1 cells and the virus
was assayed on monolayers of L2 cells in a standard
plaque assay as previously described (17).

Viral Purification

Following growth to high titers on monolayers of 17 CL1
cells, the virus was harvested by one cycle of freeze-
thawing and clarified by centrifugation at 4,500 X g
for 1 hour at 4°C as previously described (18). The
supernatant was recovered and the virus was precipated
by adding to each 10 ml., 1.1 ml. of 5 M NaCl and 5.5
ml. 30% (W/V) PEG-6000 in MOPS-saline EDTA, pH 6.8
(10mM MOPS, 1mM EDTA, 15 M NaCl, Baker Scientific
Company, Philipsburg, N.J.) (18). The solution was
stirred on ice for 30 minutes and the virus pelleted by
centrifugation at 9,250 x g at 4°C for 30 minutes as
previously described (18). The pellet was resuspended
in a small volume of MOPS-saline-EDTA and purified in
sequential 5-25% and 10-40% K-tartrate gradients (18).
The fractions containing virus were pooled, diluted to
5 ml. with MOPS-saline EDTA and pelleted at 45,000 RPM
for 30 minutes at 4°C in a SW50.1 rotor (Beckman
Scientific Co., Toronto, Canada). The virus pellet was
resuspended in 0.5 ml carbonate buffer by three bursts
of sonication at 4°C and viral protein concentration
was determined in a modified Lowry assay as previously
described (17).

Plaque Neutralization Assay

Virus was assayed on monolayers of L2 cells in a
standard plaque assay as previously described (17). For
the determination of neutralizing antibody, heat
inactivated sera was incubated with 100 PFU of MHV-3
for 30 minutes at 4°C. 200 μl of the mixture were then
layered onto confluent monolayers of L2 cells in 6
well plastic culture dishes (Linbro Plastics, McLean,
Va.) for 30 minutes at 22°C and then overlayed with 1%
agarose in DMEM supplemented with 2% FCS. The plates
were incubated for 48 hours at 37°C in a 5% CO_2
incubator and then stained with 0.1 gm % crystal violet
in 20% ethanol for enumeration of plaques. The end
point of the assay was taken as the dilution of
antibody which reduced the number of plaques to 50% of
the control value.

Solid Phase Radioimmunoassay

Flexible 96 well microtiter plates were coated with 25
ng of purified MHV-3 which was diluted in 100 μl of
carbonate buffer pH 9.6. The plates were then incubated
overnight at 4°C in a humid chamber. The antigen was
crosslinked using 10 μl of a 10 mg/ml solution of 1-
ethyl-3-(3-dimethylaminopropyl) carbodiimide HCl. The
next day the plate was washed repeatedly with 200 μl
aliquots of 1% BSA, 0.05 % Tween-20 and 0.02% sodium
azide in phosphate buffered saline (PBS pH 7.4) (SPRIA
buffer). The carbodiimide was inactivated with 0.1 M
NH_4Cl for 1 hour and then the plate was repeatedly
washed with SPRIA buffer. Mouse antisera at a dilution
of 1/200 was added for 4 hours at room temperature,
removed and the plates were washed repeatedly with
SPRIA buffer. ^{125}I-labelled affinity purified goat
anti-mouse immunoglobulin (Spec. Act. 3.2 x 10^{10}
cpm/mg) was added and following an hour incubation the
plates washed and individual wells counted in a gamma
counter. Appropriate positive and negative control sera
were included in all assays as controls.

Radioimmunoprecipitation

Confluent monolayers of DBT cells were grown on 6 well-
plastic tissue culture plates. The cells were infected

at a high multiplicity of infection (M.O.I. 10) with MHV-3 and were then incubated at 22°C for 60-90 minutes. Unabsorbed virus was removed and the monolayers were covered with 2 ml of ADME-2 containing 5 μg/ml of actinomycin D. The plates were left to incubate at 37°C until 30% syncytia were present. The media was then removed, the cells washed twice with methionine free medium and 0.5 ml of methionine free ADME-2 containing 5 μg/ml actinomycin D and 250 μCi of ^{35}S-methionine (Amersham Scientific, Toronto, Canada) were added. The plates were left to incubate until completely covered with syncytia. The plates were then rinsed gently twice with PBS and then once with reticulocyte standard buffer (RSB 10 mM Tris, 10mM NaCl, 1.5 mM $MgCl_2$) and then the cells were lysed with 200 ul of RSB containing 0.5% NP-40, 0.1% SDS and 1% aprotinin.

An aliquot of lysate (5 μl) was added to 10 μl of mouse serum for 30 minutes on ice, then 100 μl of formalin fixed 10% (V/V) protein A bearing staphylococcus aureus (Cowan I) was added for 30 minutes and the mixtures brought to 400 μl with RSB. The sample was centrifuged at 12,000 RPM x 4 minutes and the pellet recovered and washed an additional 4 times. The pellet was then dissolved in 50 μl of tracking buffer and applied to a lane of a 10% sodium dodecyl sulfate (SDS) polyacrylamide gel. Following electrophoresis, the gels were developed for fluorography and autoradiography.

Antibody Subclass Determination

In order to determine antibody class and subtype responses, a standard commercially available enzyme linked immunosorbent assay system (ELISA) was utilized. Microtiter plates were coated with 20-50 ng of purified MHV-3 as described previously (18). Following post coating with a standard bovine albumin solution, 50 μl of a dilution of a mouse serum was added. Following a 2 hour incubation, the excess serum was removed, the plates were washed and 50 μl of rabbit anti- mouse IgA (Fc), IgG_1, IgG_{2a}, IgG_{2b}, IgG_3 and IgM (Fc) were added and left for 2 hours. The plates were washed and 50 μl of peroxidase labelled goat anti-rabbit IgG antibody was added to each well and left to incubate at room temperature for 1 hour. 100 μl of freshly prepared ABTS-H-2 was added to each well and left for 30 minutes. The results were quantitated by measuring the optical density of each well at 415 nm in an automated spectrophotometer (Flow Laboratories, Mississauga, Ontario).

RESULTS

Immune Response To Infection With MHV-3

The immune response of inbred strains of mice infected intra-peritoneally (i.p.) with 10^3 plaque forming units (PFU) of MHV-3 were determined by four different assay procedures; radioimmunoassay (RIA), plaque neutralization assay, an enzyme linked immunosorbent assay (ELISA) and by radioimmunoprecipitation (RIP).
We first examined the development of antibody during the course of primary infection with MHV-3. Balb/cJ, C3H/ebFeJ and A/J male mice, 6-8 weeks of age were infected with 10^3 PFU of MHV-3 i.p.. Blood was obtained daily for up to three months following infection or until death. All mice were pre-bled and tested for antibody to MHV and positive mice were eliminated from the study. Antibody levels were determined in a standard RIA as described previously (18). No antibody was detected in the serum of Balb/cJ mice throughout the course of the infection. In contrast, antibody was detected as early as 4 days p.i. in the A/J mice and the levels increased to maximal titers by day 5-7. The antibody titers remained high for up to three months (fig 1). In the semisusceptible C3H mice, there was a marked delay in the appearance of antibody as compared to the A/J mice with no antibody detected until day 10. The titer rose to high levels by day 11-12 and remained at these high levels throughout the course of the infection (fig 1).

Nature of the Antibody Response

Neutralizing antibody was determined in a standard plaque reduction assay (17). No neutralizing antibodies were detected in sera from MHV infected Balb/cJ mice while high titers of neutralizing antibody to MHV were detected in the A/J mice by day 2-3 and this antibody persisted for 60-90 days p.i. at high levels. These results correlated well with the data obtained by RIA (fig 1). In contrast, despite the detection by RIA of high titered antibody in the C3H mice, there was only weak neutralizing antibody detected at day 12 with no increase in titer until death at 3-4 months p.i. (fig 2).

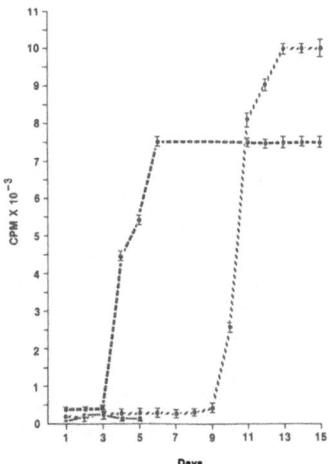

Figure 1. Antibody responses to MHV-3 infection in inbred strains of mice by radioimmunoassay (RIA). Sera at a dilution of 1/200 from Balb/cJ mice (━━━━), A/J mice (•••••••••••) and C3H mice (━▬▬▬━) were assayed in a standard RIA for the presence of antibody to MHV-3.

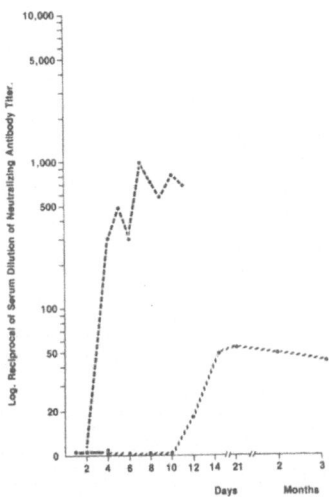

Figure 2. Neutralizing antibody titers to MHV-3 in inbred strains of mice. Heat inactivated sera from Balb/cJ (━━━━), A/J (•••••••••••) and C3H mice (▬▬▬▬) were analysed for the presence of neutralizing antibody in a standard plaque reduction assay.

The Specificity of the Response to Viral Structural
Proteins

To determine the antigenic site to which the antibodies
were directed, antisera were analysed by
radioimmunoprecipitation (RIP) to a ^{35}S-methionine
labelled MHV lysate as previously described (18). DBT
cells were infected with MHV-3 and labelled from 6-18
hours p.i. with ^{35}S-methionine. The cell lysate was
prepared as described previously and the lysate
electrophoresed on a 10% polyacrylamide gel and
fluorographs prepared as described previously (18). E2
glycoprotein (180,000 daltons), nucleocapsid protein
(50-60,000 daltons) and E1 glycoprotein (20-24,000
daltons) were easily distinguished in the MHV-3 lysates
as compared to the mock infected lysates (fig 3,4).
When A/J sera were analysed, reactivity to nucleocapsid
and E2 glycoprotein were seen as early as 2 days p.i
(fig 3). This correlated with the finding of
neutralizing antibody seen in the plaque reduction
assay on day 2-3. Increased reactivity especially to
the E2 glycoprotein was seen by day 5 and by day 13-15
p.i., antibodies to E2, E1 and nucleocapsid proteins
were found in high quantities (fig 3).
In contrast, in sera from the C3H mice, antibody could
only be detected at day 14 by RIP and was only directed
to the nucleocapsid protein (fig 4). By day 21 a strong
anti-nucleocapsid response was seen with a weak
response to E2 glycoprotein (fig 4). This correlated
well with the results both from the RIA and the plaque
neutralization assays in which a strong antibody
response was observed by day 14 but only a very weak
titer of neutralizing antibody was detected. Reactivity
to nucleocapsid protein increased by day 34 and
persisted until death of the animals at 90-120 days
p.i. At day 34 a weak E2 glycoprotein response was
found and by day 90 weak E2 and E1 responses could be
seen on the RIP (fig 4).

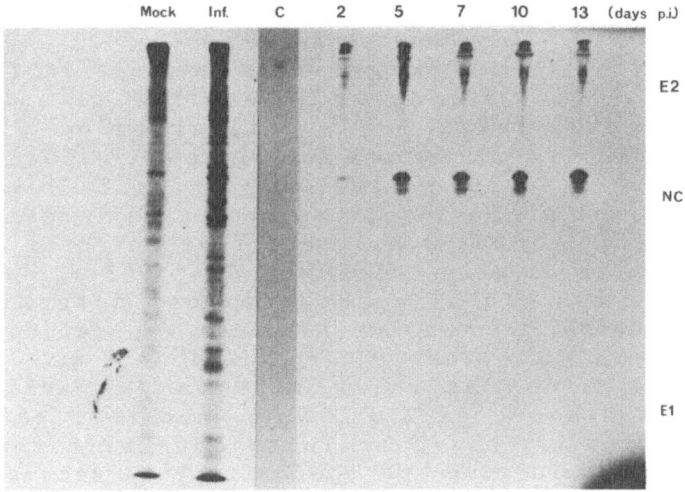

Figure 3. Polyacrylamide gel analysis of antibody response of A/J mice to MHV-3 infection. Lane 1, mock infected lysate. Lane 2 MHV-3 infected lysate demonstrating E2 glycoprotein (mw 180,000 daltons), nucleocapsid protein (nc) (mw 60,000 daltons) and E1 glycoprotein (mw 20-24,000 daltons). Lane 3-7 are radioimmunoprecipitations of sera from control, 2, 5, 7, 10 and 14 days post MHV-3 infected A/J mice.

Figure 4.
Polyacrylamide
gel analysis of
antibody re-
sponse of C3H
mice to viral
proteins fol-
lowing MHV-3
infection.
Lane 1 mock
infected ly-
sate, Lane 2
MHV-3 infec-
ted lysate

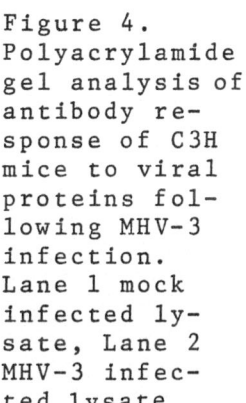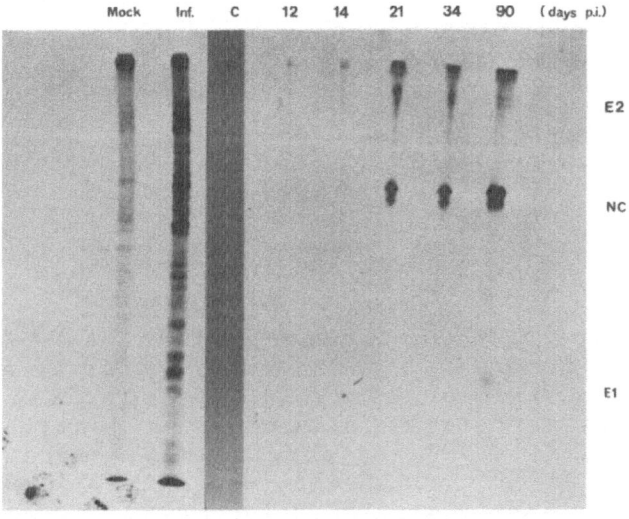

demonstrating E2 glycoprotein (mw 18,000 daltons), nucleocapsid protein (nc) (mw 60,000 daltons and E1 glycoprotein (mw 20-24,000 daltons). Lane 3-7 are radioimmunoprecipations of sera from control (C), 12, 14, 21,34 and 90 days post MHV-3 infected C3H mice.

Immunoglobulin Class Determination of Antibodies

Specificity of the immunoglobulin response in the sera
from A/J and C3H mice was determined in an enzyme
linked immunosorbent assay (ELISA) using affinity
purified rabbit anti mouse IgG_1, IgG_{2a}, IgG_{2b}, IgG_3,
IgA (Fc) and IgM (Fc) probes as previously described.
Individual wells of microtiter plates were coated with
25 ng of purified MHV-3 and sera from infected animals
was added at a dilution of 1/50. Identification of the
specific immunoglobulin response was determined as
described above. A positive response was defined as an
optical density of greater than 0.2 at 415 nm.
In the A/J mice, an early rise in IgA anti MHV-3
antibody was detected 2 days p.i. and this persisted
until 7 day p.i. This correlated both with the acute
phase of the infection and the ability to recover virus
from livers and serum of A/J mice. IgM anti-MHV-3 was
also detected at day 2 and this persisted until 13 days
p.i (fig 5). By day 25, IgM was no longer detected
(data not shown). A strong IgG_{2a} response was observed
by day 7 and by day 13 an increase in IgG_1 was noted
(fig 5).

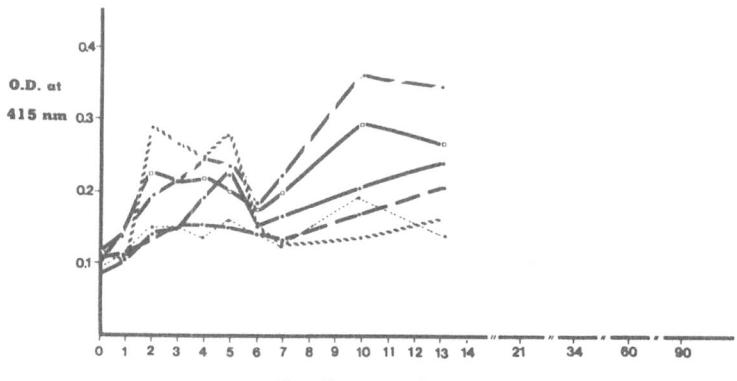

Figure 5. Immunoglobulin subclass determinations in
sera from MHV-3 infected A/J mice by an enzyme linked
immunosorbent assay (ELISA). Individual wells of 96
well microtiter plates were coated with 25 ng of
purified MHV-3 and sera from A/J mice at a dilution of
1/50 added. Rabbit anti mouse IgG_1 (━ ━ ━ ━ ━ ━),
IgG_{2a} (━ ━ ━ ━), IgG_{2b} (━━━━━), IgG_3 (-- -- -- -- --)
IgM (━━━━━) and IgA (⁄⁄⁄⁄) was added and the
optical density (O.D.) determined at 415 nm.

When sera from C3H mice was analysed, an increase in
IgA anti-MHV-3 was observed during the acute infection
(days 2-7) which returned to normal by day 10 (fig 6).
By day 3, a marked increase in IgG_1 antibody was found
that remained elevated until the death of the animal at
3-4 months p.i. The IgM anti-MHV response was delayed
as compared to the A/J mice and was first detected at
11 days p.i. (fig 6). The IgM antibody level remained
elevated until the animals died at 3-4 months p.i. No
significant amounts of IgG antibody could be detected
in the sera from C3H mice, although on day 34 a
questionable rise in IgG_{2a} and IgG_{2b} was noted. By day
90 the titers of these antibodies had not increased and
was only barely detectable (fig 6).

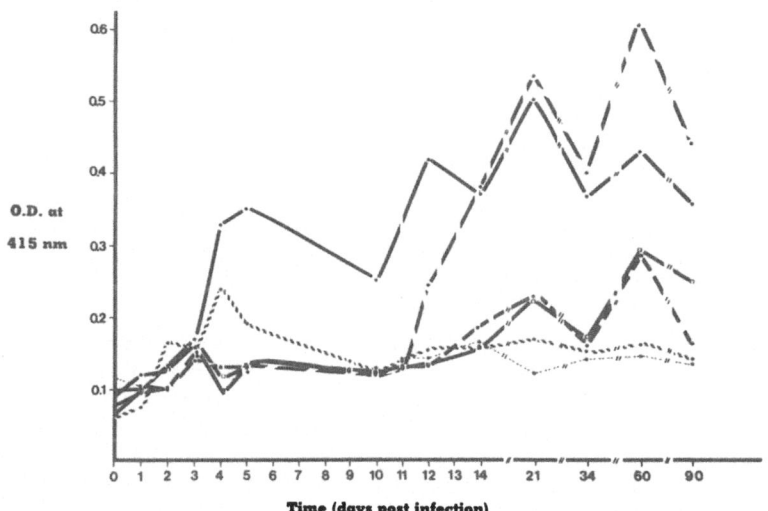

Figure 6. Immunoglobulin subclass determinations in
sera from MHV-3 infected C3H mice by ELISA. Individual
wells were coated with 25 ng of MHV-3, sera from C3H
mice added at a dilution of 1/50 and rabbit anti mouse
IgG_1 (▬ ▬ ▬ ▬), IgG_{2a} (▬▬ ▬▬), IgG_{2b} (▬▬▬▬▬▬),
IgG_3 (-- -- --), IgA (▰▰▰▰) and IgM (▬▬ ▬▬) was added
and the optical density (O.D.) determined at 415 nm.

No antibody was detected in the sera from the Balb/cJ mice in the ELISA at any time during the infection (data not shown).

Effect of Transfer of Immune Serum on MHV Infection

To determine the effects of the transfer of high titered neutralizing antisera on the course of MHV infection in the susceptible Balb/cJ mice and the semi-susceptible C3H/ebFeJ mice, antisera from A/J mice that had been infected with 10^3 PFU of MHV-3 10-14 days earlier was collected and pooled. Balb/cJ and C3H mice (6-8 weeks of age) were infected with 10^3 PFU of MHV-3 i.p. and divided into three groups of animals with 10 mice in each group. Mice in group 1 were given 100 μl of normal saline as controls; mice in group 2 were given 100 μl of sera from A/J mice 2-4 hours p.i. and mice in the third group were given 100 μl of A/J sera 2-4 hours p.i. and a second dose 24 hours p.i. Serum was given by an intravenous injection through the tail vein. Mortality was determined and the livers were removed from the animals and viral titers determined in a standard plaque assay.

Balb/cJ mice infected with 10^3 PFU of MHV-3 were given 2 hours p.i. 100 μl of normal saline I.V. All died within 5 days of infection (fig 7). In contrast, mice that were given 1 injection of 100 μl of sera from A/J mice (group 2) showed an increased survival (fig 7). At 5 days p.i. when all control Balb/cJ mice had died, only 2 of the group 2 mice had died (20%) (fig 7). However, with no further treatment, only one of the mice survived longer than 10 days and died 14 days p.i. In the animals in group 3, no animals died by day 5 p.i. but by 10 days 50% of the animals (5 mice) had died and all of the animals were dead by 21 days p.i. (fig 7).

In studies on viral recovery and growth from the livers of infected animals, a 2 log decrease in maximal virus growth was found in livers from group 2 mice as compared to the livers from control Balb/cJ mice (fig 8); whereas the livers from animals that had received 2 doses of sera from A/J mice (group 3) had a 3 log decrease in viral titers as compared to the livers of the control mice (fig 8).

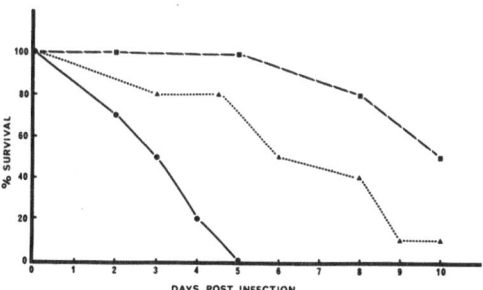

Figure 7. Effect of transfer of serum from A/J mice on the survival of susceptible Balb/cJ mice following MHV-3 infection. Balb/cJ mice were infected with 10^3 PFU of MHV-3 and then injected I.V. with 100 μl of normal saline (━━━━━━) 2 hours p.i., 100 μl of sera from A/J mice (∙∙∙∙∙∙∙∙∙∙∙∙) 2 hours p.i. or 2 injections of 100 μl of A/J sera (━∙━∙━∙━) 2 hours and 24 hours p.i.

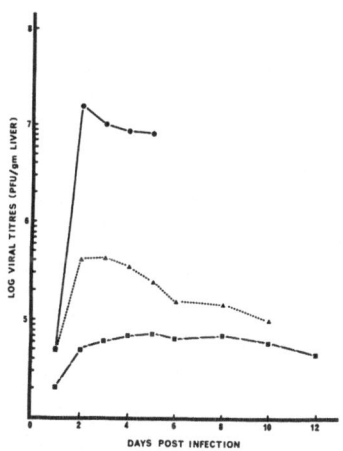

Figure 8. Effect of transfer of immune serum from A/J mice on recovery and growth of virus from the livers of MHV-3 infected Balb/cJ mice. Viral titers were determined in a standard plaque assay in homogenized livers from Balb/cJ mice which had been infected with 10^3 PFU of MHV-3 and were immunized with 100 μl of normal saline (━━━━━━), 100 μl of serum from A/J mice (∙∙∙∙∙∙∙∙∙∙) or 2 injections of 100 μl of serum from A/J mice (━━━━━━).

Control C3H mice (group 1) that were given 100 μl of
saline 2 hours p.i. had a 30% mortality during the
acute phase of the MHV-3 infection (Day 1-10) and all
of these animals developed viral persistence, chronic
liver disease and died within 3-4 months of infection.
In contrast, there were no deaths in any of the C3H
mice that had received 1 injection (group 2) or 2
injections of A/J sera p.i. All of the animals survived
and none of them developed chronic disease (fig 9).

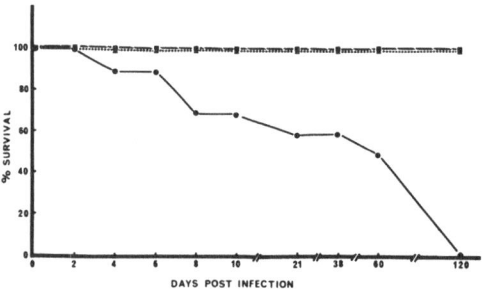

Figure 9. Effect of transfer of immune serum from A/J
mice on survival of semisusceptible C3H mice following
MHV-3 infection. C3H mice were infected with 10^3 PFU of
MHV-3 i.p. and immunized with 100 μl of normal saline 2
hours p.i. (——————), 100 μl of serum from A/J mice 2
hours p.i. (••••••••••••) or 2 injections of serum from A/J
mice 2 hours and 24 hours p.i. (————————).

Furthermore, we were unable to recover any virus from
the livers of the C3H mice that had received sera from
A/J mice in contrast to the high viral titers found in
the livers of control C3H mice (fig 10).

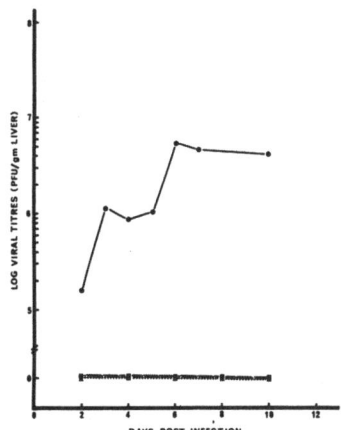

Figure 10. Effect of transfer of immune serum from A/J mice on viral titers from the livers of semisusceptible C3H mice. Viral titers were determined in livers from C3H mice infected with 10^3 PFU MHV-3 i.p. in a standard plaque assay which were immunized with 100 μl of normal saline 2 hours p.i. (━━━━━), 100 μl of serum from A/J mice 2 hours p.i. (┉┉┉┉┉) and 100 μl of serum from A/J mice 2 hours and 24 hours p.i. (━━ ━━ ━)

DISCUSSION

The results of these experiments indicate that there are major differences in the humoral response to MHV-3 in inbred strains of mice that differ in their suceptibility to MHV-3 infection. In the fully resistant A/J mice there is an early IgM response directed primarily to nucleocapsid protein followed by the production of IgG antibodies primarily of the IgG_{2a}, IgG_1 and IgG_{2b} classes. High titers of neutralizing antibody directed at E2 and E1 glycoprotein could be detected as early as 3-4 days p.i. and reached maximal titers by 7-10 days p.i. In contrast, no detectable antibody could be detected in the fully susceptible Balb/cJ mice, all of whom died within 5 days of infection. Furthermore, in the C3H mice, a strain in which there is viral persistence and chronic disease, antibody response was delayed and was primarily directed against nucleocapsid protein. Antibody appeared to be of the IgG_1 and IgM class. By 60 days, IgM remained predominant and there was very little production of IgG. Even late in the infection, the response was largely anti-nucleocapsid with very low titer of anti E2 and El detected.

The IgG subclass concentrations of an individual are determined at least in part by genetic factors (19). The four subclasses of murine IgG listed in order of concentration are IgG_{2a}, IgG_1, IgG_{2b} and IgG_3 (20). Furthermore only certain IgG subclasses are produced in response to specific antigens (21). In rodents, immunization with protein antigens results in the synthesis of IgG_1 antibodies whereas immunization with carbohydrates or mixtures of proteins and carbohydrates results in the production of predominantly IgG_{2a} and IgG_{2b} (19). Mouse IgG_{2a} and IgM activate the classic complement pathway, whereas IgG_1 fails to do so (19). Furthermore, only IgG_{2a} is cytophilic for monocyte/macrophages and the other classes of antibody fail to bind to these cells (19). Therefore, the failure of Balb/cJ mice to produce any antibody and the failure of C3H mice to maintain an appropriate IgG response may explain the lack of resistance to MHV-3 exhibited by these strains.

It is now recognized that for in-vivo B cell responses to T-dependent antigens, both thymus matured T cells as well as monocyte/macrophages are necessary for the production of antibody (22). Even with the class of antigens designated T-independent, the presence of thymus-matured T cells and antigen presenting monocyte/macrophages results in an augmented production of circulating antibodies (23,24). Furthermore the influence of T lymphocytes over B cell responses with T independent antigens is restricted to only some of the Ig isotypes namely the IgG_{2a} and IgG_{2b} subclasses.

Resistance to infection with MHV is genetically restricted and is dependent upon the ability of macrophages to control MHV infection and upon T cells and T cell factors (1,2,16). The abnormalities in synthesis in antibody could reflect accessory cell dysfunction with deficiencies in processing of viral antigens by macrophages and/or T cells resulting in both failure of cellular and humoral immunity as is seen in the fully susceptible Balb/cJ mice or the production of abnormal subclasses of antibodies and the failure of production of specific neutralizing antibodies as is seen in the C3H mice. Furthermore, the persistence of IgM antibodies and the failure of the conversion from IgM to the production of IgG antibodies may reflect abnormalities in processing and antigen handling by T cells and monocyte/macrophages or a primary B cell defect.

Similar abnormalities have been observed in patients with viral hepatitis B infection. Patients who survive and clear the virus produce large amounts of specific antibodies to both the core and surface antigens, whereas those patients who either die of acute infection or go on to a chronic disease state continue to produce high titers of anti-core IgM antibodies but fail to produce specific IgG anti-surface neutralizing antibodies (25). Chisari and co-workers have shown that the production of antibodies to the surface antigen of hepatitis B virus in inbred strains of mice is genetically controlled within the H-2 locus (26). A number of strains are high responders whereas some strains fail to generate any humoral response. This suggests that abnormalities in the immune response in MHV infection in some strains of mice may also be operative in man, resulting in the susceptibility of some patients to hepatitis B infection.

The presence of high titers of IgA early in the course of the infection in both A/J and C3H mice correlates with abnormal liver cell function. Delacroix et al have recently reported that patients with acute and chronic liver disease have abnormally high levels of polymeric and monomeric IgA in the serum (27). As the liver is believed to be the major site of removal of IgA from the circulation, he postulated that the increased levels of IgA found in these patients were due to abnormalities in binding of IgA to its liver cell receptor (secretory component) and decreased clearance through the liver (27). The presence of abnormally high levels of IgA even in the fully resistant A/J mice suggests that even in these animals there may be disruption of normal liver cell function.

We have shown here that passive transfer of high titered antisera containing neutralizing antibodies leads to the elimination of virus from semi-susceptible C3H mice and prevents the chronic disease state. Furthermore, this antibody at least partially protects the Balb/cJ mice resulting in lower viral titers in affected organs and increased survival. It is possible that the presence of high titered neutralizing antibody results in the activation of macrophages and T cells enabling a normal cellular immune response to occur. This could result in the elimination of the virus and the production of long lasting neutralizing antibodies. Future studies are required to determine the genetic requirements for both the cellular and humoral basis of the immune response to MHV infection. These studies are essential in order to determine those factors that contribute to either resistance or susceptibility in the particular host.

REFERENCES

1. Robb JS, Bond CW: Coronaviridae I. Eds. H. Fraenkel-Conrat and RR Wagner Comprehensive Virology, Vol 14. Plenum Press, 1979, pp. 193-247.

2.   Tyrell DAJ: Coronaviridae. Intervirology 10:321-336, 1978.

3.   Wege H, Sidell S and Ter Meulen V: The Biology and Pathogenesis of Coronaviruses. Ed. M Cooper Current Topics in Microbiology and Immunology. Vol 99, 1982, pp. 165-199.

4.   Levy GA, Leibowitz JL and Edgington TS: Lymphocyte Instructed Monocyte Induction of the Coagulation Pathways Parallels the Induction of Hepatitis by the Murine Hepatitis Virus. IN: Progress in Liver Diseases eds: H Popper and F Schaffner, Grune and Stratton Inc. Vol 7, 1982, pp. 393-409.

5.   Levy GA, Leibowitz JL and Edgington TS: Induction of Monocyte Procoagulant Activity by Murine Hepatitis Virus Type 3 Parallels Disease Susceptibility in Mice. J. Exp Med 154:1981:172.

6.   Levy-Leblond E and Dupuy JM: Neonatal Susceptibility to MHV Infections In Mice I. Transfer of Resistance. J. Immunol 118:1977:1219.

7.   Bang F and Warwick A: Mouse macrophages as host cells for the mouse hepatitis virus and the genetic basis of their susceptibility. Proc Nat Acad Sci 46:1960:1065.

8.   Stohlman SA, Frelinger JA and Weiner LP: Resistance to fatal central nervous system disease by mouse hepatitis virus strain JHM II. Adherent Cell Mediated Protection. J. Immunol 124:1980:1733.

9.   Mogensen SC: Genetics of macrophage controlled resistance to hepatitis induced by herpes simplex virus type 2 in mice. Infect Immun 17:1977:268.

10. Mogensen SC: Role of Macrophages in Natural Resistance to Viral Infections. Microb Rev 43:1979:1.

11. Lawman MJR, Rouse BT, Courtney RJ, and Walker RD: Cell mediated immunity against herpes simplex:Induction and cytotoxic T lymphocytes. Infect Immun 27:1980:133.

12. Pfizenmaier K, Starzinski-Powitz A, Rollinghoff M, Falke D, and Wagner H: T cell mediated cytotoxicity against herpes simplex virus infected target cells. Nature 265:1977:630.

13. Welsh RM: Mouse Natural Killer Cells. Induction Specificity and function. J. Immunol 121:1978:1631.

14. Lodmell DL and Notkins AL: Cellular Immunity to Herpes Simplex Virus Mediated By Interferons. J. Exp Med 140:1974:764.

15. Gresser I, Tovey MG, Maury C, and Bandu MT: Role of Interferon in the Pathogenesis of Herpes Simplex Virus Disease in Mice. IARC Sci Pub. 24:1978:1049.

16. Virelizier JL: Pathogenicity and Persistence of mouse hepatitis virus in inbred strains of mice IN: Biochemistry and Biology of Coronaviruses. Advances in Exp Med and Biol Ed. V. Ter Meulen, S. Sidell and H. Wege Plenum Press Vol 142:1980:349.

17. Levy GL, Leibowitz JL and Edgington TS: Induction of Monocyte Procoagulant Activity by murine hepatitis virus type 3 parallels disease susceptibility in mice. J. Exp Med 154 No 4:1981:1254.

18. Leibowitz JL, Fung LS and Levy GA: A sensitive radioimmunoassay for the detection of antibodies to MHV-3. J. Virol Methods In Press 1983.

19. Spiegelberg HL: Biological Activities of Immunoglobulins of different classes and subclasses. Adv. Immunol 19:1974:259.

20. Grey HM, Hirst JW and Cohn M: J. Exp Med 133:1971:289.

21.   Karch H, Gmeiner J and Nixdorff K: Alterations of
       the Immunoglobulin G subclass responses in mice
       to lipopolysaccharides: Effect of nonbacterial
       proteins and bacterial membrane phospholipids or
       outer membrane proteins of proteus mirabilis.
       Infect Immun 40:1983:157.

22.   Rosenberg YJ and Asofsky R: T cell regulation of
       isotype expression. The requirement for a second
       Ig-specific helper T cell population for the
       induction of IgG responses. Eur J. Immun. 11:1981
       :705.

23.   Mongini PKA, Stein KE and Paul WE: T cell
       regulation of IgG subclass antibody production in
       response to T-independant antigens. J.Exp Med
       153:1981:1.

24.   Herzenberg LA, Okumura K, Cantor H, Sato VL, Shen
       FW, Boyse EA and Herzenberg LA: T cell regulation
       of antibody responses: demonstration of allotype
       specific helper T cells and their specific
       removal by suppressor T cells. J. Exp Med
       144:1976:330 .

25.   Levy GA and Chisari FV: The immunopathogenesis of
       Hepatitis B Virus Induced Liver Disease. IN:
       Springer Seminars In Immunopathology. Eds
       Miescher PA and Muller-Eberhard HJ Springer-
       Verlag New York, N.Y. 3:1981:439.

26.   Milich DR and Chisari FV: Genetic regulation of
       the immune response to hepatitis B surface
       antigen (HBsAg) I Restriction of the murine
       humoral immune response to the a and d determinants
       of HBsAG. J. Immunol 129:1982:320.

27.   Delacroix DL, Elkon KB, Geubel AP, Hodgson HF,
       Dive C and Vaerman JP: Changes in size, subclass
       and metabolic properties of serum immunoglobulin A
       in liver diseases and in other diseases with high
       serum immunoglobulin A. J. Clin Invest.
       71:1983:358.

This work was supported by a grant from   the
Medical Research Council of Canada and by a grant from
the Canadian Liver Foundation.

PATHOGENIC DIFFERENCES BETWEEN VARIOUS FELINE CORONAVIRUS ISOLATES

Niels C. Pedersen, John W. Black, John F. Boyle,
James F. Evermann, Alison J. McKeirnan, and Richard
L. Ott

Depts. of Medicine, Schools of Veterinary Medicine,
Univ. of Calif., Davis (Pedersen, Boyle), Washington
State Univ., Pullman (Evermann, McKeirnan, Ott), and
Specialized Assays, Nashville, TN (Black)

INTRODUCTION

Coronaviruses are being isolated with increasing frequency
from cats. These various isolates can be divided into two
major groups: 1) coronaviruses that induce a disease of cats
known as feline infectious peritonitis (FIP), and 2) coronaviruses that cause a transient subclinical to severe enteritis[1,2]. The various isolates in each of these groups are morphologically and antigenically related, and probably represent
strains of a common species of virus that infects cats, dogs
(canine coronavirus or CCV), and swine[3,4].

The purpose of the report is to describe the coronavirus
strains that have been isolated from cats. The antigenic similarities of the various isolates will be compared, and the
pathogenesis of FIP virus (FIPV) and feline enteric coronavirus
(FECV) infection will be discussed.

Feline Infectious Peritonitis Virus

A number of isolates of FIPV have been made throughout the
world. Unfortunately, early isolates could only be propagated

in vivo by serial passage in cats, so comparisons of isolates were difficult to make. Within the last several years, however, at least 6 FIPV isolates have been cultivated in tissue culture. These include the isolate of O'Reilly and co-workers[5], the NW1 (UCD1) strain[1], the TN-409 (Black) strain[6], the Nor-15 isolate[7], the 79-1146 virus[8], and the UCD2 strain[9].

We have studied 4 of the 6 strains in our laboratory, including FIPV UCD1, FIPV-Black, FIPV-79-1146, and FIPV-UCD2. The UCD1, UCD2, and Black strains are very similar in regard to cytopathic effect (CPE), cell-associated growth, pathogenecity, and in their comparative neutralization by antiserum to various strains of FECV, FIPV, TGEV, and CCV. The 79-1146 strain, however, is clearly different in growth characteristics in tissue culture, pathogenecity, and because of its greater re-semblance to CCV.

The UCD1, UCD2, and Black strains of FIPV produce slow CPE in culture. Tissue culture supernatants will rarely yield more than 4,000 to 40,000 $TCID_{100}$ of non-cell associated virus per ml. Cell sonicates will contain 10 times more infectious virus than culture supernatants. These 3 strains grow best in certain cat cell lines, such as fcwf-4 or fc-0009 (fc9) cells[1]. They grow less well on Crandell feline kidney (CRFK) cells. Foci appear slowly over a period of 36 to 96 hours and consist initially of refractile angular shaped or multinucleated cells. Primary foci enlarge slowly from the peripheries. Secondary foci of infection are seen only occasionally, indicating that infection proceeds mainly by cell to cell contact. As the foci grow, cells in the middle of the plaque slough into the media or remain adhered to the plastic in a stellate, multinucleate, or lace-like form. The infection is most readily propagated by co-passing infected with normal cells.

The 79-1146 strain of FIPV was originally isolated from a 4 day old kitten by McKeirnan and associates[8]. It was later found to induce FIP in cats[9]. FIPV-79-1146 closely resembles canine coronavirus in its growth in cell culture. It grows well in most cat cell lines, including CRFK cells, and yields up to 10^6 to 10^7 TCID$_{100}$ of infectious virus per ml of culture supernatants. Small foci of CPE appear in cultures within 12 to 24 hours. Cells within the foci become retracted, refractile, and angular or rounded in appearance. Multinucleated giant cells are prominent. Secondary foci of infection appear very rapidly, and by 24-72 hours the entire cell sheet will be destroyed.

The various strains of FIPV are antigenically related to each other and to FECV isolates. The similarities are more pronounced when the isolates are compared by indirect fluorescent antibody than by virus neutralization assays (Table I, II). Antiserum to FECV-UCD and FIPV-Black cross reacts strongly in virus neutralization tests against FIPV-Black but weakly with FIPV-79-1146, FECV-79-1683 and CCV (Table II). Antiserum to FECV-79-1683 reacts weakly with FIPV-Black but strongly with FIPV-79-1146, FECV-79-1683 and CCV (Table II).

Table I. Indirect fluorescent antibody cross-reactions between FIPV-like (Type I) and CCV-like (Type II) feline coronaviruses. Titers are expressed as the highest inverse dilution of serum that still produced 1+ fluorescence.

Virus Substrate

Antiserum	FIPV-BLACK (Type I)	FECV-79-1683 (Type II)
Anti-FIPV-Black (Type I)	50,000	1,250
Anti-FECV-79-1683 (Type II)	1,500	26,600

Table II. Virus neutralization titers (inverse dilution) of serum samples collected from cats with experimentally induced feline coronavirus infection.

Serum #	Immunizing Strain	Virus Neutralization Titer Against:			
		FIPV-Black	FIPV-79-1146	FECV-79-1683	CCV
1	FIPV-Black	48	<2	<2	2
2	FIPV-Black	64	<2	<2	8
3	FECV-UCD	16	2	<2	<2
4	FECV-UCD	64	4	<2	<2
5	FECV-79-1146	4	100	400	200
6	FECV-79-1683	4	400	600	800

The CCV-like isolates of FIPV clearly represent a different strain, whereas FIPV-Black, FIPV-UCD1 and FIPV-UCD2 are very similar if not identical to each other[10]. In the field, strains similar to FIPV-Black account for the majority of cases of FIP (Table III). CCV-like strains of FIPV, such as FIPV-79-1146, are an infrequent cause of FIP in nature.

The pathogenecity of the UCD1 and Black strains of FIPV are similar on an infectious particle to particle basis[11]. They both have a relatively low infectivity for cats by oronasal instillation. Doses of virus in the range of 4,000 $TCID_{100}$ produce infection in a small number of animals, while doses of 40,000 $TCID_{100}$ or more will infect most cats. The initial febrile response, indicating the onset of fatal disease, occurs about 8-14 days after infection in coronavirus antibody free cats. Death usually occurs within 7 to 21 days from the onset of fever. If cats have been preimmunized with FECV or high passage avirulent FIPV-Black, fever is seen within 12 to 48 hours and the cats are usually moribund by day 7 to $10^{1,11,12}$.

FIPV-79-1146 has a comparatively high infectivity by oro-nasal instillation, and clinical signs in coronavirus negative cats appear around day 8 to 14. Previous exposure with other related coronaviruses, however, does not shorten the incubation period. A slight fever is seen in coronavirus antibody negative and positive cats around 24-48 hours after infection with FIPV-79-1146.

Table III. Virus neutralization titers (inverse dilution) of serum samples collected from cats with naturally occurring feline infectious peritonitis.

		Virus Neutralization Titer Against:			
Serum #	FIPV Type	FIPV-Black	FIPV-79-1146	FECV-79-1683	CCV
1	I	3200	<10	<10	20
2	I	3200	<10	<10	<10
3	I	640	<20	<10	<10
4	I	1600	<10	<10	10
5	I	2400	20	<10	80
6	II	40	6400	6400	12,800
7	I	320	<10	10	20
8	I	640	<10	<10	<10
9	I	160	<10	<10	<10
10	I	500	10	<10	10
11	I	80	<10	<10	<10
12	I	160	<10	<10	<10
13	I	640	<10	<10	<10
14	I	320	<10	<10	<10
15	I	128	<4	<4	4
16	I	64	<4	<4	8
17	I	160	N.T.*	<10	<10
18	I	640	<10	N.T	N.T
19	I	320	<10	<10	<10
20	I	1600	<10	<10	10

*N.T. = not tested

The temperature returns to normal in 12 to 24 hours and the cats appear healthy until day 8-14, when a sustained fever appears. Cats infected with FIPV-79-1146, whether presensitized or not, survive longer with clinical signs than cats infected with FIPV-UCD1 or FIPV-Black.

Pathogenesis of FIPV infections - The pathogenesis of FIPV infection is complex and not completely understood. There is enough known about the disease, however, to speculate on its pathogenesis (Fig. 1). The primary route of infection is probably oral, and virus replication is thought to occur initially in the mature apical epithelium of the intestinal tract[13]. In support of this assumption, orally administered FIPV will infect the intestinal epithelium of neonatal pigs in a manner identical to TGEV[14]. Clinical signs are not associated with the initial intestinal infection of cats. In cats serologically negative for coronavirus infection, the earliest signs of illness occur from 8 to 14 days after exposure. Clinical illness appears to be associated with dissemination of virus from the mucous membranes and regional lymph nodes, probably by way of blood-borne phagocytes[15]. This is one essential difference between FIPV and FECV infections. FECV does not spread further than the intestinal epithelium and the regional lymph nodes[2]. Disseminated FIPV is found preferentially within phagocytic cells in the target tissues, which include the liver, visceral peritoneum and pleura, uveal tract of the eyes, and the meninges and ependyma of the brain and spinal cord. The form of the disease that follows dissemination is dependent on the type of immunity that develops (Fig. 1).

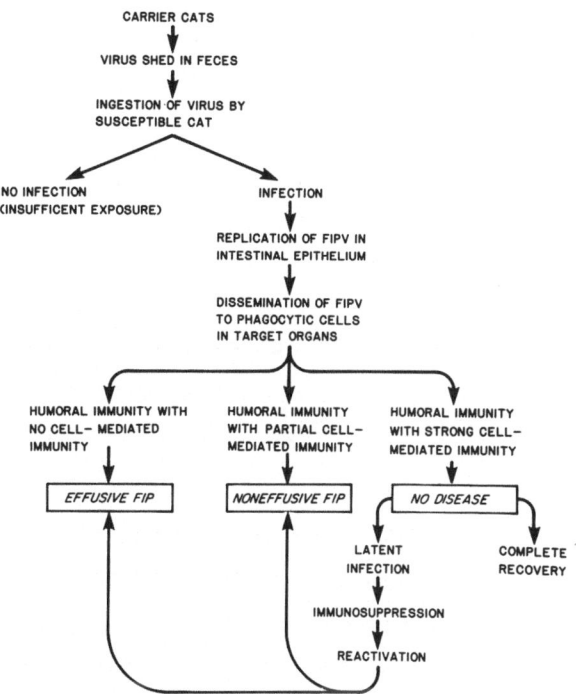

Fig. 1 - The possible pathogenesis of Feline Infectious Peritonitis as formulated from current knowledge.

FIP occurs in two distinct forms[16,17]. The first form is essentially a peritonitis or pleuritis, or both. The target tissues are the visceral peritoneum and pleura, and the omentum. Inflammation in these tissues results in a great outpouring of fluid into either or both of these body cavities, hence the name "wet" or "effusive" FIP. Meningeal and ependymal involvement is usually clinically inapparent in the effusive form of FIP. A second form of FIP was subsequently recognized by Montali and Strandberg[18]. Lesions in this form are more granulomatous in nature and localized primarily in parenchymatous organs such as the mesenteric lymph nodes, kidneys, uveal tract, and the meninges and ependyma of the brain and spinal cord. There is minimal or no exudation of fluid into the body cavities, and this form of the disease is, therefore, called "dry" or noneffusive FIP. Under experimental conditions, effusive FIP is about 2 to 3 times more common than noneffusive FIP.

Effusive FIP is characterized by a pyogranulomatous type of reaction around small venules in the target organs[19,20,21]. This vasculitis is responsible for the outpouring of protein and fibrin-rich fluid into the chest or abdomen. The lesions of effusive FIP develop simultaneously with the appearance of humoral immunity. Humoral immunity is not protective, but in fact, is actually harmful. Cell-mediated immunity appears to be the only beneficial protective response[11]. Antibody seems to enhance virus uptake by phagocytic cells, a preferred site for virus replication[1,12]. The net effect is to enhance rather than decrease the level of virus proliferation. Antibody also reacts with antigen and complement, possibly resulting in a localized arthus-like response [12,15,22-24]. The presence of circulating immune complexes is also suggested by the fluctuating complement levels and the development of glomerulonephritis in cats with FIP[25,26]. Complement mediated activation of terminal clotting factors, coupled with vascular lesions that consume platelets and clotting factors, causes a coagulopathy in cats with effusive FIP[22].

It is theorized that the noneffusive form of FIP occurs in cats that develop only partial cell-mediated immunity[11]. Partial cellular immunity will limit the virus to localized sites in target organs, but is insufficient to destroy or contain the infection. The resulting granulomatous reaction surrounds small accumulations of virus-laden phagocytic cells in the center of the lesions. The granulomatous reactions seen in noneffusive FIP are, therefore, equivalent to similar reactions seen in diseases such as coccidioidomycosis, histoplasmosis, or tuberculosis.

Cats that develop strong cell-mediated immunity do not show signs of illness, or will demonstrate a transient fever and localized mesenteric lymphadenopathy. Cell-mediated immunity does not always lead to complete elimination of the virus. Virus apparently persists in the body of some cats in a walled-off form. With deterioration of immune responsiveness, usually associated with aging or diseases such as FeLV infection, the FIPV infection may become active again.

Heterotypic immunity to non-FIP-inducing coronaviruses (FECV's) may be involved in the pathogenesis of FIP. Cats with cross reacting serum antibodies are often more sensitive to intraperitoneal challenge with FIPV[1,2,12]. Cats with sensitizing heterotypic coronavirus immunity will develop effusive FIP after 24 to 72 hours, versus 8 to 14 days or more for cats without previous coronavirus exposure. This enhancement is more consistently seen when FIPV strains such as UCD1 or Black are used for the challenge. FIPV-79-1146 infection is not appreciably influenced by heterotypic immunity in one way or the other. Aerosol inoculation with FIPV-UCD1 of cats with prior coronavirus exposure causes a severe fulminating pneumonia[15,22-24]. The enhancement of illness caused by a prior exposure to an antigenically related virus is reminiscent of dengue hemorrhagic shock syndrome of man. This similarity has been described by Horzinek and Osterhaus[27], Pedersen and Boyle[12], and Weiss and Scott[23].

Initial attempts to immunize cats using TGEV of swine have been unsuccessful[28,29]. Immunization with modified live FIPV has also failed to protect cats[11]. Kittens immunized oronasally with the modified live FIPV-Black developed both IFA and virus neutralizing antibodies. Following challenge with virulent FIPV-Black, however, the infection rate was increased, latency period reduced, and disease severity enhanced in vaccinated as compared to nonvaccinated kittens. Apparently, avirulent virus does not confer a protective type immunity, but elicits humoral immunity that is actually deleterious. The failure of avirulent FIPV to immunize might be due to its failure to persist in the body[11]. Cats have been successfully immunized against FIPV using sublethal doses of virulent virus[11]. Unfortunately, this is not of clinical relevance because the dose that immunized some cats caused fatal FIP in others.

Feline Enteric Coronavirus Infection

Feline enteric coronaviruses are the cause of inapparent to mild, infrequently severe, intestinal infections in kittens between birth and 12 weeks of age. Although they are morphologically and antigenically similar to FIPV, FECV strains do not cause FIP. To date, 2 different strains of FECV have been characterized. The first isolate, designated FECV-UCD, was described by Pedersen and coworkers[2]. A second isolate was identified by McKeirnan and associates[8], and has been designated FECV-79-1683. FECV-79-1683 was isolated from a fatal case of peracute hemorrhagic enteritis in an adult cat. Like FECV-UCD, this strain produced mild to inapparent enteritis in specific pathogen free cats[9]. Coronavirus particles identical to those described for FECV-UCD have been identified in the stools of a cat with diarrhea by Dea and coworkers[30]. This isolate shared some antigens with calf diarrhea coronavirus. Hayashi and coworkers[13] also observed a coronavirus in the intestine of a cat with diarrhea. This virus was antigenically similar to FIPV, and was probably another FECV. Hoshino and Scott[31] have demonstrated coronavirus-like particles in the stool of normal cats, but they appear morphologically and antigenically different from other FECV isolates.

Repeated attempts to grow FECV-UCD in cell culture have failed. The virus is currently maintained by in vivo passage in kittens. FECV-79-1683 grows readily in cell culture, and in regard to cytopathic effect, cell tropism and level of free virus production, it is similar to FIPV-79-1146. It also seems to be more closely related to CCV than to FECV-UCD.

Pathogenesis

The target tissue for FECV-UCD infection is the mature columnar epithelium of the small intestine[2]. Virus replication also occurs to a lesser extent in the tonsils and mesenteric lymph nodes. Clinical signs occur when a large percentage of the apical intestinal villous epithelium is damaged. Signs began between 2 and 7 days after oronasal infection. Vomiting is the first sign observed, preceding diarrhea by 12 to 48 hours. The diarrhea is seldom severe and lasts for 48 to 96 hours. Fever, when it occurs, is mild. Many recovered cats will become asymptomatic virus shedders.

FECV-79-1683 causes an almost identical disease syndrome to FECV-UCD, although perhaps milder in nature. Following oral infection, virus replication is seen in the mature apical columnar epithelium of the small intestine, mesenteric lymph nodes, tonsils, and to a lesser extent in the lungs. Virus shedding, as detected by cell culture infectivity of fecal supernatants, is only apparent for the first 13-16 days. Recovered cats, however, remain infectious to susceptible contact animals for a much longer period of time.

Classification of Feline Coronaviruses

We propose that feline coronaviruses be classified using the following critera: 1) morphological, structural, and antigenic relationship to TGEV and CCV, 2) type of disease that they cause, e.g. FIP, enteritis, etc., 3) growth characteristics in cell culture (ease of isolation in cell culture, ease of adaptability to various cell-lines, cell-associated growth characteristics), and 4) degree of relatedness to CCV in virus neutralization tests. In such a scheme, the 5 characterized isolates can be categorized as listed in the following outline:

I.   Feline Coronaviruses

    A.   Non TGEV-like (theoretical existence)
    B.   TGEV-like

        1.   FIP inducing
            a.   Type I (difficult to grow in cell culture, grow best in selective cell lines, cell associated growth, antiserum to these strains reacts weakly in virus neutralization with heterologous strains such as CCV).

                1)   FIPV-UCD1
                2)   FIPV-UCD2
                3)   FIPV-Black

      b.   Type II (easily isolated in cell culture, grows in many different cell lines, produces large amounts of non-cell associated virus, antiserum to these strains reacts strongly in virus neutralization with heterologous viruses such as CCV).

            1)   FIPV-79-1146

  2.   Non-FIP inducing

      a.   Enteritis causing agents

            1)   Type I (criteria as listed above for type I FIPV strains)
               a)   FECV-UCD
            2)   Type II (criteria as listed above for type II FIPV strains)
               a)   FECV-79-1683

REFERENCES

1.   Pedersen NC, Boyle JF, Floyd K: Infection studies in kittens utilizing feline infectious peritonitis virus propagated in cell culture. Am J Vet Res 42:363-367, 1981a.

2.   Pedersen NC, Boyle JF, Floyd K: An enteric coronavirus infection of cats, and its relationship to feline infectious peritonitis.   Am J Vet Res 42:368-377, 1981b.

3.   Horzinek MC, Lutz H, Pedersen NC: Antigenic relationship among homologous structural polypeptides of porcine, feline, and canine coronavirus. Infect Immun 37:1148-1155, 1982.

4.   Pedersen NC, Ward J, Mengeling WL: Antigenic relationship of the feline infectious peritonitis virus to corona-virus of other species. Arch Virol 58:45-53, 1978.

5.   O'Reilly KJ, Fishman LM, Hitchcock LM: Short communication: Feline infectious peritonitis; isolation of a coronavirus. Vet Rec 104:348, 1979.

6.   Black JW: Recovery and in-vitro cultivation of a corona-
     virus from laboratory-induced cases of feline infec-
     tious peritonitis (FIP). VM SAC 75:811-814, 1980.

7.   Evermann JF, Baumgartner L, Ott RL, et al: Characteristics
     of a feline infectious peritonitis virus isolate. Vet
     Path 18:256-265, 1981.

8.   McKeirnan AJ, Evermann JF, Hargis A, et al: Isolation of
     feline coronaviruses from two cats with diverse
     disease manifestations.   Feline Pract 11(3):16-20,
     1981.

9.   Pedersen NC: unpublished observations, 1983.

10. Black JW: Unpublished observations, 1983.

11. Pedersen NC, Black JW: Attempted immunization of cats
     against feline infectious peritonitis using either
     avirulent live virus or sublethal amounts of virulent
     virus. Am J Vet Res 44:229-234, 1983.

12. Pedersen NC, Boyle JF: Immunologic phenomena in the
     effusive form of feline infectious peritionitis. Am J
     Vet Res 41:868-876, 1980.

13. Hayashi T, Watabe Y, Nakayama H, Fujiwara K: Enteritis due
     to feline infectious peritonitis virus. Jpn J Vet
     Sci 44:97-106, 1982.

14. Woods RD, Cheville NF, Gallagher JE: Lesions in the small
     intestine of newborn pigs inoculated with porcine,
     feline, and canine coronaviruses.   Am J Vet Res
     42:1163-1169, 1981.

15. Weiss RC, Scott FW: Pathogenesis of feline infectious
     peritonitis: Nature and development of viremia. Am J
     Vet Res 41:382-390, 1981a.

16. Holmberg CA, Gribble DH: Feline infectious peritonitis:
     Diagnostic gross and microscopic lesions.   Feline
     Pract 3(4):11-14, 1973.

17. Pedersen NC: Feline infectious peritonitis: Something
     old, something new. Feline Pract 6:42-51, 1976.

18. Montali RJ, Strandberg JD: Extraperitoneal lesions in
     feline infectious peritonitis. Vet Pathol 9:109-121,
     1972.

19. Feldman BM, Jortner BS: Clinicopathologic conference:
    Feline systemic proliferative and exudative vasculi-
    tis. J Am Vet Med Assoc 144:1409-1420, 1964.

20. Hayashi T, Goto N, Takahashi R, Fujiwara K: Systemic
    vascular lesions in feline infectious peritonitis.
    Jpn J Vet Sci 39:365-377, 1977.

21. Ward JM, Munn RJ, Gribble DH, Dungworth DL: An observation
    of feline infectious peritonitis. Vet Rec 83:416-417,
    1968.

22. Weiss RC, Dodd WJ, Scott FW: Disseminated intravascular
    coagulation in experimentally induced feline infec-
    tious peritonitis. Am J Vet Res 41:663-671, 1980.

23. Weiss RC, Scott FW: Antibody-mediated enhancement of
    disease in feline infectious peritonitis: Comparison
    with dengue hemorrhagic fever. Comp Immunol Microbiol
    Infect Dis 4:175-189, 1981b.

24. Weiss RC, Scott FW: Pathogenesis of Feline Infectious
    Peritonitis: Pathologic changes and immunofluores-
    cence. Am J Vet Res 42:2036-2048, 1981c.

25. Jacobse-Geels HEL, Daha MR, Horzinek MC: Isolation and
    characterization of feline C3 and evidence for the
    immune complex pathogenesis of feline infectious
    peritonitis. J Immunol 125:1606-1610, 1980.

26. Jacobse-Geels HEL, Daha MR, Horzinek MC: Antibody, immune
    complexes, and complement activity. Fluctuations in
    kittens with experimentally induced feline infectious
    peritonitis. Am J Vet Res 43:666-670, 1982.

27. Horzinek MC, Osterhaus ADME: The virology and pathogenesis
    of feline infectious peritonitis. Brief review. Arch
    Virol 59:1-15, 1979.

28. Toma B, Duret C, Chappuis G, Pellerin B: Echec de
    L'immunisation contre la peritonite infectieuse feline
    par infection de virus de la gastro-enterite transmis-
    sible du porc. Rec Med Vet 155:799-803, 1979.

29. Woods RD, Pedersen NC: Cross-protection studies between
    feline infectious peritonitis and porcine transmissi-
    ble gastroenteritis viruses. Vet Microbiol 4:11-16,
    1979.

30. Dea S, Roy RS, Elazhary MASY: Coronavirus-like particles
        in the feces of a cat with diarrhea.   Can Vet J
        23:153-155, 1982.

31. Hoshino Y, Scott FW: Coronavirus-like particles in the
        feces of normal cats. Arch Virol 63:147-152, 1980.

    Support for this work was obtained from the Robert H. Winn
Foundation for Cat Research of the Cat Fancier Association, Red
Bank, NH, Save our Cats and Kittens (SOCK) Corp., Walnut Creek,
CA, and the Ralston Purina Co., St. Louis, Mo.

EXPRESSION OF FELINE INFECTIOUS PERITONITIS (FIP) CORONAVIRUS

ANTIGENS ON THE SURFACE OF FELINE MACROPHAGE-LIKE CELLS

H.E.L. Jacobse-Geels and M.C. Horzinek

Institute of Virology, Veterinary Faculty
State University
Yalelaan 1, 3508 TD Utrecht, The Netherlands

Indications for the involvement of the immune system in the pathogenesis of Feline Infectious Peritonitis (FIP) have been reported (1,2). A major role is attributed to the macrophage, the predominant if not the only target cell of FIP Virus (FIPV) in vivo.

FIPV has been propagated in vitro in several organ and cell cultures of feline origin, e.g. the FCWF cell line (felis catus whole foetus) (3). These cells are able to phagocytose latex and carbon particles and stain strongly positive for aspecific esterases. Fc receptors are present on their membrane. They can therefore be identified as macrophage-like. FIPV grows readily in FCWF cells but more than 99% of the infectivity is cell-associated at 15 hours postinfection when cytopathological effects (syncytia) are pronounced. By immunofluorescence, granular accumulations of viral antigen could first be detected on cell membranes by 16 h.p.i. Surface labeling with ^{125}I followed by immunoprecipitation and SDS-PAGE analysis revealed a protein pattern as shown in Fig.1. Antiserum against FIPV recognized four proteins with apparent molecular weights of 225.5, 175, 138, and 25 K (lane a). No corresponding proteins were seen in mock-infected control cells (lane c) nor were they precipitated by normal cat serum in infected (lane b) or in mock-infected cells (lane d). When detergent disrupted, FIPV infected cells were labeled an additional protein of 44 K (lane e) was recognized and a protein of 34 K which was also seen in mock-infected cells (lane g). The larger proteins (225.5 K, 175 K and 138 K) are considered as the peplomer protein and its precursors, respectively. The intracellular 44 K protein can be identified as the nucleoprotein on the basis of its molecular weight as determined recently in electroblotting experiments of gradient purified FIPV; the 25 K protein corresponds to the envelope protein (3).

Expression of viral antigen on the cell membrane may be an important factor in the immune pathogenesis of FIP (1,2). Immune mediated lysis of infected cells may be of particular pathogenic importance since surface expression of FIPV antigens is seen late in infection when virus progeny is already formed. The activity of the complement system is reduced in terminal FIP cases, possibly as a result of its activation during antibody mediated lysis of viral antigen-bearing cells. A pronounced increase in T lymphocytes is also seen which may be an indication of enhanced direct lymphocyte-mediated cytotoxicity.

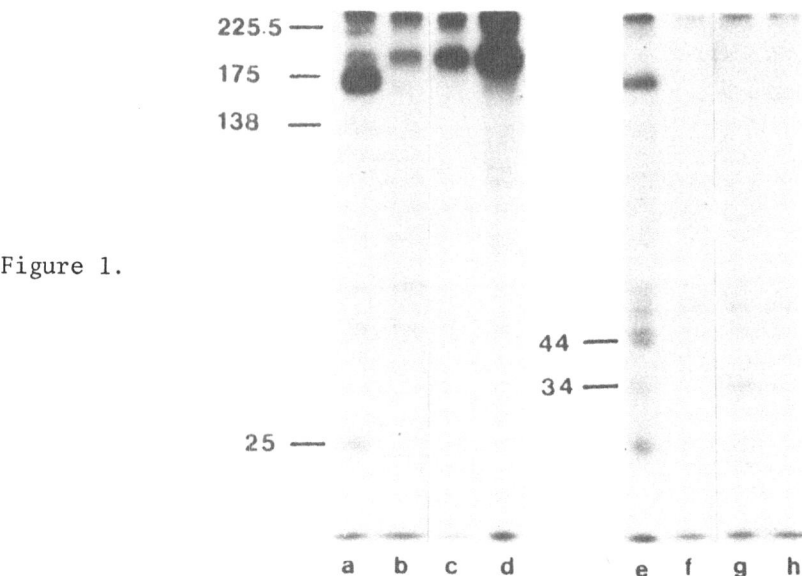

Figure 1.

REFERENCES

1. H.E.L.Jacobse-Geels, M.R.Daha and M.C.Horzinek, Isolation and characterization of feline C3 and evidence for the immune complex pathogenesis of feline infectious peritonitis, J.Immunol. 125:1606-1610 (1980).
2. H.E.L. Jacobse-Geels, M.R. Daha and M.C.Horzinek, Antibody, immune complexes, and complement activity fluctuations in kittens with experimentally induced feline infectious peritonitis, Am.J.Vet.Res. 43:666-670 (1982).
3. N.C. Pedersen, J.F. Boyle and K. Floyd, Infection studies in kittens, using feline infectious peritonitis virus propagated in cell culture, Am.J.Vet.Res. 42:363-367, (1981).
4. M.C. Horzinek, H. Lutz and N.C. Pedersen, Antigenic relationships among homologous structural polypeptides of porcine, feline and canine coronaviruses, Inf.& Immun. 37:1148-1155 (1982).

ROLE OF CIRCULATING ANTIBODIES AND THYMUS-DEPENDENT LYMPHOCYTES IN PRODUCTION OF EFFUSIVE TYPE FELINE INFECTIOUS PERITONITIS AFTER ORAL INFECTION

Toshiharu Hayashi, Kunio Doi*, and Kosaku Fujiwara

Department of Veterinary Pathology, and *Department of Biomedical Science, Faculty of Agriculture, University of Tokyo, 1-1-1 Yayoi, Bunkyo, Tokyo 113, Japan

Seropositive or antibody-transferred kittens have been reported to have an overt disease after parenteral challenge with virulent feline infectious peritonitis (FIP) virus, suggesting that the effusive type FIP[2,3] might result from an interaction between the virus and host response.   On the other hand, feline leukemia virus infection was suggested to enhance the infection of FIP virus[1].   The present study deals with roles of circulating antibodies as well as thymus-dependent lymphocytes in pathogenesis after oral infection of FIP virus.

Fibrinous serositis was produced in 4 of 20 seropositive kittens or those having received transfer of anti-FIP cat antibody after intragastric inoculation with FIP virus, whereas 30 seronegative animals had no signs of illness but some enteritis. Lesions produced in the serosa and abdominal organs were characterized by fibrinous inflammation with necrotic and pyogranulomatous vasculitis as well as necrosis in lymphoreticular tissues(Fig.1).   Viral antigen was detected within macrophages and enterocytes in those lesions by immunofluorescence assay(Fig.2).

In another experiment, 3 kittens were thymectomized (Tx). One of them received normal cat serum (Tx+Ab -)); the other 2 remained non-treated(Nt).   Another group of 5 kittens received anti-FIP cat antibody, and 2 of them were thymectomized(Tx+Ab) while 3 were sham-operated(Sh+Ab).   Shortly after the operation all 8 kittens were challenged orally with FIP virus.   All of Nt, Tx or Tx+Ab(-) cases were shown to have enteritis without serosal and visceral affections.   Enteritis in Tx or Tx+Ab(-) cases was more profound than in Nt cases.   Virus antigen was detected mostly within macrophages in the former whereas within enterocytes in the latter,suggesting that infection of macrophages in the tunica propria might be important in the subsequent

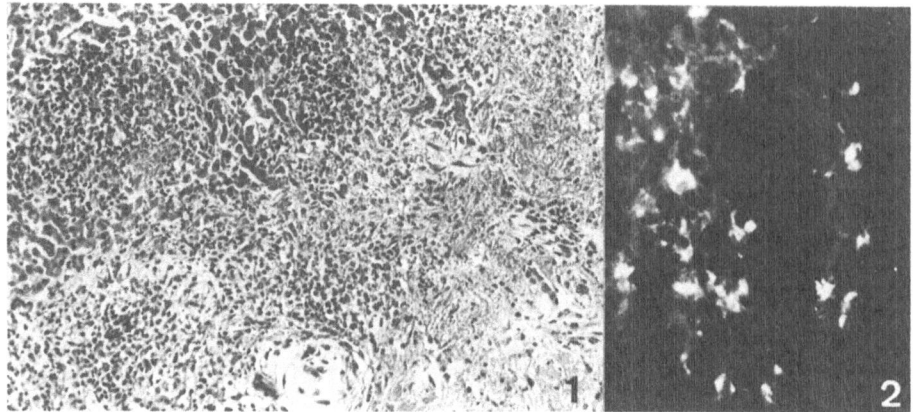

Antibody-transferred and intragastrically inoculated case
dead on day 19 postinoculation.

Fig. 1. Severe coagulative necrosis,   Fig. 2. Viral antigen
    focal infiltration of inflam-   within the cytopla-
    matory cells and proliferation   sm of macrophages
    of fibroblasts in the liver.   accumulated in and
    HE stain x620.   around an inter-
                                                 lobular artery.

production of lesions in abdominal organs. On the other hand, all
cases of both Tx+Ab and Sh+Ab groups showed fibrinous serositis,
which was developed more severe in Tx+Ab. Also in Tx+Ab cases
virus antigen-positive cells were more numerous than in Sh+Ab.

    These results suggest that the humoral antibody and T lympho-
cytes might play an important role in enhancing and supressing,
respectively, the production of serositis as well as parenchymatous
lesions.

REFERENCES

1. S. M. Cotter, C. E. Gilmore, and C. Rollins. Multiple cases
    of feline leukemia and feline infectious peritonitis in a
    household, J.Am.Vet.Med.Assoc. 162, 1054-1058, (1973).

2. N. C. Pedersen, and J. F. Boyle. Immunologic phenomena in the
    effusive form of feline infectious peritonitis, Am.J.Vet.Res.
    41, 868-876, (1980).

3. R. C. Weiss, and F. W. Scott. Pathogenesis of feline
    infectious peritonitis : Pathologic changes and
    immunofluorescence, Am.J.Vet.Res. 42, 2036-2048, (1980).

INTERACTIONS OF PORCINE ENTERIC CORONAVIRUS TGEV

WITH MACROPHAGES AND LYMPHOCYTES

H. Laude, B. Charley & C. La Bonnardiere

I.N.R.A., Station de Recherches de Virologie et

d'Immunologie, F-78850 Thiverval–Grignon

Enterocytes covering the microvilli of small intestine are the only target cell of transmissible gastroenteritis (TGEV) that have been characterized until now. Such a tropism has been shown to explain the severe intestinal disorders affecting infected animals. However, several authors mentioned isolation of TGEV from respiratory tract (1, 2, 3), and the possibility of extra-intestinal sites of replication was strenghtened by recent studies on the systemic interferon (IFN) response of newborn piglets infected by wild or cell-adapted strains (H. Laude & C. La Bonnardière, to be published).

a) Multiplication of TGEV in alveolar macrophages. Adherent phagocytic cells derived from lungs of 6 months old pigs and maintained in culture are able to support TGEV replication, as proved by positive immunofluorescence, infectious virus release and IFN synthesis.

Table 1. Multiplication of cell-adapted strains of TGEV in macrophage cultures.

Virus Strain (1-3pfu/cell)	Cell viability[*] (% of control)		Infectivity titer (pfu / ml)		IFN titer[**] (MDBK units/ml)	
	Batch n°1	n°2	n°1	n°2	n°1	n°2
D_{52-5}	39	42	1.2×10^5	9.5×10^4	470	250
6386-5	37	48	4.5×10^4	7×10^4	270	170
Purdue 115	26	35	4.5×10^5	1.1×10^5	1400	510
" +antiserum	>95	n.t.	$< 10^1$	n.t.	n.t.	n.t.
UV-inactivated	>95	n.t.	$< 10^1$	n.t.	≤ 10	n.t.

[*] *Measured by O.D. at 460 nm of neutral red intake (alcohol extract)*
[**] *Determined as previously reported (4).*

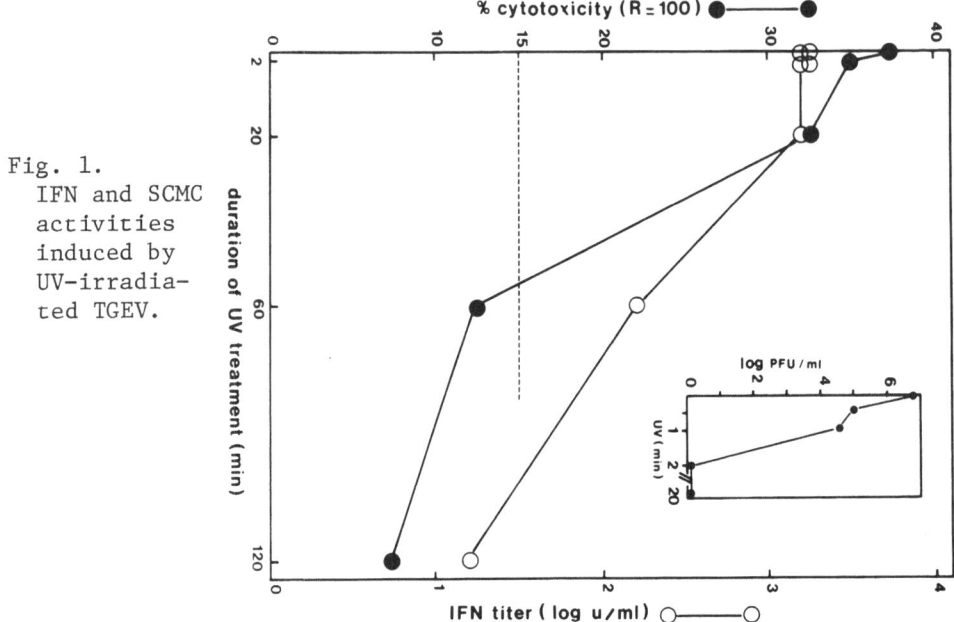

Fig. 1.
  IFN and SCMC
  activities
  induced by
  UV-irradia-
  ted TGEV.

Extensive cell death was observed at virus input > 0.1 p.f.u./cell
whereas prolonged and limited virus production occured at lower
m.o.i., indicating that TGEV replication may be controlled in this
particular kind of cells. These *in vitro* results are in agreement
with *in vivo* studies showing that both virus and IFN are associated
to the cells collected by washing the lungs of infected animals
(90 per cent being macrophages).

     b) Effect of TGEV on lymphocytes : In contrast, no virus pro-
duction could be induced in leucocyte preparations originating from
blood, spleen or intestine. Nevertheless an IFN-activity was consistently present in TGEV-inoculated lymphocyte cultures, at a concentration which was shown to efficiently stimulate their spontaneous cell-mediated cytotoxicity (SCMC test performed as in 5).
Equivalent interferon induction was obtained when using UV-irradia-
ted non-infectious virus (Fig. 1).

     These interactions of TGEV with immunocompetent cells call
further attention because of their virtual implications in natural
and acquired defence mechanisms.

REFERENCES

1. Underdahl et al., Am. J. vet. Res. 35, 1209 (1974).
2. Kemeny et al., Cornell. vet. 65, 352 (1975).
3. Furuuchi et atl, Vet. Microbiol. 3, 169 (1978/9).
4. La Bonnardière and Laude, Inf. Immun. 32, 28 (1981).
5. Charley et al., Ann. Virol 134E, 119 (1983).

EFFECT OF STOMACH AND GUT JUICES ON INFECTIVITY OF LOW AND HIGH PASSAGED STRAINS OF T.G.E. CORONAVIRUS: PROPERTIES OF A VIRUS MUTANT RESISTANT TO INACTIVATION BY STOMACH JUICE OBTAINED BY CYCLES OF SURVIVOR SELECTION IN TISSUE CULTURE

J.M. Aynaud, E. Bottreau and A. Brun*

INRA Laboratoire de Pathologie Porcine,
37380 Monnaie, France
*IFFA-MERIEUX, 254 rue M. Mérieux, 69007 Lyon, France

The coronavirus causing transmissible gastroenteritis (T.G.E.) of swine is considered a major etiologic agent of the neonatal enteritis. Sows orally immunized with virus strains modified by serial passages in cell culture confer little or no protection to their suckling pigs (lactogenic immunity), in contrast to the protection seen in piglets milking sows given field virus strains. Improvement of immunisation methods of pregnant sows by oral route using live virus vaccine is the main objective of the present work. Induction of an efficient lactogenic immunity (passive protection of young piglets by milk) is strongly dependant of local antigenic stimulation of the maternal gut before farrowing. Stability of virus vaccine infectivity in digestive fluids (during the transit between mouth and gut epithelium) is a critical parameter for oral immunization of adult swine. Viruses, pig cell lines (RP.TG and S.T.) plaque assay are previously described (1). Virus is diluted 10-fold in i) stomach juice (18 samples or ii) gut juice (22samples) collected from adult pigs or iii) in Mcilvaine buffer (0.1 M, pH 2 and 3). The mixture is placed in stirring water bath at 37°C. T.G.E. virus is highly fragile in digestive fluids. No significant differences are observed between low passaged and high passaged strains. The amount of virucidal activity of digestive fluids is variable according the physiologic status of the digestive tract. These results suggest that virus infectivity of the vaccine dose given orally could be dramatically reduced during transit in stomach and gut lumen. This feature can partly explain the disappointing results of numerous attempts to immunize pregnant sows by oral route with live virus vaccine against T.G.E.

The "152-SG" virus mutant was selected in tissue culture after
152 cycles of survivor selection in stomach juice. This mutant is
characterized by a high resistance to acidity (pH = 2.0) and by
small plaques (0.5 mm) in a swine testis cell line (S.T.). In
contrast, normal plaques (1.5 - 2.0 mm) are observed in RP.TG
cell line. Other T.G.E. virus strains (L.P. and H.P. strains)
show normal plaques both in S.T. and in RP.TG cells.
Two litters of 4 days old S.P.F. piglets were inoculated by oral
route with 4.10^6 and 4.10^7 P.F.U. of the "152-SG" mutant of T.G.E.
virus. Mortality was nil and mild diarrhea was observed between
4th and 7th day post inoculation only in the litter given 4×10^7
P.F.U. An immune response (neutralizing antibodies) was also
observed in serum and in secretions. These results suggest that
the "152-SG" mutant is attenuated for the newborn S.P.F. piglet.
Testing of immunogenic activity in the pregnant sow is in progress.

Table I

Stability of T.G.E. coronavirus infectivity in low pH buffer

(10 minutes/37°C in Mc.Ilvaine Buffer)

Virus strain	pH = 7.0	pH = 3.0	pH = 2.0
152 SG	$4 \times 10^{6*}$	2×10^6	1×10^6
Purdue 115	3×10^7	4×10^7	1×10^4

* P.F.U./0.3 ml

REFERENCES

1. H. LAUDE, J. GELFI and J.M. AYNAUD. In vitro properties of
   low and high passaged strains of transmissible gastroenteritis
   coronavirus of swine. Am. J. Vet. Res., 42:447 (1981).

PATHOGENICITY OF MOUSE HEPATITIS VIRUS, MHV-2cc, FROM A PERSISTENTLY INFECTED DBT CELL LINE

Naoaki Goto, Norio Hirano*, and Akio Sato

Department of Veterinary Pathology, Faculty of
Agriculture, Yamaguchi University, and *Department
of Microbiology, Faculty of Agriculture, Iwate
University, 1677-1 Yoshida, Yamaguchi 753, Japan

Pathogenicity of a small plaque mutant of mouse hepatitis virus, MHV-2cc, from persistently infected DBT cell culture for nude mice (BALB/c) was studied. The mutant virus was purified by the same procedure as described previously[1] by serial cultures of resistant DBT cells carrying MHV-2.

After inoculation with 10^5 PFU of MHV-2cc, adult ICR mice, which were highly susceptible to the original MHV-2, showed no signs of illness, while suckling ICR mice died of fulminant hepatitis. Adult athymic nude mice, however, were found to have subacute or chronic hepatitis resulting in death between 18 and 90 days after inoculation. Grossly they showed remarkable nodular hyperplastic changes in the liver (Fig.1). By direct immunofluorescence MHV antigen was demonstrated within the cytoplasm of hepatocytes. Though the times-to-death were varied, changes of the liver were common to all cases until one week postinfection. The viral antigen was demonstrated as early as 48 hr postinoculation followed by production of many focal necrotic lesions. Specific fluorescence mostly faded at 7 days postinoculation when some inflammatory reactions appeared around the lesions. By electron microscopy, a small number of virions was seen outside of hepatocytes at 72 hr postinoculation but many virions still existed in the cytoplasm of degenerated hepatocytes (Fig.2). Some hepatocytes containing virions were phagocytized by macrophages, and recurrent inflammatory reactions as well as fibrosis were observed later.

Chronic active hepatitis has been experimentally produced in some nude mice[2] after infection with low virulent MHV, MHV-NuU, but the pathogenicity of this virus for nude mice is not uniform enough to be a model for subacute or chronic hepatitis. MHV-2cc virus seems to be of much lower virulence producing a

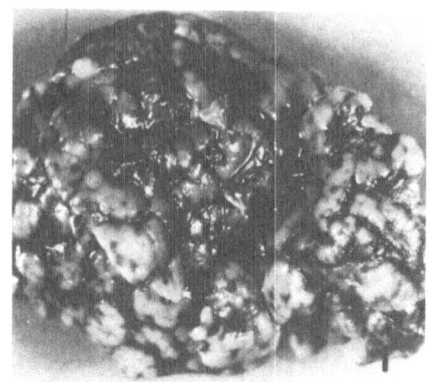

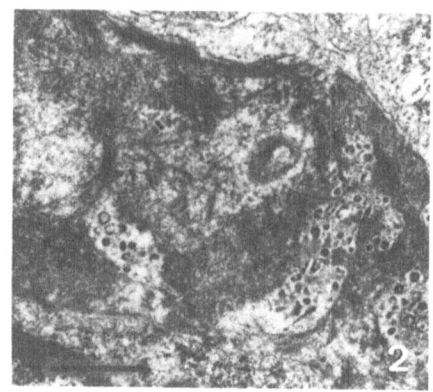

Fig.1. The liver of an MHV-2cc
       infected athymic nude
       mouse. 42 days post-
       inoculation.

Fig.2. MHV-2cc virons in the
       cytoplasm of a degerated
       hepatocyte of an athymic
       nude mouse. 96 hr post-
       inoculation. Bar=1μ

more typical chronic active hepatitis with recurrent inflammatory
reactions. Such type of MHV mutant retaining high hepatotropism
has never been reported, while various neurotropic mutants of MHV
have been shown to cause persistent infection in the nervous system
[1,3]. The system of MHV-2cc and athymic nude mice may provide a
good model for progressive hepatitis with virus persistence.

REFERENCES

1. N. Hirano, N. Goto, S. Makino, and K. Fujiwara. Persistent
   infection with mouse hepatitis virus, JHM strain in DBT cell
   culture. In Biochemistry and Biology of Coronavirus, Plenum
   Publishing, New York (1981).

2. T. Tamura, K. Ueda, N. Hirano, and K. Fujiwara. Response of
   nude mice to a mouse hepatitis virus isolated from a wasting
   nude mouse. Jpn. J. Exp. Med. 46, 19-30, (1967).

3. S. A. Stohlman, and L. P. Weiner. Stability of neurotropic
   mouse hepatitis virus (JHM strain) during chronic infection
   of neuroblastoma cells. Arch. Virol. 57, 53-61, (1978).

THE PATHOGENESIS AND AGE RELATED SUSCEPTIBILITY OF OC43 VIRUS IN MICE

J. Pearson and C.A. Mims

Dept. of Microbiology, Guy's Hospital Medical School

London SE1, England

Coronavirus OC43 is a human respiratory virus which was isolated in organ culture. It has since been adapted to grow in suckling mouse brain but no further work on the pathogenesis of this virus has been described.

CD1.mice infected intracerebrally or extraneurally with OC43 virus develop a lethal neurotropic infection. Organs and tissues were removed from infected mice and tested for the presence of viral antigen and/or infectious virus. Replication of OC43 is confined solely to the nervous system, neither infectious virus nor viral antigen could be detected in any extraneural tissue tested including heart, liver, lungs, spleen, thymus and adrenals.

Examination of the brains of infected mice by FAT revealed that by 48 hours post infection there was extensive infection of the brain and particularly of the cerebral cortex. Infection of the cerebellum, however, was restricted to Purkinje cells. Spinal cord; ganglia and retina were also positive by FAT.

Histological examination of extensively infected brain by H&E stain revealed very little necrosis and luxol fast blue staining did not demonstrate any demyelination.

Infected mice develop an age related susceptibility to the virus becoming resistant to infection by ic inoculation by 20 days of age and by ip inoculation by 15 days of age.

We have carried out experiments to investigate which of the following possible mechanisms were responsible for the resistance to OC43 infection in adult mice.

A)   Injected virus does not reach the brain - this could not be
responsible as the mice remain resistant even when inoculated with
large doses of virus ic.

B)   Differences in interferon production of sensitivity - 12
adult (resistant) mice were inoculated intravenously with Anti-
interferon globulin (AIG) followed 1 hour later by ic inoculation
with 10^6SMic LD$_{50}$ OC43. At 3 days pi the animals were given a
second dose of AIG. Eleven of the mice treated with AIG remained
well and examination of their brains by FA at 7 dpi did not reveal
any viral antigen. We conclude therefore that interferon is not
responsible for the resistance in adult mice.

C)   Inability of macrophages to support infection - Cultures of
peritoneal macrophages from 2 day old and 12 week old mice were
infected with 10^5TCID$_{50}$ OC43 per ring culture. The cultures were
examined by FA for the presence of viral antigen at 48, 72 hours
and 7 days after infection and were negative at all times.

    Likewise peritoneal MØ removed from 2 day old and 12 week old
mice infected with OC43 were negative for viral antigen. There is
no difference in the ability of macrophages from mice of different
ages to support infection.

D)   Maturation of the cell mediated immune system - Experiments
were carried out to investigate what effect immunosuppression of
adult mice and the transfer of adult spleen cells to suckling mice
would have on the outcome in infection with OC43.

    Immunosuppression of adult mice with cyclophosphamide does
not increase their susceptibility to OC43, a proportion of 15 day
old mice given a previously sub-lethal dose died. The brains of
the dead mice were positive for viral antigen.

    The immune system, whilst being partially protective in 15
day old mice, was not the sole factor in this resistance.
Neither immune or non-immune spleen cells were capable of
protecting the suckling mice.

E)   Inability of the virus to grow in adult brain cells - as
mechanisms A-D are not responsible for the resistance the ability
or otherwise of the virus to grow in brain cells must play an
important role.

    In order to better understand the interaction between OC43
and neural cells - cultures of neural cells have been established
and the effect of the virus on the different cell types is being
investigated.

FAILURE TO DETECT CORONAVIRUS SK ANTIGEN IN MULTIPLE SCLEROSIS

BRAIN TISSUE BY AUTORADIOGRAPHY

J.S. Burks, B.L. DeVald, J.C. Gerdes, I.T. McNally,
and M.C. Kemp

Center for Neurological Diseases/Rocky Mountain Multiple
Sclerosis Center, Veterans Administration Medical Center
University of Colorado School of Medicine
Denver, Colorado, U.S.A.

Illnesses such as subacute sclerosing panencephalitis (SSPE) are known to be induced by a virus which is present in a non-infectious state. Measles virus antigen and IgG are present in the brains of SSPE patients as shown by immunofluorescent techniques (1). Autoradiography techniques using I^{125} have been useful in demonstrating viral antigen and IgG in the brain and spinal cords of coronavirus SD infected mice in areas of demyelination when infectious virus cannot be recovered (2). Autoradiography is more sensitive than immunofluorescence in this coronavirus system.

This study utilizes autoradiography in an attempt to detect coronavirus SK antigen in mutiple sclerosis (MS) autopsy brain tissue (3). Coronavirus SK was isolated while working with MS autopsy material. Antibody to SK was produced by immunizing guinea pigs by repeated inoculations with an SK infected cell extract.

We studied 17 areas of the brain (14 from demyelinated areas and 3 from normal appearing white matter) from 10 MS patients. Also, we examined white matter autopsy tissue from 6 patients without neurologic disease. We did not detect coronavirus SK antigen in any of the tissue from MS or control patients.

Possible reasons for our inability to detect SK virus antigen in MS tissue include: (1) SK antigen is not present in MS brain tissue; (2) SK antigen may be present in brain areas other than those evaluated since we studied only a very few small areas of the brain; (3) The autoradiography technique may not have the sensitivity to detect latent SK virus in human brain. More sensitive technology such as coronavirus nucleic acid hybridization studies are needed before drawing final conclusions.

REFERENCES

1. ter Meulen, V., G. Enders-Ruckle, D. Muller and G. Joppich. 1968. Immunohistological, Microscopial and Neurochemical Studies on Encephalitis. Acta Neuropath. 12:244-259.
2. Gerdes, J.C., I. McNally, L. Hileman, J.S. Burks, 1982. Autoradiographic Detection of IgG and Viral Antigens. J. Immunol. Meth. 54:191-202.
3. Burks, J.S., B.L. DeVald, L.D. Jankovsky, J.C. Gerdes, 1980. Two Coronaviruses Isolated from Central Nervous System Tissue of Two Multiple Sclerosis Patients. Science. 209:933-934.

ACKNOWLEDGMENT

This study supported by the Kroc Foundation, the Veterans Administration, and the National MS Society.

ANTIVIRAL ACTION OF INTERFERON IN THE BOVINE SPECIES: STUDY <u>IN</u>
VITR<u>O</u> AND <u>IN VIVO</u>

C.Vanden Broecke[1], P.P.Pastoret[2], A.Schwers[2], A.
Goossens[1], B.Lansival[3], L.Bugyaki[4], L.Dagenais[2],
J.Werenne[1]

1. Faculty of Sciences, University of Brussels
2. Faculty of Veterinary Medicine, University of Liège
3. Laboratory of Virology, Marloie
4. Institute of Hygiene and Epidemiology, Brussels

Awaiting a multipotent antiviral vaccine preparation, perhaps
a feasible goal for the future, there is still at the present time,
we believe, enough room left for alternative ways to control viral
diseases. Given the recent developments of bacterial production of
interferon, the cost/benefits ratio of its possible use as antiviral has significantly increased. There is no more objective reason
at this time to limit the investigations using interferon exclusively to the field of human health. Indeed , considerable economical interest could reside in an efficient way to control domestic
animal viral diseases. We have undertaken the present study to evaluate interferon activity in the bovine species. As enough bovine
interferon cannot be obtained for this purpose using our bovine
cell system, we decided to use bacterially produced human interferon (Hu-IFNα_2). It is readily available now and has been provided to us by Dr.C.WEISSMANN (Zürich University). This interferon
was shown to cross the species barrier, using <u>in vitro</u> cell systems.

We also showed that rotavirus[1] is sensitive to interferon. We
also demonstrated that other bovine virus species responsible for
economically important cattle diseases like Bovine Rhinotracheitis
(Bovine Herpes virus I) or pseudorabies (Suid Herpes virus I)
are inhibited by interferon[2]. As Bovine enteric coronavirus was
associated with important economical losses, we decided to screen
also <u>in vitro</u> for its susceptibility to interferon despite the
fact that the HRT cells in which the cytopathogenicity of the vi-

rus is easy to follow express a moderate antiviral effect only under interferon treatment.

As it was shown recently that the administration of α interferon to human volunteers protected them against a respiratory
coronavirus challenge[3], we have started in vivo investigations in
the bovine species also. Twelve calves were intramuscularly injected with different doses of interferon using a double blind proto-
cole. We have been able to achieve an efficient protection of the
animals against an experimental infection with vaccinia virus
which causes lesions very easy to follow in a quantitative manner.
A total protection can be reached at the higher dose used (10^6
Units/kg).[4] Nevertheless, individual variation in sensitivity
to the treatment was observed. Our experimental system appeared
therefore a convenient model to approach the study of the mechanism of action of interferon in vivo we have already been able
to follow in a couple of animals the biochemical modifications
known to occur in cell culture under the action of interferon.

Moreover, we have obtained strong evidence for a role of
endogenous interferon in the control of pathogenicity of rotavi-
ruses in newborn calves.

We may therefore predict on the basis of our study, the first
evidence ever for the efficiency of interferon in a viral infection in the bovine species, a broad perspective for its use in
the veterinary field, at least in situations where proper vacci-
nation has not been used.

References

1. L.Dagenais, P.P.Pastoret, C.Vanden broecke, and J.Werenne
      Susceptibility of bovine rotavirus to interferon, Arch.
      of Virol., 70, 377-379 (1981)
2. A.Goossens, A.Schwers, C.Vanden Broecke, L.Dagenais,M.Maenhoudt
      R.Duwijn, B.Van Camp, P.P.Pastoret, and J.Werenne.
      Sensibilité des virus de la Rhinotracheite infectieuse bovi-
      ne (Bovine herpes virus I) et de la maladie d'Aujeszky (Suid
      herpes virus I) à l'interféron humain produit par des bacté-
      ries, Ann.Méd.Vét., 135-139 (1983)
3. G.M.Scott, R.J.Phillpotts, P.G.Higgins and D.J.Tyrell. Intra-
      nasal interferon against common colds. In "The biology of
      the interferon system" H.Schellekens Ed. Elsevier 1983 in
      press
4. A.Goossens,A.Schwers,C.Vanden broecke, M.Maenhoudt, E.Bugyaki,
      P.P.Pastoret, J.Werenne. Antiviral efficiency of IFN in the
      bovine species: preliminary data on the activity in calves
      of bacterially produced human interferon (Hu-IFNα_2)

THE EFFECTS OF MOUSE HEPATITIS VIRUS TYPE 3 ON THE MICROCIRCULATION OF THE LIVER IN INBRED STRAINS OF MICE

G.A. Levy, P.J. MacPhee, L.S. Fung, M.M. Fisher and A.M.Rappaport

Liver Disease Unit, Department of Medicine
Sunnybrook Medical Center, University of Toronto
Toronto, Ontario, Canada

Mouse Hepatitis Virus Type 3 (MHV-3) infection results in strain dependant liver disease. The acute effects of MHV-3 on the in vivo microcirculation of the liver in fully susceptible (Balb/cJ), fully resistant (A/J) mice and the chronic effects on C3H mice were studied. In Balb/cJ mice by 6 to 12 hours following infection, granular flow and sinusoidal microthrombi were present predominantly in periportal areas. By 24 to 48 hours, liver cell edema and small focal necrotic lesions were prominent. After 48 hours, thrombi and hepatocellular necrosis were widespread. The animals succumbed to the infection within 5 days.

In C3H mice, during the acute phase of the infection granular flow and areas of focal necrosis were noted similar to the Balb/cJ mice. The acute phase was followed by persistent lesions and abnormal flow was seen adjacent to these focal areas of necrosis. By 2 months, a large number of granulomatous lesions were distributed throughout the liver parenchyma with concommitant distorted flow patterns.

These abnormalities were in sharp contrast to the normal flow studies in the resistant A/J mice despite the presence of virus as demonstrated by both immunofluorescence and recovery and growth of virus in all strains studied.

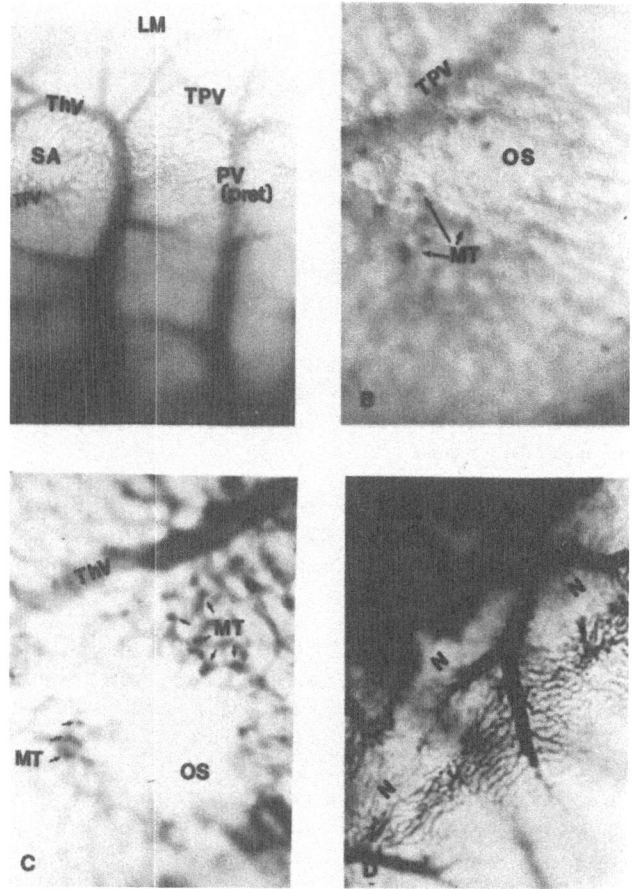

Figure 1

Studies of the In-Vivo Microcirculation in
Balb/cJ mice:
(A) Normal microvascular pattern at liver
    margin (LM) x 60.
(B) Areas devoid of sinusoidal flow (OS)
    with microthrombi (MT) at the perip-
    hery of the lesion as seen 24 to 48
    hours post infection x 200.
(C) Microthrombi and microcirculatory
    defect extend towards ThV, x 200.
(D) Confluent perivenular necrosis (N)
    x 125.
SA=Simple acinus TPV=Terminal portal venule
ThV=Terminal hepatic venule PV (pret)=
Preterminal branch of portal vein.

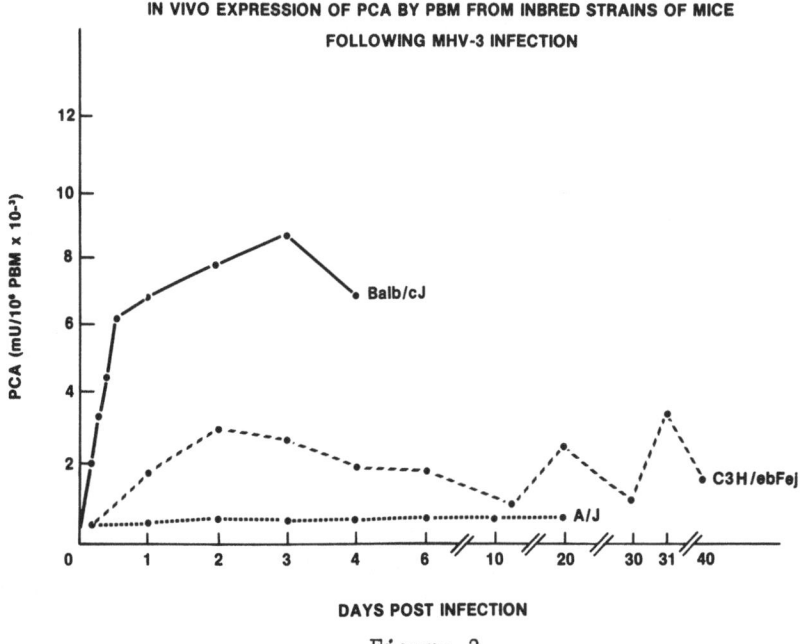

IN VIVO EXPRESSION OF PCA BY PBM FROM INBRED STRAINS OF MICE
FOLLOWING MHV-3 INFECTION

Figure 2

CONCLUSIONS

This study demonstrates:

1.Virus is present within the livers of resistant, semi-susceptible and susceptible mice.

2.Monocyte PCA is expressed within 4 hours following infection in susceptible animals. No PCA is expressed in resistant mice.

3.MHV-3 infection induces severe and progressive hepatic microcirculatory abnormalities in susceptible Balb/cJ mice and in the semi-resistant C3H mice. They consist of granular flow, microthrombi, liver cell edema and necrosis. No microcirculatory changes were noted in the fully resistant A/J mice.

We postulate that monocytes expressing surface PCA could initiate microcirculatory flow abnormalities with resultant microthrombi, endothelial cell injury and hepatocellular necrosis and are an important factor in the pathogenesis of tissue injury.

CONTRIBUTORS

Anderson, R., University of Western Ontario, Department of Microbiology and Immunology, London, Ontario, Canada N6A 5C1

Armstrong, J., European Molecular Biology Laboratory, Postfach 10.2209,D-6900 Heidelberg, FRG

Aynaud, J.M., I.N.R.A., Laboratoire de Pathologie Porcine, 37380 Nouzilly, France

Baird, G.D., Agricultural Research Council, Institute for Research on Animal Diseases, Compton, Newbury, Berkshire RG16 0NN, England

van Berlo, M.F., Institute of Virology, Veterinary Faculty, State University Utrecht, Yalelaan 1, 3508 TD Utrecht, The Netherlands

Bountiff, L., Agricultural Research Council, Institute for Research on Animal Diseases, Compton, Newbury, Berkshire RG16 0NN, England

Boursnell, M.E.G., Department of Microbiology, Houghton Poultry Research Station, Huntingdon, Cambridgeshire PE17 2DA, England

Boyle, J.F., Department of Medicine, School of Veterinary Medicine, University of California, Davis, CA 95616, USA

Brown, T.D.K., Houghton Poultry Research Station, Houghton, Huntingdon, Cambridgeshire PE17 2DA, England

Burks, J.S., Center for Neurological Diseases, Rocky Mountain M.S. Center, Box B-181, 4200 E.9th Ave., Denver, Co. 80262, USA

Cavanagh, D., Houghton Poultry Research Station, Houghton, Huntingdon, Cambridgeshire PE17 2DA, England

Dales, S., University of Western Ontario, Department of Microbiology and Immunology, Health Sciences Centre, London, Ontario, Canada N6A 5C1

DeVald, B.L., Center for Neurological Diseases, Rocky Mountain M.S. Center, Box B-181, 4200 E.9th Ave. ,Denver CO 80262, USA

Doi, K., Department of Biomedical Science, Faculty of Agriculture, University of Tokyo, Yayoi 1-1, Bunkyo-ku, Tokyo 113, Japan

Dupuy, J.M., Université de Québec, Institut Armand-Frappier, 531,Boulevard des Prairies, Ville de Laval, Québec, Canada H7N 4Z3

Flintoff, W., University of Western Ontario, Department of Microbiology and Immunology, London, Ontario, Canada N6A 5C1

Fujiwara, K., Department of Veterinary Pathology, Faculty of Agriculture, University of Tokyo, Yayoi 1-1, Bunkyo-ku, Tokyo 113 Japan

Garwes, D.J., Agricultural Research Council, Institute for Research on Animal Diseases, Compton, Newbury, Berkshire RG16 ONN, England

Goto, Department of Veterinary Pathology, Faculty of Agriculture, Yamaguchi University, Yoshida 1677-1, Yamaguchi-shi, Yamaguchi 753, Japan

Hayashi, T., Department of Veterinary Pathology, Faculty of Agriculture, University of Tokyo, Yayoi 1-1, Bunkyo-ku, Tokyo 113, Japan

Hirano, N., Department of Veterinary Microbiology, Iwate University, Morioka 020, Japan

Holmes, K.V. Uniformed Services University of the Health Sciences, 4301 Jones Bridge Road, Bethesda, Maryland 20814, USA

Horzinek, M.C., Institute of Virology, Veterinary Faculty, State University Utrecht, Yalelaan 1, 3508 TD Utrecht, The Netherlands

Jacobse-Geels, H.E.L., Institute of Virology, Veterinary Faculty, State University Utrecht, Yalelaan 1, 3508 TD Utrecht, The Netherlands

Kemp, M.C., Center for Neurological Diseases, Rocky Mountain M.S. Center, Box B-181, 4200 E.9th Ave., Denver CO 80262, USA

Klenk, H.-D., Institut fuer Virologie, Justus-Liebig-Universitaet Giessen, Fachbereich Humanmedizin, Frankfurter Str.107, 6300 Giessen, FRG

Koolen, M.J.M., Institute of Virology, Veterinary Faculty, State University Utrecht, Yalelaan 1, 3508 TD Utrecht, The Netherlands

Lai, M.M.C., Department of Microbiology, University of Southern California, 2025 Zonal Ave. HMR-401, Los Angeles, California 90333, USA

Laporte, J., INRA, Station de Recherches de Virologie et d'Immunologie, Route de Thiverval, 78850 Thiverval-Grignon, France

Laude, H., INRA, Station de Recherches de Virologie et d'Immunologie, Route de Thiverval, 78850 Thiverval-Grignon, France

Lavi, E., Department of Neurology, Hospital of the University of Pennsylvania, 3400 Spruce Street, Philadelphia, PA 19104, USA

Levy, G.A., Sunnybrook Medical Centre, University of Toronto, 2075 Bayview Ave., Toronto, Ontario, Canada M4N 3M5

Mahy, B.W.J., University of Cambridge, Department of Pathology, Division of Virology, Addenbrooke's Hospital, Hills Road, Cambridge CB2 2QQ, England

ter Meulen, V., Institut fuerVirologie und Immunbiologie der Universitaet Wuerzburg, Versbacher Str.7, 8700 Wuerzburg, FRG

Niemann, H., Institut fuer Virologie, Justus-Liebig-Universitaet Giessen, Frankfurter Str.107, 6300 Giessen, FRG

Pearson, J., Department of Microbiology, Guy's Hospital Medical School, London Bridge SE1 9RT,England

Pedersen, N.C., Department of Medicine, School of Veterinary Medicine, University of California, Davis, CA 95616, USA

Repp, R., Institut fuer Virologie, Justus-Liebig-Universitaet Giessen, Frankfurter Str.107, 6300 Giessen, FRG

Rottier, P.J.M., Institute of Virology, Veterinary Faculty, State University Utrecht, Yalelaan 1, 3508 TD Utrecht, The Netherlands

Siddell, S.G., Institut fuer Virologie und Immunbiologie der Universitaet Wuerzburg, Versbacher Str.7, 8700 Wuerzburg, FRG

Skinner, M., Institut fuer Virologie und Immunbiologie der Universitaet Wuerzburg, Versbacher Str.7, 8700 Wuerzburg, FRG

Spaan, W.J.M., Institute of Virology, Veterinary Faculty, State University Utrecht, Yalelaan 1, 3508 TD Utrecht, The Netherlands

Stern, D.F., Center for Cancer Research, Massachusetts Institute of Technology, E17-517, 77 Massachusetts Ave., Cambridge, MA 02139 USA

Stohlman, S.A., University of Southern California, School of Medicine, Department of Neurology, 2025 Zonal Ave., Los Angeles CA 90033, USA

Sturman, L.S. Center for Laboratories and Research, N.Y.State Department of Health, Empire State Plaza, Albany, N.Y. 12201, USA

Vautherot, J.F., Station de Recherches de Virologie et d'Immunologie, Route de Thiverval, 78850 Thiverval–Grignon, France

Watanabe, R., Institut fuer Virologie und Immunbiologie der Universitaet Wuerzburg, Versbacher Str.7, 8700 Wuerzburg, FRG

Wege, H., Institut fuer Virologie und Immunbiologie der Universitaet Wuerzburg, Versbacher Str.7, 8700 Wuerzburg, FRG

Werenne, J., Université Libre de Bruxelles, Faculté des Sciences (CP 160), Chimie Générale, Ave.F.D.Roosevelt, 50, B–1050 Brussels, Belgium

van der Zeijst, B.A.M., Institute of Virology, Veterinary Faculty, State University Utrecht, Yalelaan 1, 3508 TD Utrecht, The Netherlands